DYSLEXIA: OVERVIEW, ABSTRACTS AND GUIDE TO BOOKS

DYSLEXIA: OVERVIEW, ABSTRACTS AND GUIDE TO BOOKS

OLIVER P. MOYNIHAN (EDITOR)

Nova Science Publishers, Inc.
New York

Senior Editors: Susan Boriotti and Donna Dennis
Coordinating Editor: Tatiana Shohov
Office Manager: Annette Hellinger
Graphics: Wanda Serrano
Editorial Production: Jennifer Vogt, Matthew Kozlowski,
               Jonathan Rose and Maya Columbus
Circulation: Ave Maria Gonzalez, Vera Popovich, Luis Aviles, Melissa Diaz,
          Nicolas Miro and Jeannie Pappas
Communications and Acquisitions: Serge P. Shohov
Marketing: Cathy DeGregory

Library of Congress Cataloging-in-Publication Data
Available Upon Request

ISBN 1-59033-456-6

CONTENTS

PREFACE

Researchers have devoted considerable attention to how people learn to read, specifically how they recognize, pronounce, and understand printed words. These studies are helping to illuminate not only the normal process of learning to read but also the problems that may underlie dyslexia, a condition in which people are unable to acquire a high degree of reading skill despite adequate intelligence and training. When reading instruction begins, children (as well as adult learners) already possess large spoken-word vocabularies. Their initial task is to learn how these spoken words correspond to written alphabetic symbols. Mastering the correspondence between the written and spoken forms of language is a key step in becoming literate; impairments in this reading skill are often seen among children who have problems learning in school.

Dyslexia is a brain-based type of learning disability that specifically impairs a person's ability to read. These individuals typically read at levels significantly lower than expected despite having normal intelligence. Although the disorder varies from person to person, common characteristics among people with dyslexia are difficulty with phonological processing (the manipulation of sounds) and/or rapid visual-verbal responding.

This new book presents an overview of dyslexia, current abstracts of the literature which have been carefully selected and edited, and a guide to the books in the field. Easy-to-use indexes by subject, author and title are provided.

OVERVIEW[*]

Dyslexia is a brain-based type of learning disability that specifically impairs a person's ability to read. These individuals typically read at levels significantly lower than expected despite having normal intelligence. Although the disorder varies from person to person, common characteristics among people with dyslexia are difficulty with phonological processing (the manipulation of sounds) and/or rapid visual-verbal responding.

The main focus of treatment should be on the specific learning problems of affected individuals. The usual course is to modify teaching methods and the educational environment to meet the specific needs of the individual with dyslexia.

For those with dyslexia, the prognosis is mixed. The disability affects such a wide range of people, producing different symptoms and varying degrees of severity, that predictions are hard to make. The prognosis is generally good, however, for individuals whose dyslexia is identified early, who have supportive family and friends and a strong self-image, and who are involved in a proper remediation program.

The NINDS and other institutes of the National Institutes of Health, including the National Institute of Child Health and Human Development and the National Institute of Mental Health, conduct research on dyslexia. Current research avenues focus on developing techniques to diagnose and treat dyslexia and other learning disabilities, increasing the understanding of the biological basis of learning disabilities, and exploring the relationship between neurophysiological processes and cognitive functions with regard to reading ability.

MODELING READING AND DYSLEXIA

Researchers have devoted considerable attention to how people learn to read, specifically how they recognize, pronounce, and understand printed words. These studies are helping to illuminate not only the normal process of learning to read but the problems that may underlie dyslexia, a condition in which people are unable to acquire a high degree of reading skill despite adequate intelligence and training.

When reading instruction begins, children (as well as adult learners) already possess large spoken-word vocabularies. Their initial task is to learn how these spoken words correspond to written alphabetic symbols. Mastering the correspondence between the written and spoken

---

[*] This article consists of an amalgam of public information derived from various websites and other sources.

forms of language is a key step in becoming literate; impairments in this reading skill are often seen among children who have problems learning in school.

Neural-network models provide a powerful approach for understanding both normal reading and reading difficulties. These computer-simulation models start out like naive children knowing nothing about the correspondence between spelling and sound. After exposure to many spelled words, with feedback about their pronunciations, the models gradually learn these correspondences. After sufficient training, a model can correctly pronounce a wide range of written words, even though many English words have irregular spellings (e.g, have/gave, sign/line, yacht/dot).

Experiments with these models have provided clues to the underlying sources of reading impairment. For example, in one type of dyslexia, people err when reading words with irregular spellings but retain knowledge of the more general spelling-sound correspondences. They make other errors as well, but until recently, it was not clear how these other errors were related to their difficulty with irregular spellings. Much of the entire range of errors can be seen to stem from damage to a single part of the neural network. Thus, the model illustrates how one small area of brain damage could cause the exact pattern of behavioral deficits. [1]

NEW DEVELOPMENTS[2]

Using a novel technique to examine how different brain regions interact during reading, National Institutes of Health (NIH) scientists have found that people with dyslexia do not use the same neural networks as normal readers. For millions who struggle with dyslexia, a disorder that causes problems with reading, writing, and spelling, this controlled study shows a lack of communication between regions of the brain involved in reading. The scientists have discovered an absence of the strong functional links between the left angular gyrus and other left hemisphere regions of the brain. Their finding suggests a functional disconnection of the left angular gyrus—part of the brain thought to play a critical role in relating letters to speech—from the occipital and temporal lobes, brain areas involved in visual and language processing. In normal readers, these regions interact strongly during reading.

"These results explicitly demonstrate that the brain circuits mediating reading in dyslexia are abnormal," reports Barry Horwitz, Ph.D, of the National Institute on Aging. Horwitz and National Institute of Mental Health colleagues Judith Rumsey, Ph.D, and Brian Donohue used positron emission tomography (PET) to find that in the good readers, regional cerebral blood flow (rCBF) in the left angular gyrus shows strong correlations with rCBF in occipital and temporal lobes during single word reading. In the men with dyslexia, the PET data show an absence of these relationships, indicating that as a group they were not using the same reading networks as the normal readers.

"A major strength of this study," explains Rumsey, "is that it examined dyslexic men while they were actually reading aloud, a task that activates posterior brain circuits critical to reading."

Because written language is a relatively recent addition to human communication, and because most of a typical individual's day is not spent reading, it is unlikely that a neural

---

[1] From "Basic Behavioral Science Research for Mental Health. A National Investment. A Report Of The National Advisory Mental Health Council. 1995, NIH Publication No. 96-3682."

[2] This section consists of excerpts from various NIH press releases

network evolved that is solely dedicated to reading, according to Horwitz. Neurons that are activated during reading are also engaged by other cognitive tasks. While previous studies have compared scans obtained during reading to those during performance of other tasks, such as visual matching, the researchers say it is not surprising that individual functional neuroimaging studies have shown activation of some but not all of the crucial nodes of the neural network. Because this study examined correlations within tasks, its results are not confounded by what neurons in the angular gyrus might be doing in other tasks used for the comparison.

To examine the functional connectivity of the angular gyrus during single word reading, the researchers measured rCBF using PET in 14 good readers and in 17 men with persistent developmental dyslexia. Each subject read two types of material, nonsense words that need to be sounded out using phonological rules (e.g, "phalbap," "chirl") and words that do not follow the rules (e.g., "choir," pharaoh"), requiring the reader to rely on experience. Two scans during each type of reading were used in the analysis. All subjects read continuously, although those with dyslexia read less accurately and more slowly.

If men with dyslexia who have learned to read to some degree are not using the normal circuits, they may have developed pathways to compensate for their impairment. Improved understanding of what various parts of the brain normally do during reading may lead to neural-based diagnosis of the nature of each individual's dyslexia. Determining alternate pathways that are successfully used may provide clues for better treatment.

Brain imaging studies at the National Institute of Mental Health (NIMH) have revealed dramatic evidence of a deficit in the brain's visual system in people with dyslexia, a disorder that affects the reading ability of millions of American school children and adults. While it has been commonly believed that only the language related areas of the brain are affected in dyslexia, this study adds to the growing body of research pointing to dysfunction of another portion of the brain known as V5/MT.

Using functional magnetic resonance imaging (fMRI), NIH scientists Guinevere Eden, D.Phil, and colleagues demonstrated in a small controlled study of adult males that people with dyslexia showed no activation in the *V5/MT brain area,* which specializes in movement perception. Dr. Eden's research confirms that people with dyslexia, hobbled by problems with reading, writing, and spelling, have trouble processing specific visual information. "We found that maps of brain activity measured while subjects were given a visual task of looking at moving dots were very different in individuals with dyslexia compared to normal control subjects," said Dr. Eden.

The eight control subjects showed robust activity in brain region V5/MT when viewing a moving dot pattern. Almost no activity was present in those areas in people with dyslexia. In fact, a clear finding in all six subjects showing no response in the V5/MT area is a step toward improving the understanding, diagnosis, and eventually, treatment for the disorder.

"This research confirms that dyslexia is a discrete brain disorder, not, as some people have believed, a by-product of a poor education," said NIMH Director Steven H. Hyman, M.D. Furthermore, if confirmed by additional research, functional brain imaging may be used as a tool for early and accurate diagnosis of this common and disabling disorder.

Whether the motion perception deficit uncovered by this study contributes to the reading disability characteristic of dyslexia is still unknown. "It is possible that the visual disturbances we found and the reading disturbances others have found may be caused by an underlying, common information processing deficit," said Dr. Eden. According to the research team, the anatomical changes underlying these functional differences are thought to occur during the early stages of development, when regional functional specialization occurs. Abnormal function in the specialized brain area V5/MT explains previously reported visual behavioral problems in dyslexia.

Future research will provide further insights into the details of visual and language deficits and their effects on reading. Dr. Eden's study suggests a broader definition of the underlying mechanisms of dyslexia, thus opening the way for development of special help and effective treatment for more people with the disorder.

All of the dyslexic subjects in this study had a childhood history of reading disability, a measurable reading deficit, a discrepancy of at least 2 standard deviations between their reading and verbal IQ, and poorer phonological awareness compared to controls, and none had neurological disorders. Normal controls were closely matched to dyslexics in age, education, socio-economic status, and IQ.

The technique of functional magnetic resonance imaging is based on the principle that blood flow, rich in oxygen, increases locally in active areas of the brain. Usually used to obtain information on structural details of the brain, fMRI can also pinpoint regions where oxygenation levels are changing as a result of neural activity. The procedure is noninvasive, as it exploits a magnetic tracer, namely hemoglobin, that is a normal constituent of blood.[3]

A Yale research team funded by the National Institute of Child Health and Human Development (NICHD) has used sophisticated brain imaging technology to show that there is decreased functioning while performing reading tasks in certain brain regions of individuals with the most common form of dyslexia. The study appears in the March 3 issue of the *Proceedings of the National Academy of Sciences*.

In their study, the researchers used a technology known as functional magnetic resonance imaging (fMRI), which produces computer-generated images of the brain while it is performing intellectual tasks. With fMRI, the team produced images of an impairment in the brains of dyslexic readers that became apparent when they tried to perform tasks which would require a firm command of the ability to decipher words phonetically.

"If you have a broken arm, we can see that on an X-ray," said the study's first author, Sally E. Shaywitz, MD, of the Yale University School of Medicine. "These brain activation patterns now provide us with hard evidence of a disruption in the brain regions responsible for reading--evidence for what has previously been a hidden disability."

Dr. Shaywitz explained that the words we speak are made up of individual sounds called phonemes. In spoken language, the brain automatically combines these sounds to form words. To make normal conversation possible, such sound pieces are strung together rapidly--about 8 to 10 per second--and blended so thoroughly that it's often impossible to separate them.

For people with dyslexia, the problem arises in converting this natural process to print. Written English is a kind of code: The 26 letters of the alphabet, either singly or in combination with other letters, stand for the 44 letter phonemes in spoken English. Dyslexic readers have extreme difficulty with phonological awareness (breaking spoken words into their component sounds) and with phonetics (the ability to match these letter sounds to the letters that represent them).

---

[3] The study, "Abnormal Processing of Visual Motion Processing in Dyslexia Revealed by Functional Brain Imaging," was published July 4 in *Nature*. Coauthors are Judith M. Rumsey, Ph.D, and Jose Ma. Masog,

In their study, Dr. Shaywitz and her coworkers presented 29 dyslexic readers (14 men and 15 women, ages 16-54) and 32 normal readers (16 men and 16 women, ages 18-63) with a battery of reading tasks while observing their brain functioning with the fMRI scanner. Most of these tasks required the readers to manipulate and understand phonologic principals-- the skills needed to consciously manipulate the letter sounds in words.

The dyslexic readers found it difficult to read nonsense rhyming words, such as "lete" and "jeat." This task is designed to measure the phonologic principals underlying reading and is far more difficult for dyslexic readers to complete than rhyming actual words, which they may have previously memorized.

When performing such tasks, the dyslexic readers in the study showed less activation in a brain region linking print skills to the brain's language areas, in comparison to normal readers. Specifically, dyslexic readers showed reduced activity in a large brain region that links the visual cortex and visual association areas (angular gyrus) to the language regions in the superior temporal gyrus (Wernike's area).

In the article, the authors noted that their findings are consistent with those of earlier studies of acquired inability to read (alexia). In both alexia and dyslexia, the same brain regions appear to be affected; however, in people with dyslexia, the study shows the impairment is a functional one, whereas in alexia, it has been attributed to a tumor or brain injury due to a stroke.

When they performed phonologic tasks, the dyslexic readers also showed activation in the brain region known as Broca's area, which has been associated with spoken language. In contrast, the normal readers did not show any increased activity in Broca's area when reading. Dr. Shaywitz explained that the dyslexic readers may have used this brain region in an attempt to compensate for impairments in the brain regions normally used for phonological skills.

"In summary, for dyslexic readers, these brain activation patterns provide evidence of an imperfectly functioning system for segmenting words into their phonologic constituents; accordingly, this disruption is evident when dyslexic readers are asked to respond to increasing demands on phonologic analysis," the authors wrote. "The pattern of relative underactivation in posterior brain regions contrasted with relative overactivation in the anterior regions may provide a neural signature for the phonologic difficulties characterizing dyslexia."

Dr. Shaywitz explained that it is too early to use fMRI as a method for diagnosing dyslexia. Nonetheless, the findings have important implications. First, they provide neurologic evidence for the critical role that lack of phonological awareness plays in dyslexia. They also confirm the fundamental neurobiologic nature of dyslexia and provide a neural signature for the phonologic difficulties accompanying the disorder.

ORGANIZATIONS

International Dyslexia Association
8600 LaSalle Road

M.D, of NIMH, Thomas A. Zeffiro, M.D, Ph.D, and John W. VanMeter, Ph.D, of Sensor Systems, Inc, and Roger Woods, M.D, of U.C. L.A.

Chester Building, Ste. 382
Baltimore, MD 21286-2044
info@interdys.org
http://www.interdys.org
Tel: 410-296-0232 800-ABCD123
Fax: 410-321-5069

Learning Disabilities Association of America
4156 Library Road
Pittsburgh, PA 15234-1349
ldanatl@usaor.net
http://www.ldanatl.org
Tel: 412-341-1515 412-341-8077
Fax: 412-344-0224

National Center for Learning Disabilities
381 Park Avenue South
Suite 1401
New York, NY 10016
http://www.ld.org
Tel: 212-545-7510 888-575-7373
Fax: 212-545-9665

National Institute of Child Health and Human Development (NICHD)
National Institutes of Health
Bldg. 31, Rm. 2A32
Bethesda, MD 20892-2425
NICHDClearinghouse@mail.nih.gov
http://www.nichd.nih.gov
Tel: 301-496-5133 800-370-2943

National Institute of Mental Health (NIMH)
6001 Executive Blvd.
Rm. 8184, MSC 9663
Bethesda, MD 20892-9663
nimhinfo@nih.gov
http://www.nimh.nih.gov
Tel: 301-443-4513 TTY: 301-443-8431
Depression Info: 800-421-4211
Anxiety Info: 88-88-ANXIETY (269-4389)
Panic Info: 888-64-PANIC (64-72642)
Fax: 301-443-4279

BIBLIOGRAPHY

100 years research in reading and spelling--what do we know today? von Suchodoletz W Z Kinder Jugendpsychiatr Psychother 1999 Aug;27(3):199-206.

30 years rehabilitation preparatory courses and their role in the future exemplified by the Hamburg vocational promotion center Abstract: Over the last 30 years, some 12,000 disabled people have participated in the pre-rehabilitation courses ("Rehabilitationsvorbereitungslehrgange", RVL) offered by the Hamburg Vocational Training Centre (on average, some 75% of all rehabilitees have attended RVLs prior to their specific vocational retraining); 90% of them successfully, hence able to start their retraining as scheduled Butzer B Rehabilitation (Stuttg) 1998 Nov;37(4): 210-5.

A biological marker for dyslexia. Frith C Frith U Nature 1996 Jul 4;382(6586):19-20.

A candidate phenotype for familial dyslexia. Abstract: The probative analysis of genotype-phenotype relations in familial dyslexia requires operationally defined psychobiological outcome variables that are not confounded by cultural differences of orthography or other factors that may influence the clinical ascertainment and diagnosis of dyslexia. Timing precision, as expressed in coordinated motor action, was used as an objective behavioral measure that can be mapped on current knowledge of central nervous system functions as well as on the most salient non-reading deficits in developmental dyslexia. Dyslexia families with four distinct pedigrees and a normally reading reference group were the study subjects. Wolff PH Eur Child Adolesc Psychiatry 1999;8 Suppl 3:21-7.

A case of concomitant impairment of operational signs and punctuation marks. Abstract: A patient affected by amnestic aphasia, E.B, presented with a prevailing impairment in the use of operational signs and punctuation marks. His performance on tasks exploring his knowledge of these symbols is compared with that of two other patients suffering from similar aphasic disturbances. This comparison enables us to reject the hypothesis that E.B.'s defects arise from aphasia per se. A possible cognitive link between operational signs and punctuation marks is discussed. Laiacona M Lunghi A Neuropsychologia 1997 Mar;35(3):325-32.

A case of pure alexia whose writing ability with eyes closed was superior to that with eyes open Abstract: We compared the writing ability between eyes open (looking at one's writing) and eyes closed (without looking) in a case of pure alexia. The patient is a 84-year-old right handed man who developed pure alexia following an infarction in the distribution of the left posterior cerebral artery. He showed right homonymous hemianopsia, slight memory disorder and slight anomia. He could not read any kinds of letters and words at all though he could categorize letters: Kana (phonograms), Kanji (morphograms) and Arabic numbers, and he could distinguish the real letters from false ones. He could achieve almost 60-70% of Kana and Kanji dictation, though it was not perfect. Otsuki M Soma Y Tsuji S Aizawa F Yamazaki M Onishi Y No To Shinkei 1995 Sep;47(9):905-10.

A case study of an English-Japanese bilingual with monolingual dyslexia. Abstract: We report the case of AS, a 16 year-old English/Japanese bilingual boy, whose reading/writing difficulties are confined to English only. AS was born in Japan to a highly literate Australian father and English mother, and goes to a Japanese selective senior high school in Japan. His spoken language at home is English. AS's reading in logographic Japanese Kanji and syllabic Kana is equivalent to that of Japanese undergraduates or graduates. Wydell TN Butterworth B Cognition 1999 Apr 1;70(3):273-305.

A case study of transient dyslexia Abstract: This paper presents a case study of a seizure-induced transient dyslexic episode experienced by a radio presenter while reading a script live on air. An analysis of the recording of the episode in conjunction with the script being read yields a number of interesting observations. There is, for example, a distinct temporal pattern of breakdown from what can be characterized as orthographic errors through to semantic confusions. Many of the orthographic errors can be explained as a form of repetition blindness. Reilly RG Brain Lang 1999 Dec;70(3):336-46.

A chain of editorial reflections. Miles TR Dyslexia 2001 Apr-Jun;7(2):57-61.

A child with a learning disability: navigating school-based services. Stein MT Lounsbury B J Dev Behav Pediatr 2001 Jun;22(3):188-91; discussion 191-2.

A comparison of phonological skills in children with reading comprehension difficulties and children with decoding difficulties. Abstract: This paper examines phonological skills in children with two distinct forms of reading difficulty:

comprehension problems and decoding problems. In the first study a group of children with normal decoding skills but poor reading comprehension skills was studied. These children were found to have age-appropriate phonological skills. It is argued that normal phonological skills have enabled them to develop proficient decoding skills. A second study assessed the phonological skills of a group of children with decoding difficulties. Stothard SE Hulme C J Child Psychol Psychiatry 1995 Mar;36(3):399-408.

A comparison of temporal integration in children with a specific reading disability and normal readers. Abstract: Previous research has suggested that whereas some techniques show that subjects with a specific reading disability (SRD) have greater visible persistence than controls, a temporal integration of form technique does not. It has been suggested that the failure of the temporal integration task to show a difference results from the spatial separation between stimuli used in the technique. In this study SRD and control subjects were compared on a new version of a temporal integration task, under two conditions varying the spatial separation of elements in the display. Hogben JH Rodino IS Clark CD Pratt C Vision Res 1995 Jul;35(14):2067-74.

A comparison of the cognitive deficits in reading disability and attention-deficit/hyperactivity disorder. Abstract: This study used a nonreferred sample of twins to contrast the performance of individuals with reading disability (RD; n = 93), attention-deficit/hyperactivity disorder (ADHD; n = 52), RD and ADHD (n = 48), and neither RD nor ADHD (n = 121) on measures of phoneme awareness (PA) and executive functioning (EF). Exploratory factor analysis of the EF measures yielded underlying factors of working memory, inhibition, and set shifting. Results revealed that ADHD was associated with inhibition deficits, whereas RD was associated with significant deficits on measures of PA and verbal working memory. Willcutt EG Pennington BF

Boada R Ogline JS Tunick RA Chhabildas NA Olson RK J Abnorm Psychol 2001 Feb;110(1):157-72.

A complex background in children and adolescents with psychiatric disorders: developmental delay, dyslexia, heredity, slow cognitive processing and adverse social factors in a multifactorial entirety. Abstract: A consecutive cohort of 112 children, 42 girls and 70 boys, aged 5-17 years, receiving child psychiatric inpatient care, was investigated regarding the probability of a complex background of concomitant biological and social factors. Most of the subjects showed maladjustment and depressive states, school problems, problems with peers, psychosomatic complaints and anxiety. A very high rate of factors indicating neurodevelopmental dysfunctions was found particularly in boys, who exhibited developmental delay, dyslexia, heredity for dyslexia, and a slow complex reaction time (CRT) - suggesting slow cognitive processing - considered an impairment in itself. Frisk M Eur Child Adolesc Psychiatry 1999 Sep;8(3):225-36.

A computational model of neglect dyslexia. Abstract: This paper presents a straightforward theory of neglect (a pre-attentive salience system selects objects' centers for the focus of an attentional "spotlight") as a computational model. This construction permits simulations of model "lesions" and allows checking unequivocally the model's implications. The current model can account for some of the common patterns of observations of neglect dyslexia: that errors increase with word length and that short words may be read as "too long". Anderson B Cortex 1999 Apr; 35(2):201-18.

A connectionist approach to making the predictability of English orthography explicit to at-risk beginning readers: evidence for alternative, effective strategies. Abstract: A case is made (and illustrated with empirical data with children) for connectionist models that are not only computationally explicit but instructionally explicit. First-graders (N = 128) at the bottom of their classes in reading (average 11.5 percentile on nationally normed tests) participated in a 3-layer intervention. In the first layer, kept constant for all treatment groups, the alphabet principle was taught, making functional spelling units and alternations explicit Berninger VW Abbott RD Brooksher R Lemos Z Ogier S Zook D Mostafapour E Dev Neuropsychol 2000;17(2):241-71.

A connectionist multiple-trace memory model for polysyllabic word reading. Abstract: A connectionist feedforward network implementing a mapping from orthography to phonology is described. The model develops a view of the reading system that accounts for both irregular word and pseudoword reading without relying on any system of explicit or implicit conversion rules. The model assumes, however, that reading is supported by 2 procedures that work successively: a global procedure using knowledge about entire words and an analytic procedure based on the activation of word syllabic segments. Ans B Carbonnel S Valdois S Psychol Rev 1998 Oct;105(4):678-723.

A dissociation between developmental surface and phonological dyslexia in two undergraduate students. Abstract: This study compares the nature of the reading deficit that was observed in two dyslexic undergraduate students who were severely impaired at reading and spelling compared with normal undergraduates. They both achieved the same (below average) score on the National Adult Reading Test and on the Schonell spelling test. One of them, however, was good at reading and spelling nonwords, had good phonological awareness skills, was better at reading regular than irregular words, and made phonologically accurate reading and spelling errors (i.e. was a surface dyslexic). Hanley JR Gard F Neuropsychologia 1995 Jul;33(7):909-14.

A dominant gene for developmental dyslexia on chromosome 3. Abstract: Developmental dyslexia is a neuro-functional disorder characterised by an unexpected difficulty in learning to read and write despite adequate intelligence, motivation, and education. Previous studies have suggested mostly quantitative susceptibility loci for dyslexia on chromosomes 1, 2, 6, and 15, but no genes have been identified yet. We studied a large pedigree, ascertained from 140 families considered, segregating pronounced dyslexia in an autosomal dominant fashion. Nopola-Hemmi J Myllyluoma B Haltia T Taipale M Ollikainen V Ahonen T Voutilainen A Kere J Widen E J Med Genet 2001 Oct;38(10):658-64.

A family with a grand-maternally derived interstitial duplication of proximal 15q. Abstract: About 1% of individuals with autism or types of pervasive develop-mental disorder have a duplication of the 15q11-q13 region. These abnormalities can be detected by routine G-banded chromosome study, showing an extra marker chromosome, or demonstrated by fluorescence in situ hybridization (FISH) analysis, revealing an interstitial duplication. We report here the molecular, cytogenetic, clinical and neuropsychiatric evaluations of a family in whom 3 of 4 siblings inherited an interstitial duplication of 15q11-q13. Boyar FZ Whitney MM Lossie AC Gray BA Keller KL Stalker HJ Zori RT Geffken G Mutch J Edge PJ Voeller KS Williams CA Driscoll DJ Clin Genet 2001 Dec;60(6):421-30.

A functional lesion in developmental dyslexia: left angular gyral blood flow predicts severity. Abstract: Functional imaging studies have shown reduced regional cerebral blood flow (rCBF) in temporal and inferior parietal regions in dyslexia. To relate such abnormalities to the severity of dyslexia, correlations between reading skill and rCBF during a series of reading tasks and visual fixation were mapped for 17 right-handed dyslexic men, ages 18-40, and 14 matched controls. These correlations uniquely identified the left angular gyrus as the most probable site of a functional lesion in dyslexia: Here, higher rCBF was associated with better reading skill in controls (p <.01), but with worse reading skill in dyslexia (p <.01 Rumsey JM Horwitz B Donohue BC Nace KL Maisog JM Andreason P Brain Lang 1999 Nov;70(2):187-204.

A functional magnetic resonance imaging study during sentence reading in Japanese dyslexic children. Abstract: A functional magnetic resonance imaging (fMRI) study during Japanese 'kana' readings was performed on Japanese dyslexic children. Five dyslexic children (aged 9-12 years) and five healthy children (aged 9-11 years) were investigated. The fMRI examination was performed by getting these children to read sentences constructed from Japanese phonograms, 'kana', compared with staring at meaningless figures as a control task. All control subjects showed activation of the left middle temporal gyrus Seki A Koeda T Sugihara S Kamba M Hirata Y Ogawa T Takeshita K Brain Dev 2001 Aug;23(5):312-6.

A functional neuroimaging description of two deep dyslexic patients. Abstract: Deep dyslexia is a striking reading disorder that results from left-hemisphere brain damage and is characterized by semantic errors in reading single words aloud (e.g, reading 'spirit' as 'whisky'). Two types of explanation for this syndrome have been advanced. One is that deep dyslexia results from a residual left-hemisphere reading system that has lost the ability to pronounce a printed word without reference to meaning. Price CJ Howard D Patterson K Warburton EA Friston KJ Frackowiak SJ J Cogn Neurosci 1998 May;10(3):303-15.

A genomewide linkage screen for relative hand skill in sibling pairs. Abstract: Genomewide quantitative-trait locus (QTL) linkage analysis was performed using a continuous measure of relative hand skill (PegQ) in a sample of 195 reading-disabled sibling pairs from the

United Kingdom. This was the first genomewide screen for any measure related to handedness. The mean PegQ in the sample was equivalent to that of normative data, and PegQ was not correlated with tests of reading ability (correlations between minus sign0.13 and 0.05). Relative hand skill could therefore be considered normal within the sample. Francks C Fisher SE MacPhie IL Richardson AJ Marlow AJ Stein JF Monaco AP Am J Hum Genet 2002 Mar;70(3):800-5.

A genome-wide search strategy for identifying quantitative trait loci involved in reading and spelling disability (developmental dyslexia). Abstract: Family and twin studies of developmental dyslexia have consistently shown that there is a significant heritable component for this disorder. However, any genetic basis for the trait is likely to be complex, involving reduced penetrance, phenocopy, heterogeneity and oligogenic inheritance. This complexity results in reduced power for traditional parametric linkage analysis, where specification of the correct genetic model is important. One strategy is to focus on large multigenerational pedigrees with severe phenotypes and/or apparent simple Mendelian inheritance, as has been successfully demonstrated for speech and language impairment. Fisher SE Stein JF Monaco AP Eur Child Adolesc Psychiatry 1999;8 Suppl 3:47-51.

A lack of cerebral lateralization in schizophrenia is within the normal variation in brain maturation but indicates late, slow maturation. Abstract: The planum temporale (PT) bias, PT leftward, PT symmetry, and PT rightward reversal and sidedness preference, consistent right-handedness, ambilaterality, and consistent left-handedness are placed on a continuum mirroring the normal variation in rate of brain maturation. Maturational rate declines as we pass from PT leftward bias and consistent right-handedness to PT reversal and consistent left-handedness. Concomitantly, we expect an increased prevalence of males due to their pubertal age being about 2 years later than that of females, and a shift in cognitive profile from higher verbal scores than performance scores on the WAIS to higher performance than verbal scores. Saugstad LF Schizophr Res 1999 Oct 19;39(3):183-96.

A letter is a letter is a letter: pure alexia for kana. Grossman M Nakada T Neurology 2001 Mar 27;56(6):699-701.

A living legend in pediatric oncology nursing: Jean Fergusson. Interview by Kathy Ruccione. Abstract: Jean Fergusson is a true pioneer in pediatric oncology nursing. Her many professional accomplishments include working alongside Dr. Sidney Farber and others in the first pediatric Tumor Therapy Clinic in the United States, establishing a model pediatric nurse practitioner program that graduated an influential cadre of pediatric oncology nurse practitioners, publishing landmark papers about late sequelae of childhood cancer treatment, and serving as a role model and mentor to countless nurses over the past 50 years. Fergusson J J Pediatr Oncol Nurs 2001 Sep-Oct;18(5):229-38.

A longitudinal study of reading ability in patients suffering from dementia. Abstract: The aim of this study was to investigate whether reading is a preserved ability in patients suffering from dementia, as was first suggested by Nelson and McKenna (1975). The 57 patients included in the study had possible or probable Alzheimer's disease or similar degenerative conditions and were assessed longitudinally. Their performance on the National Adult Reading Test [(NART); Nelson, 1982, 1991] is compared to that on a shortened version of the WAIS-R. Paque L Warrington EK J Int Neuropsychol Soc 1995 Nov;1(6):517-24.

A magnetic resonance imaging study of planum temporale asymmetry in men with developmental dyslexia. Abstract: Imaging studies have suggested anomalous anatomical asymmetries in language-related regions of the temporal and parietal lobes in individuals with developmental dyslexia. Autopsy studies have reported unusual symmetry of the planum temporale (PT) in patients with dyslexia. Methodological limitations characterize much of this literature, however. To examine the size and asymmetry of the PT and its extension into the parietal lobe (planum parietale [PP]) in men with well-characterized, persistent dyslexia by using magnetic resonance imaging and 3-dimensional surface rendering techniques. These results challenge the notion that anomalous asymmetry of the PT is strongly associated with developmental dyslexia. Given the heterogeneity of the dyslexic population, some subgroup of dyslexic individuals (i.e, those with developmental language disorders) may show unusual symmetry or reversed asymmetry in this region. However, anomalous asymmetry of the planum did not contribute to functional abnormalities demonstrated in these patients by positron emission tomography. Rumsey JM Donohue BC Brady DR Nace K Giedd JN Andreason P Arch Neurol 1997 Dec;54(12):1481-9.

A miracle cure? 'tonight with Trevor McDonald', ITV, 21/01/02. Wilsher CR Dyslexia 2002 Apr-Jun;8(2):116-7.

A modality-specific mapping impairment: spoken versus written production. Abstract: A 29 year-old dysphasic woman (AF) presented with superior ability in written over spoken sentences. In contrast, her comprehension showed the reverse trend. Cognitive neuropsychological investigations revealed that her double dissociation was more apparent than real. AF's superior auditory comprehension was attributed to suspected dyslexic factors impeding written comprehension. However, an account of a strong dissociation between her written and spoken production was less obvious. Fillingham J Lum C Int J Lang Commun Disord 1998;33 Suppl:196-201.

A multimodal language region in the ventral visual pathway. Abstract: Reading words and naming pictures involves the association of visual stimuli with phonological and semantic knowledge. Damage to a region of the brain in the left basal posterior temporal lobe (BA37), which is strategically situated between the visual cortex and the more anterior temporal cortex, leads to reading and naming deficits. Additional evidence implicating this region in linguistic processing comes from functional neuroimaging studies of reading in normal subjects and subjects with developmental dyslexia Buchel C Price C Friston K Nature 1998 Jul 16;394(6690):274-7.

A neo-Lurian approach to assessment and remediation. Abstract: The first part of this article presents an operational battery of tasks for measuring the four cognitive processes of Planning, Arousal-Attention, and Simultaneous and Successive processing (PASS) not only based on the qualitative data provided in Luria's syndrome analysis, but taken from tasks in experimental cognitive psychology and neuropsychology. The second part of the article presents a remedial program based on PASS for enhancement of reading. Because this part provides in some detail the efficacy of the remedial procedure, it simultaneously validates the PASS constructs as well. Das JP Neuropsychol Rev 1999 Jun;9(2):107-16.

A neural instantiation of the motor theory of speech perception. Ivry RB Justus TC Trends Neurosci 2001 Sep;24(9):513-5.

A neurodevelopmental approach to specific learning disorders / edited by Kingsley Whitmore, Hilary Hart, Guy Willems. London: Mac Keith: Distributed by Cambridge University Press, 1999. Whitmore, Kingsley. Hart, Hilary. Willems, Guy. Description: ix, 304 p.: ill. (some col.); 25 cm. ISBN: 1898683115 LC Classification: RJ496.L4 N46 1999 Dewey Class No.: 616.85/889 21 Other System No.: (DLC) 99231944 (OCoLC)41017682

A neuronal model of attentional spotlight: parietal guiding the temporal. Abstract: Recent studies have reported an attentional feedback that highlights neural responses as early along the visual pathway as the primary visual cortex. Such filtering would help in reducing informational overload and in performing serial visual search by directing attention to individual locations in the visual field. The magnocellular (M) and parvocellular (P) subdivisions are two of the major parallel pathways in primate vision that originate in the retina and carry distinctly different types of information. Vidyasagar TR Brain Res Brain Res Rev 1999 Jul;30(1):66-76.

A new gene (DYX3) for dyslexia is located on chromosome 2. Abstract: Developmental dyslexia is a specific reading disability affecting children and adults who otherwise possess normal intelligence, cognitive skills, and adequate schooling. Difficulties in spelling and reading may persist through adult life. Possible localisations of genes for dyslexia have been reported on chromosomes 15 (DYX1), 6p21.3-23 (DYX2), and 1p over the last 15 years. Only the localisation to 6p21.3-23 has been clearly confirmed and a genome search has not previously been carried out. Fagerheim T Raeymaekers P Tonnessen FE Pedersen M Tranebjaerg L Lubs HA J Med Genet 1999 Sep;36(9):664-9.

A new look at dyslexia-dysorthography. Plea for an early recognition of that handicap Abstract: Dyslexia is a primary development disorder characterized by reading and writing disability. Although frequent, it remains underdetected at school and badly known by practitioners. As a consequence, many children remain severely handicapped in their school life, and later on in their adult social life, although being fairly intelligent. Pediatricians must be involved in its early detection and management. ERTL4 test is a useful test of detection to be applied in 5-7-year-old children. Leroy D Arch Pediatr 1998 Dec;5(12):1383-6.

A new model of letter string encoding: simulating right neglect dyslexia. Whitney C Berndt RS Prog Brain Res 1999;121:143-63.

A new protocol for the optometric management of patients with reading difficulties. Abstract: Research by Evans et al. (Ophthal. Physiol. Opt. 15, 481-487, 1995) has demonstrated a correlation between visual processing and ocular motor factors in people with specific reading difficulties (dyslexia). In addition, research by Wilkins et al. (Ophthal. Physiol. Opt. 14, 365-370, 1994) has shown that some people with dyslexia will benefit from a reduction of perceptual symptoms of discomfort and distortion if they use individually prescribed coloured filters. Lightstone A Evans BJ Ophthalmic Physiol Opt 1995 Sep;15(5):507-12.

A pictographic method for teaching spelling to Greek dyslexic children. Abstract: In the Greek orthography every letter consistently represents the same sound, but the same sound can be represented by different letters or pairs of letters. This makes spelling more difficult than reading. Two methods of teaching spelling to Greek dyslexic children are compared. The first involved pictograms (specially drawn pictures) for use when alternative spellings are possible. This is referred to as the 'PICTO' method. Mavrommati TD Miles TR Dyslexia 2002 Apr-Jun;8(2):86-101.

A positron emission tomographic study of impaired word recognition and phonological processing in dyslexic men. Abstract: Developmental dyslexia is characterized by impaired word recognition, which is thought to result from deficits in phonological processing. Improvements during the course of development are thought to disproportionately involve orthographic components of reading; phonological deficits persist into adulthood. These, along with prior findings, are compatible with a hypothesis of bilateral involvement of posterior temporal and parietal cortices in dyslexia. Rumsey JM Nace K Donohue

B Wise D Maisog JM Andreason P Arch Neurol 1997 May;54(5):562-73.

A preliminary investigation into the aetiology of Meares-Irlen syndrome. Abstract: A recent double-masked placebo-controlled trial has confirmed that some children experience a reduction in symptoms of eyestrain and headache when they read through individually prescribed coloured filters and has shown that this benefit cannot be solely attributed to a placebo effect. People who are helped by coloured filters in this way have been described as having "Meares-Irlen syndrome'. We investigated the mechanism of this benefit by studying the optometric and visual perceptual characteristics of the children in the double-masked study. Evans BJ Wilkins AJ Brown J Busby A Wingfield A Jeanes R Bald J Ophthalmic Physiol Opt 1996 Jul;16(4):286-96.

A preliminary version of a computerized naming test for preschool children with language impairment. Abstract: The most prevailing hypothesis regarding mechanisms behind specific language impairment today is the hypothesis of general limitations of processing capacity. Such an hypothesis can hardly be tested by available language assessment tools, especially not by instruments in use for clinical assessment of the lexical-semantic domain in children. Reduced naming speed is by some researchers considered as a core deficit in dyslexia and a better predictor of some aspects of reading proficiency than phonological processing. Sahlen B Radeborg K Reuterskiold Wagner C Friberg C Rydahl L Logoped Phoniatr Vocol 2000;25(3):115-21.

A problem with auditory processing? Abstract: Recent studies have found associations between auditory processing deficits and language disorders such as dyslexia; but whether the former cause the latter, or simply co-occur with them, is still an open question. Rosen S Curr Biol 1999 Sep 23;9(18):R698-700.

A quantitative-trait locus on chromosome 6p influences different aspects of developmental dyslexia. Abstract: Recent application of nonparametric-linkage analysis to reading disability has implicated a putative quantitative-trait locus (QTL) on the short arm of chromosome 6. In the present study, we use QTL methods to evaluate linkage to the 6p25-21.3 region in a sample of 181 sib pairs from 82 nuclear families that were selected on the basis of a dyslexic proband. We have assessed linkage directly for several quantitative measures that should correlate with different components of the phenotype, rather than using a single composite measure or employing categorical definitions of subtypes. Fisher SE Marlow AJ Lamb J Maestrini E Williams DF Richardson AJ Weeks DE Stein JF Monaco AP Am J Hum Genet 1999 Jan;64(1):146-56.

A randomized double-blind, placebo-controlled study of the effects of supplementation with highly unsaturated fatty acids on ADHD-related symptoms in children with specific learning difficulties. Abstract: (1) The authors tested the prediction that relative deficiencies in highly unsaturated fatty acids (HUFAs) may underlie some of the behavioral and learning problems associated with attention-deficit hyperactivity disorder (ADHD) by studying the effects of HUFA supplementation on ADHD-related symptoms in children with specific learning difficulties (mainly dyslexia) who showed ADHD features. (2) Forty-one children aged 8-12 years with both specific learning difficulties and above-average ADHD ratings were randomly allocated to HUFA supplementation or placebo for 12 weeks. (3) At both baseline and follow-up, a range of behavioral and learning problems associated with ADHD was assessed using standardized parent rating scales. (4) At baseline, the groups did not differ, but after 12 weeks mean scores for cognitive problems and general behavior problems were significantly lower for the group treated with HUFA than for the placebo group; there were significant improvements from baseline on 7 out of 14 scales for active treatment, compared with none for placebo. RichardJournalAJ Puri BK Prog Neuropsycho-pharmacol Biol Psychiatry 2002 Feb;26(2):233-9.

A review of the management of 323 consecutive patients seen in a specific learning difficulties clinic. Abstract: Visual correlates of specific learning difficulties (SpLD) include: binocular instability, low amplitude of accommodation, and Meares-Irlen Syndrome. Meares-Irlen Syndrome describes asthenopia and perceptual distortions which are alleviated by using individually prescribed coloured filters. Data from 323 consecutive patients seen over a 15 month period in an optometric clinic specialising in SpLD are reviewed. Visual symptoms and headaches were common. 48% of patients were given a conventional optometric intervention (spectacles, orthoptic exercises) and 50% were issued with coloured filters, usually for a trial period. 40% of those who were given orthoptic exercises were later issued with coloured overlays. 32% of those who were issued with coloured overlays were ultimately prescribed Precision Tinted lenses Evans BJ Patel R Wilkins AJ Lightstone A Eperjesi F Speedwell L Duffy J Ophthalmic Physiol Opt 1999 Nov;19(6):454-66.

A review of the role of visual problems in reading disabilities. Abstract: In this review we discuss the etiology of reading disturbances in children and adults. The majority of reading problems in children are either due to primary causes (dyslexia) or secondary to a variety of nonophthalmologic disorders or diseases. In adults the nature of reading difficulties is different to that in children and is defined as asthenopia. Asthenopia can develop as a result of uncorrected refractive errors or due to an imbalance of extraocular muscle action. Spierer A Desatnik H Metab Pediatr Syst Ophthalmol 1998;21(1-4):15-8.

A revision of the Abel and Becker Cognition Scale for intellectually disabled sexual offenders. Abstract: The Abel and Becker Cognition Scale (ABCS) measures cognitive distortions supportive of sexually assaultive behavior by child molesters. Research has shown that ABCS items may be too complex to be comprehended by offenders with intellectual disabilities. A modification of the ABCS to increase its readability may be one way to facilitate the valid assessment of the cognitive distortions of intellectually disabled offenders. In addition, a dichotomous scoring system was found to be helpful in the reduction of extremity bias by such offenders. Kolton DJ Boer A Boer DP Sex Abuse 2001 Jul;13(3):217-9.

A school-aged child with delayed reading skills. Abstract: During a health supervision visit, the father of a 7.5-year-old African American second-grader asked about his son's progress in reading. He was concerned when, at a recent teacher-parent conference to review Darren's progress, the teacher remarked that Darren was not keeping up with reading skills compared with others in his class. She said that he had difficulty sounding out some words correctly. In addition, he could not recall words he had read the day before. The teacher commented that Darren was a gregarious, friendly child with better-than-average verbal communication skills. Stein MT Zentall S Shaywitz SE Shaywitz BA J Dev Behav Pediatr 1999 Oct;20(5):381-5.

A school-aged child with delayed reading skills. University of California, San Diego, USA. Stein MT Zentall S Shaywitz SE Shaywitz BA J Dev Behav Pediatr 2001 Apr;22(2 Suppl):S111-5.

A sibling-pair based approach for mapping genetic loci that influence quantitative measures of reading disability. Abstract: Family and twin studies consistently demonstrate a significant role for genetic factors in the aetiology of the reading disorder dyslexia. However, dyslexia is complex at both the genetic and phenotypic levels, and currently the nature of the core deficit or deficits remains uncertain. Traditional approaches for mapping disease genes, originally developed for single-gene disorders, have limited success when there is not a simple relationship between genotype and phenotype. Recent advances in high-throughput genotyping technology and quantitative statistical methods have made a new approach to identifying genes involved in complex disorders possible. Francks C Fisher SE Marlow AJ Richardson AJ Stein JF Monaco AP Prostaglandins Leukot Essent Fatty Acids 2000 Jul-Aug;63(1-2):27-31.

A student discovers she is dyslexic. Lane ME Hayes C Imprint 1996 Nov-Dec;43(5):56.

A study and meta-analysis of lay attributions of cures for overcoming specific psychological problems. Abstract: Lay beliefs about the importance of 24 different contributors to overcoming 4 disorders that constitute primarily cognitive deficits were studied. A meta-analysis of previous programmatic studies in the area was performed Journalthat 22 different psychological problems could be compared. In the present study, 107 participants completed a questionnaire indicating how effective 24 factors were in overcoming 4 specific problems: dyslexia, fear of flying, amnesia, and learning difficulties. Furnham A Hayward R J Genet Psychol 1997 Sep;158(3):315-31.

A systematic procedure for identifying and classifying children with dyscalculia among primary school children in India. Abstract: This paper describes the procedures adopted by two independent studies in India for identifying and classifying children with dyscalculia in primary schools. For determining the presence of dyscalculia both inclusionary and exclusionary criteria were used. When other possible causes of arithmetic failure had been excluded, figures for dyscalculia came out as 5.98% (15 cases out of 251) in one study and 5.54% (78 out of 1408) in the second. It was found in the latter study

that 40 out of the 78 (51.27%) Journal had reading and writing problems. Ramaa S Gowramma IP Dyslexia 2002 Apr-Jun;8(2):67-85.

A test of a hypothesis of automatic phonological processing of Kanji words Abstract: This paper aims to examine a hypothesis that phonological processing should occur in Japanese Kanji words as well as in Kana words, but automatic in Kanji words. In Experiment 1, subjects performed concurrent articulation or finger tapping during a semantic processing task of Kana words with 2 to 4 phonemes, for which phonological processing should be indispensable. Concurrent articulation was found to eliminate the phoneme number effect found in the control condition, but finger tapping was not. Mizuno R Shinrigaku Kenkyu 1997 Apr;68(1):1-8.

A twin and family study of the association between immune system dysfunction and dyslexia using blood serum immunoassay and survey data. Abstract: We conducted a study of the association between developmental reading disability (DRD) and immune disorders (ID) using both survey and immunoassay data in two separate samples of families. One sample was made up of twins and their parents and was ascertained through a population-based sampling scheme. The other sample was a set of extended pedigrees selected for apparent autosomal dominant transmission of DRD. We failed to find an association between DRD and ID in either sample, regardless of the method used to assess immune system function. H Brain Cogn 1998 Apr;36(3):310-33.

A twin MRI study of size variations in human brain. Abstract: Although it is well known that there is considerable variation among individuals in the size of the human brain, the etiology of less extreme individual differences in brain size is largely unknown. We present here data from the first large twin sample (N=132 individuals) in which the size of brain structures has been measured. As part of an ongoing project examining the brain correlates of reading disability (RD), whole brain morphometric analyses of structural magnetic response image (MRI) scans were performed on a sample of adolescent twins. Pennington BF Filipek PA Lefly D Chhabildas N Kennedy DN Simon JH Filley CM Galaburda A DeFries JC J Cogn Neurosci 2000 Jan;12(1):223-32.

A writing fool. Cannell SJ Newsweek 1999 Nov 22;134(21):79.

Aaron, P. G. Dyslexia and hyperlexia: diagnosis and management of developmental reading disabilities / P.G. Aaron. Dordrecht; Boston: Kluwer Academic Publishers, c1989. Description: xvii, 302 p.: ill.; 25 cm. ISBN: 1556080794 (U.S.: alk. paper) LC Classification: RJ496.A5 A27 1989 NLM Class No.: WM 475 A113 Dewey Class No.: 616.85/53 19

Abnormal callosal morphology in male adult dyslexics: relationships to handedness and phonological abilities. Abstract: The classical notion that developmental dyslexia may somehow relate to impaired communication between hemispheres has not yet received convincing support. Sixteen dyslexic adults and 12 controls received a high resolution brain MRI scan for morphometric study of the corpus callosum. Automatized measurements of callosal area and calculation of indices defining the general morphology of the callosal mid-surface were performed. Each participant received global intelligence and reading achievement evaluation; dyslexics were further proposed specific neuropsychological tests specially designed to explore the mechanisms of reading impairment. Robichon F Habib M Brain Lang 1998 Mar;62(1):127-46.

Abnormal cerebral phospholipid metabolism in dyslexia indicated by phosphorus-31 magnetic resonance spectroscopy. Abstract: It has recently been suggested that many of the features of dyslexia may be explicable in terms of an abnormality of membrane phospholipid metabolism. To investigate this we studied 12 dyslexic and 10 non-dyslexic adults using in vivo cerebral phosphorus-31 magnetic resonance spectroscopy (31P MRS), as the phosphomonoester (PME) and phosphodiester (PDE) peaks include indices of membrane phospholipid turnover. Spectral localization was achieved using four-dimensional chemical shift imaging methods. Richardson AJ Cox IJ Sargentoni J Puri BK NMR Biomed 1997 Oct;10(7):309-14.

Abnormal functional activation during a simple word repetition task: A PET study of adult dyslexics. Abstract: Eight dyslexic subjects, impaired on a range of tasks requiring phonological processing, were matched for age and general ability with six control subjects. Participants were scanned using positron emission tomography (PET) during three conditions: repeating real words, repeating pseudowords, and rest. In both groups, speech repetition relative to rest elicited widespread bilateral activation in areas associated with auditory processing of speech; there were no significant differences between words and pseudowords McCrory E Frith U Brunswick N Price C J Cogn Neurosci 2000 Sep;12(5):753-62.

Abnormal processing of visual motion in dyslexia revealed by functional brain imaging. Abstract: It is widely accepted that dyslexics have deficits in reading and phonological awareness, but there is increasing evidence that they exhibit visual processing abnormalities that may be confined to particular portions of the visual system. In primate visual pathways, inputs from parvocellular or magnocellular layers of the lateral geniculate nucleus remain partly segregated in projections to extrastriate cortical areas specialized for processing colour and form versus motion. Eden GF VanMeter JW Rumsey JM Maisog JM Woods RP Zeffiro TA Nature 1996 Jul 4;382(6586):66-9.

Abnormal saccadic eye movements in autistic children. Abstract: The saccadic eye movements, generated during a visual oddball task, of autistic children, normal children, children with attention deficit disorder and hyperactivity (ADDH), and dyslexic children were examined to determine whether autistic children differed from these other groups in saccadic frequency. Autistic children made more saccades during the presentation of frequent stimuli (than normals and ADDH children), and between stimulus presentations. Also, unlike the normal and dyslexic groups, their saccadic frequency did not depend on stimulus type. Kemner C Verbaten MN Cuperus JM Camfferman G van Engeland H J Autism Dev Disord 1998 Feb;28(1):61-7.

Absence of an association between insulin-dependent diabetes mellitus and developmental learning difficulties. Abstract: For several years, investigators have been examining the relationship between learning difficulties and a variety of immunological disorders. Two recent studies by Hansen and colleagues reported a negative association between Type 1 diabetes and reading disabilities (dyslexia): subjects with Type 1 diabetes had a lower prevalence of dyslexia than their nondiabetic relatives. In order to control for the impact of environmental variables on learning, we investigated the relationship between Type 1 diabetes and learning problems in 27 sibling pairs, ranging in age from 6 to 20 years. Crawford SG Kaplan BJ Field LL Hereditas 1995;122(1):73-8.

Absence of ear advantage on the consonant-vowel dichotic listening test in adolescent and adult dyslexics: specific auditory-phonetic dysfunction. Abstract: The present study investigated auditory-phonetic processing in a group of adolescent and adult reading disabled subjects. Right- and left-handed dyslexic subjects were compared with an age, sex, and handedness matched control group. All subjects were studied with a consonant-vowel version of the dichotic listening task with repeated presentations of dichotically presented pairs of CV-

syllables. Left and right ear correct scores were compared for ear advantage in each of the different subgroups of subjects. Hugdahl K Helland T Faerevaag MK Lyssand ET Asbjornsen A J Clin Exp Neuropsychol 1995 Dec;17(6):833-40.

Absence of linkage of phonological coding dyslexia to chromosome 6p23-p21.3 in a large family data set. Abstract: Previous studies have suggested that a locus predisposing to specific reading disability (dyslexia) resides on chromosome 6p23-p21.3. We investigated 79 families having at least two siblings affected with phonological coding dyslexia, the most common form of reading disability (617 people genotyped, 294 affected), and we tested for linkage with the genetic markers reported to be linked to dyslexia in those studies. No evidence for linkage was found by LOD score analysis or affected-sib-pair methods. Field LL Kaplan BJ Am J Hum Genet 1998 Nov;63(5):1448-56.

Absence of significant linkage between phonological coding dyslexia and chromosome 6p23-21.3, as determined by use of quantitative-trait methods: confirmation of qualitative analyses. Abstract: We recently reported the absence of significant linkage of phonological coding dyslexia (PCD) to chromosome 6p23-p21.3 in 79 families with at least two affected siblings, even though linkage of dyslexia to this region has been found in four other independent studies. Whereas, in our previous analyses, we used a qualitative (affected, unaffected, or uncertain) PCD phenotype, here we report a reanalysis of linkage to the chromosome 6p region, by use of four quantitative measures of reading disability: phonological awareness, phonological coding, spelling, and rapid-automatized-naming (RAN) speed. Petryshen TL Kaplan BJ Liu MF Field LL Am J Hum Genet 2000 Feb;66(2):708-14.

Academic outcomes in children with histories of speech sound disorders. Abstract: Tests of phonology, semantics, and syntax were administered to 52 preschool children (19 girls and 33 boys, age 4-6 years) with moderate to severe speech sound disorders. The children's performance on these tests was used to predict language, reading, and spelling abilities at school age (age 8-11 years). Language impairment at school age was related to poor performance on preschool tests of syntax and nonsense word repetition, while reading impairment was predicted by poor performance in all preschool test domains (phonology, semantics, and syntax). Lewis BA Freebairn J Commun Disord 2000 Jan-Feb;33(1):11-30.

Acalculia. Neurological bases, evaluation and disorders. Abstract: To make a review of the literature on alterations in mathematical ability secondary to structural cerebral lesions. We refer to the initial classification of acalculia of Berger (secondary acalculia when this is due to broader neuropsychological deficits and primary acalculia when it occurs alone) to the classical division of Hecaen (alexia and numerical agraphia with or without alterations in reading and writing of letters and words, visuo-spatial acalculia due to alterations in the spatial organization of multi-digit figures and the partial results of arithmetical operations, anarithmetia or primary failure in mathematical ability) and the most recent classifications based on neurocognitive models, which subdivide the acalculias into those secondary to changes in the system for processing numbers and those due to changes in the cognitive system for mathematics (McCloskey and Caramazza). Similarly, we review the correlations between the clinical changes in mathematics and the cerebral localization of the causative lesions (left parieto-temporal, right and including frontal and subcortical associative areas) together with the association of acalculia and other neuropsychological deficits. Finally we review the neuropsychological instruments available for the evaluation of acalculias, with particular reference to the tools validated and scaled for our language and sociocultural setting. Dobato JL Hernandez-Lain A Caminero AB Rev Neurol 2000 Mar 1-15;30(5):483-6.

Ackerman, Adrienne. Dyslexia: motivation / Adrienne Ackerman. London: Helen Arkell Dyslexia Centre, 1974. Description: [2], 13 p.: ill.; 21 cm. ISBN: 0950362611: LC Classification: LB1050.5.A72 Dewey Class No.: 371.9/14 National Bib. No.: GB75-02778

Acquired alexia in multilingual aphasia and computer-assisted treatment in both languages: issues of generalisation and transfer. Abstract: This single-subject study addresses the issue of investigation and remediation of an acquired reading impairment observed in a Spanish-English bilingual speaker. Detailed bilingual reading testing showed parallel disturbances in the two languages, both from a qualitative and a quantitative point of view, with characteristics of letter-by-letter and aphasic alexia. On the basis of this mixed pattern, common to both languages, a two-step computer-assisted remediation programme was designed for English, then for Spanish, using a crossover AB-AB design. Laganaro M Overton Venet M Folia Phoniatr Logop 2001 May-Jun;53(3):135-44.

Acquired alexia: lessons from successful treatment. Abstract: Two individuals with anomic aphasia and acquired alexia were each provided treatment for their reading impairment. Although reading of single words in isolation was fairly accurate, their text reading was slow and effortful, including functor substitutions and semantic errors. Prior to treatment, reading reaction times for single words showed grammatical class and word-length effects. Both patients responded positively to a treatment protocol that included two phases: (1) multiple oral rereading of text, and (2) reading phrase-formatted text that had increased spacing between phrasal clauses. Beeson PM Insalaco D J Int Neuropsychol Soc 1998 Nov;4(6):621-35.

Acquired dysgraphia in alphabetic and stenographic handwriting. Abstract: We report the unusual case of AZO, who professionally used handwritten shorthand writing, and became dysgraphic after a stroke. AZO suffered from a complex cognitive impairment, and part of her spelling errors resulted from damage to auditory input processing, to phonology-orthography conversion procedures and to the ortographic output lexicon. However, analysis of her writing performance showed that the same variables affected response accuracy in alphabetic and shorthand writing; and, that the same error types, including transpositions, were observed in all tasks in the two types of writing. These observations are consistent with damage to the graphemic buffer. They suggest that, Miceli G CapasJournalR Ivella A Caramazza A Cortex 1997 Jun;33(2):355-67.

Acquired dysgraphia with selective damage to the graphemic buffer: a single case report. Abstract: We describe one patient with acquired dysgraphia who showed spelling errors (mainly deletions and substitutions), both for words and non-words, across all output modalities (oral and written spelling, and delayed copying). Spelling accuracy was not affected by lexical factors, but was a function of word length. The patient's performance in oral and written tasks suggests the hypothesis of selective damage to the Graphemic Buffer. Cantagallo A Bonazzi S Ital J Neurol Sci 1996 Jun;17(3):249-54.

Acquired dyslexia. Abstract: Disorders of reading are frequently encountered in patients with acquired cerebral lesions. Investigations in the past few decades have improved our understanding of these disorders. In this article we review the peripheral dyslexias, including neglect dyslexia, attentional dyslexia, and pure alexia (or alexia without agraphia), as well as the "central" dyslexias, including deep, surface, and phonological dyslexia. Current accounts of acquired dyslexia are discussed. Finally, we briefly describe the reading tasks that serve to differentiate the different reading disorders. Coslett HB Semin Neurol 2000;20(4):419-26.

Acquired dyslexias and dysgraphias under the prism of cognitive neuropsychology: a model for the Spanish language. Abstract: The present paper discusses the different clinical manifestations of acquired disorders of reading and writing from a neurocognitive viewpoint. Based on a specific functional architecture of reading and writing--a cognitive model; presented as well--the different syndromes of acquired dyslexias and dysgraphias, that have been described in the specialized literature during the last 25 years, will be reviewed. The different pathologies are distributed along three different functional axes: a plurimodal component, including the semantic system, for the description of peripheric disorders of reading and writing; a lexical block which is justified by the findings in patients with surface dyslexia/dysgraphia; and a third, sublexical component, in order to illustrate the different functional impairments in phonological dyslexia/dysgraphia. Bohm P Dieguez-Vide F Pena-Casanova J Tainturier MJ Lecours AR Neurologia 2000 Feb;15(2):63-74.

Activation of the phonological lexicon for reading and object naming in deep dyslexia. Abstract: Poor oral reading in some cases of deep dyslexia could be due to difficulty in inhibiting the phonological lexical entries of words semantically related to the correct reading responses. If this is the case, then additional activation of the correct phonological entries should improve reading performance, whereas additional activation of competing entries should lead to errors. This should hold true for object naming as well as for reading, since both depend on a semantically mediated lexical route. Katz RB Lanzoni SM Brain Lang 1997 Jun 1;58(1):46-60.

Adult outcomes of verbal learning disability. Abstract: Although it is currently generally accepted that, in most cases, verbal learning disability (VLD) can persist into adulthood, adult outcomes of learning disability are still under much discussion. The adult outcomes of two types of VLD (dyslexia and dysgraphia) will be the focus of this article. The defining characteristics of VLD and what constitutes these types of VLD are provided in detail elsewhere in this issue (see Jones and Eberling). Sanchez PN Coppel D Semin Clin Neuropsychiatry 2000 Jul;5(3):205-9.

Adults with severe reading and learning difficulties: a challenge for the family physician. Abstract: An estimated 40 to 44 million adults living in the United States have severe difficulty reading, writing, spelling, and doing arithmetic. These deficiencies interfere with their receiving adequate health care. Many of these adults have reading or other learning disabilities that further compromise their ability to understand their medical conditions and to participate fully in their own care. characteristics of this patient population make it difficult for the family physician to provide optimal medical services. Suggestions are given to make medical care more accessible and appropriate for these patients. Kelly MS Gottesman RL J Am Board Fam Pract 1997 May-Jun;10(3):199-205.

Afhild Tamm--an early expert on speech disorders in children Nettelbladt U Samuelsson C Lakartidningen 1998 Dec 16;95(51-52):5918-20.

Albertslund projekt I. Eksp.: Pædagogisk Central, Kanalens Kvarter 68, [1971?] Håkonsson, Erik. [from old catalog] Description: p. cm. LC Classification: LB1028.5.A357

Alexia and agraphia in posterior cortical atrophy. Abstract: A 65-year-old woman with progressive visuospatial dysfunction for 2 years complained of later-onset associated memory impairment. MRI revealed diffuse cerebrocortical atrophy, which was especially severe in both parieto-occipital regions but spared the calcarine and pericalcarine cortices. Examination 5 years after onset revealed left visual hemi-neglect, oculomotor apraxia, optic ataxia, simultanagnosia, verbal alexia, lexical and spatial agraphia, and anterograde amnesia. Ardila A

Rosselli M Arvizu L Kuljis RO Neuropsychiatry Neuropsychol Behav Neurol 1997 Jan;10(1):52-9.

Alexia caused by a fusiform or posterior inferior temporal lesion. Abstract: We evaluated the alexia and agraphia of three patients with different lesions using Japanese kanji (morphograms) and kana (phonograms) and made a lesion-to-symptom analysis. Patient 1 (pure alexia for both kanji and kana and minor agraphia for kanji after a fusiform lesion) made more paragraphic errors for kanji, whereas patient 2 (alexia with agraphia for kanji after a posterior inferior temporal lesion) showed severe reading and writing disturbances and more agraphic errors for kanji. Brodmann Area 37 was affected in both patients, but in patient 2 the lesion was located lateral to that in patient 1. Patient 3 showed agraphia without alexia after restricted lesion to the angular gyrus. Sakurai Y Takeuchi S Takada T Horiuchi E Nakase H Sakuta M J Neurol Sci 2000 Sep 1;178(1):42-51.

Alexia for Braille following bilateral occipital stroke in an early blind woman. Abstract: Recent functional imaging and neurophysiologic studies indicate that the occipital cortex may play a role in Braille reading in congenitally and early blind subjects. We report on a woman blind from birth who sustained bilateral occipital damage following an ischemic stroke. Prior to the stroke, the patient was a proficient Braille reader. Following the stroke, she was no longer able to read Braille yet her somatosenory perception appeared otherwise to be unchanged. Hamilton R Keenan JP Catala M Pascual-Leone A Neuroreport 2000 Feb 7;11(2):237-40.

Alexia without agraphia due to the lesion in the right occipital lobe in a right-handed man. Detection of hemispheric lateralization of handedness and language in a right-handed patient Alexia without agraphia has been reported in right-handed patients with left occipital lesions and in right occipital regions in left-handed patients but rarely if ever in right occipital lesions in right-handed patients. Estanol B Vega-Boada F Corte-Franco G Juarez S Hernandez R Garcia-Ramos G Rev Neurol 1999 Feb 1-15;28(3):243-5.

Alexia without agraphia in multiple sclerosis. Dogulu CF Kansu T Karabudak R J Neurol Neurosurg Psychiatry 1996 Nov;61(5):528.

Alexia without agraphia: a century later. Abstract: A case of alexia without agraphia is presented. It is a rare but classic disconnection syndrome, first described by Dejerine in 1892. Recent advances in modern neuroimaging techniques such as F Int J Clin Pract 2001 Apr;55(3):225-6.

Alexia without either agraphia or hemianopia in temporal lobe lesion due to herpes simplex encephalitis. Abstract: We report a case of alexia without either agraphia or hemianopia following herpes simplex encephalitis. The patient had a temporal lobe lesion with involvement of the occipitotemporal gyrus. This is an unusual cause of alexia without agraphia. The location of the lesion supports the view that transcallosal fibers from the right hemisphere to the left angular gyrus course inferior to the posterior horn of the left lateral ventricle and pass close to the left occipitotemporal gyrus. Erdem S Kansu T J Neuroophthalmol 1995 Jun;15(2):102-4.

Alexia-agraphia of kanji (Japanese morphogram) after left posterior-inferior temporal lesion Abstract: Several cases of selective alexia with agraphia of kanji have been reported in Japan in this decade. It is well known that the lesion in the posterior inferior temporal lobe of the dominant hemisphere is responsible for this cognitive syndrome. Data in our patient suggest that the postero-inferior region of the temporal lobe of the dominant hemisphere may be the visuo-verbal association area for the analysis of the complex visuo-verbal information. Hamasaki T Yasojima K Kakita K Masaki

H Ishino S Murakami M Yamaki T Ueda S Rev Neurol (Paris) 1995 Jan;151(1):16-23.

All developmental dyslexic subtypes display an elevated motion coherence threshold. PG - 510-7Abstract: Psychophysical studies indicate that many dyslexics have a motion-processing deficit. The purpose of this study was to determine whether elevated motion coherence thresholds correlate with the specific dyslexic subtypes as defined by the Boder classification scheme. Methods: Twenty-one dyslexics (seven dyseidetics, six dysphonetics, and eight dysphoneidetics) and 19 age- and gender-matched controls participated in the study. Motion-coherence deficits are not correlated with a specific dyslexic subtype, but, rather, are common to all subtypes. However, some individuals in each of the dyslexic subtypes were found to have normal motion coherence thresholds, suggesting that other factors must be considered to predict the motion sensitivity deficits found in dyslexia. Ridder WH 3rd Borsting E Banton T Optom Vis Sci 2001 Jul;78(7):510-7.

Allocation of attention during word recognition by good and poor readers. Abstract: The current study investigated differences in allocation of attention between good and poor readers, using dual task methodology. For 54 undergraduates classified as Good Readers and 54 classified as Poor Readers, based on their Nelson-Denny reading comprehension scores, significant main effects and interactions were found for word frequency, lexicality, and stimulus onset asynchrony, but no significant group differences (either in the form of main effects or interaction effects) were found between Good and Poor Readers. Possible explanations include task demands in the conditions and speed-accuracy trade-offs made by some subjects. Gillund B Ferraro FR Percept Mot Skills 1996 Jun;82(3 Pt 1):899-902.

Alpha and beta band power changes in normal and dyslexic children. Abstract: Previous research with healthy subjects suggests that the lower alpha band reflects attentional whereas the upper alpha band semantic processes. The aim of the present study was to investigate whether dyslexics show deficits in attentional control and/or semantic encoding Dyslexics have a lack of attentional control during the encoding of words at left occipital sites and a lack of a selective topographic activation pattern during the semantic encoding of words. Because only in controls reading of words is associated with a strong beta-1b desynchronization at those recording sites which correspond to Broca's area (FC5) and the angular gyrus (CP5, P3), we may conclude that this frequency band reflects the graphemicphonetic encoding of words. Klimesch W Doppelmayr M Wimmer H Gruber W Rohm D Schwaiger J Hutzler F Clin Neurophysiol 2001 Jul;112(7):1186-95.

Alterations in the functional anatomy of reading induced by rehabilitation of an alexic patient. Abstract: The goal of the study was to measure regional cerebral blood flow (CBF) in a stroke patient with acquired phonologic alexia before and after therapy using the Auditory Discrimination in Depth (ADD) program After rehabilitation of acquired language disorders, functional imaging can detect activity in brain structures that do not mediate language during normal conditions. However, the anatomic correlates of recovery or rehabilitation from acquired reading disorders are largely undescribed Dyslexia rehabilitation may facilitate right-hemisphere cortical networks in the reading process and increase engagement of phonologic articulatory motor representations in Broca's area. Adair JC Nadeau SE Conway TW Gonzalez-Rothi LJ Heilman PC Green IA Heilman KM Neuropsychiatry Neuropsychol Behav Neurol 2000 Oct;13(4):303-11.

Ameliorating neglect with prism adaptation: visuo-manual and visuo-verbal measures. Abstract: Previous studies have shown that adaptation to rightward displacing prisms improves performance of neglect patients

on visuo-manual (VM) tasks such as line cancellation, figure copying, and line bisection [Nature 395 (1998) 166]. The present study further evaluated the effect of prism adaptation (PA) on neglect symptoms by investigating: (a) the range of beneficial effects on common visuo-spatial deficits as well as less frequent phenomena like neglect dyslexia; (b) the duration of improvement following a single exposure to the right optical deviation; (c) the extent to which visuo-spatial performance can be comparatively ameliorated in VM tasks and visuo-verbal (VV) tasks (i.e. involving or not the adapted arm, respectively) and (d) the presence and duration of the manual visuo-motor bias induced by the prismatic adaptation (i.e. the after-effect Farne A Rossetti Y Toniolo S Ladavas E Neuropsychologia 2002;40(7):718-29.

Amplification of sign language in severe dyslexia. The hand-alphabet of the sign language makes the connection sound-letters-words easier Melhus H Melhus E Johansson U Lakartidningen 1998 Jul 22;95(30-31):3304-5.

An audit of the processes involved in identifying and assessing bilingual learners suspected of being dyslexic: a Scottish study. Abstract: The Commission for Racial Equality (Special Educational Needs Assessment in Strathclyde: Report of a Formal Investigation, CRE, London, 1996) highlighted the significant under-representation of bilingual children among pupils assessed as having specific learning difficulties/dyslexia. In this present study an audit was undertaken in order to explore issues arising from the Commission's report, initially using 53 schools from one education authority Deponio P Landon J Mullin K Reid G Dyslexia 2000 Jan-Mar;6(1):29-41.

An electrophysiological study of dyslexic and control adults in a sentence reading task. Abstract: Event-related potentials and cued-recall performance were used to compare dyslexic and control adult subjects. Sentences that ended either congruously or incongruously were presented visually, one word at a time, at fast (stimulus onset asynchrony (SOA)= 100 ms) or slow (SOA=700 ms) rates of presentation. Results revealed (1) a large effect of presentation rate that started with the N1-P2 components and lasted for the entire recording period, (2) larger N400 components for dyslexic than control subjects, at slow presentation rates, to both congruous and incongruous endings and (3) a large ERPs difference related to memory (Dm effect) that did not differentiate controls from dyslexics but was larger at slow than at fast rates of presentation. Robichon F Besson M Habib M Biol Psychol 2002 Feb;59(1):29-53.

An evaluation of the dyslexia training program: a multisensory method for promoting reading in students with reading disabilities. Abstract: The development of reading and spelling skills in students with dyslexia, by definition, is delayed and often remains delayed despite years of instruction. Three qualities are thought to facilitate reading development in these children: the provision of a highly structured phonetic-instruction training program with heavy emphasis on the alphabetic system, drill and repetition to compensate for short-term verbal memory deficits, and multisensory methods to promote nonlanguage mental representations Oakland T Black JL Stanford G Nussbaum NL Balise RR J Learn Disabil 1998 Mar-Apr;31(2):140-7.

An examination of the relationship between dyslexia and offending in young people and the implications for the training system. Abstract: A screening study was undertaken which involved 50 young offenders, serving sentences of various lengths, all from the largest young offenders' institution in Scotland. All 50 were screened for dyslexia and a number received a more detailed follow-up assessment. The results of the screening showed that 25 of the young offenders (50%) were dyslexic to some degree. This finding has implications for professionals, particularly in respect of follow-up

assessment and support, and for politicians in relation to issues such as school experience, prison education and staff training. Kirk J Reid G Dyslexia 2001 Apr-Jun;7(2):77-84.

An example of how to measure the relation between developmental dyslexia and illiteracy Abstract: The ability to read and the phonological fitness of 89 youth (average age of 21.3 years) having difficulty with social and professional integration were examined. We observed that 64% of them (n = 57) had difficulty in reading. The results of the phonological and reading tests showed that developmental dyslexia constitutes, for 56% of the subjects (n = 32), or for 36% of the population of youth with difficulties, the explanatory framework for the delay of acquisition of these capacities. Delahaie M Billard C Calvet C Gillet P Tichet J Vol S Sante Publique 1998 Dec;10(4):369-83.

An open, nonrandomized clinical comparative study evaluating the effect of epilepsy on learning. Abstract: Children with epilepsy, as a group, have a greater risk for developing learning problems as comorbid disorders. It is unknown which factors contribute to the development of such learning problems; therefore, our current knowledge does not allow the prediction of educational delay in an individual child with epilepsy. This study aimed at excluding as many factors as possible that could interfere with the analysis of the impact of epilepsy on learning. From patients referred to us in 1997 (N = 123), children were included with mild global learning impairment, defined as educational delay between 6 months and 1 year and no other apparent reason for learning impairment except for epilepsy (ie, excluding children with dyslexia, attention-deficit hyperactivity disorder, or mental handicap Aldenkamp AP Overweg-Plandsoen WC Arends J J Child Neurol 1999 Dec;14(12):795-800.

Analysis of perceptual confusions between nine sets of consonant-vowel sounds in normal and dyslexic adults. Abstract: It is widely accepted that most developmental dyslexics perform poorly on tasks that assess phonological awareness. One reason for this association might be that the early or "input" phonological representations of speech sounds are distorted or noisy in some way. We have attempted to test this hypothesis directly. In Experiment 1, we measured the confusions that adult dyslexics and controls made when they listened to nine randomly presented consonant-vowel (CV) segments [sequence: see text] under four conditions of increasing white noise masking. Cornelissen PL Hansen PC Bradley L Stein JF Cognition 1996 Jun;59(3):275-306.

Anastasiou, Demetres. Dyslexia: theoria kai ereuna, opseis praktikes Athena: Atrapos, 1998- Description: v. <1: ill.; 24 cm. ISBN: 9607412796 LC Classification: RJ496.A63 1998

Anatomical risk factors for phonological dyslexia. Abstract: Successful behavioral genetic studies require precise definition of a homogenous phenotype. This study searched for anatomical markers that might restrict variability in the reading disability phenotype. The subjects were 15 college students (8 male/7 female) diagnosed with a reading disability (RD) and 15 controls (8 males/7 females). All subjects completed a cognitive and reading battery. Only 11 of the RD subjects had a phonological deficit [phonological dyslexia (PD): pseudo word decoding scores < 90 (27th percentile Leonard CM Eckert MA Lombardino LJ Oakland T Kranzler J Mohr CM King WM Freeman A Cereb Cortex 2001 Feb;11(2):148-57.

Angermaier, Michael. Legasthenie, pro und contra: d. Kritik am Legastheniekonzept u. ihre fatalen Folgen / Michael J. W. Angermaier. Edition Information: 1. Aufl. Weinheim; Basel: Beltz, 1977. Description: 102 p.: ill.; 19 cm. ISBN: 3407500599: LC Classification: LB1050.5.A62 National Bib. No.: GFR77-A

Annals of dyslexia: [an interdisciplinary journal of the Orton Dyslexia Society]. Annals of dyslexia Ann. dyslexia Baltimore, Md.: The Society, c1982-Orton Dyslexia Society. Description: v.: ill, ports.; 23 cm. Vol. 32 (1982)- Current Frequency: Annual Continues: Bulletin of the Orton Society 0474-7534 (OCoLC)1638876 (DLC) 72626458 ISSN: 0736-9387 Incorrect ISSN: 0474-7534 Cancel/Invalid LCCN: sc 83007026 LC Classification: RJ496.A5 O78 NLM Class No.: W1 AN574 Dewey Class No.: 616.85/53/005 19 Other System No.: (OCoLC)ocm08872116 Repro./Stock No.: Orton Dyslexia Society, 724 York Road, Baltimore, MD 21204 Serial Record Entry: Annals of dyslexia. Baltimore, Md. 83-641415 Repository: universal pattern

Annotation: contemporary approaches to the teaching of reading. Snowling MJ J Child Psychol Psychiatry 1996 Feb;37(2):139-48.

Annotation: long-term outcomes of developmental reading problems. Maughan B J Child Psychol Psychiatry 1995 Mar;36(3):357-71.

Anosognosia for hemiplegia, neglect dyslexia, and drawing neglect: clinical findings and theoretical considerations. Abstract: In this paper different models of anosognosia are confronted and data concerning denial behaviors are presented that were collected on a selected population of right brain-damaged patients affected by motor and neglect disorders. Anosognosia for motor impairment and anosognosia for cognitive impairments were found to be dissociated, as well as anosognosia for the upper and lower limb motor impairments. These findings are then discussed in an attempt to choose the more suitable theoretical framework for interpreting the various disorders related to denial of illness. Berti A Ladavas E Della Corte M J Int Neuropsychol Soc 1996 Sep;2(5):426-40.

Application of ChromaGen haploscopic lenses to patients with dyslexia: a double-masked, placebo-controlled trial. Abstract:

Many patients with dyslexia report distortion to text when they are reading. After a successful pilot trial of an improvement in reading rate using ChromaGen haploscopic filters in comparison with the Intuitive Colorimeter, a full-scale, randomized, cross-over, double-masked, placebo-based trial was undertaken. The significant increase in the reading rate amongst those who reported distortion suggests that by decreasing the distortion to text, a substantial proportion of dyslexic patients--in combination with their normal reading programs--would benefit from this aid. Harris D MacRow-Hill SJ J Am Optom Assoc 1999 Oct;70(10):629-40.

Approach to learning disability. Abstract: Learning disabilities (LD) is one of the important causes of poor academic performance in school going children. Learning disabilities are developmental disorders that usually manifest during the period of normal education. These disabilities create a significant gap between the true potential and day to day performance of an individual. Dyslexia, dysgraphia and dyscalculia denote the problem related to reading, writing and mathematics. Perinatal problems are certain neurological conditions, known to be associated with LD; however, genetic predisposition seems to be the most probable etiological factors. Kulkarni M Kalantre S Upadhye S Karande S Ahuja S Indian J Pediatr 2001 Jun;68(6):539-46.

Approaches to gene mapping in complex disorders and their application in child psychiatry and psychology. Abstract: Twin studies demonstrate the importance of genes and environment in the aetiology of childhood psychiatric disorders. Advances in molecular genetics enable the identification of genes involved in complex disorders and enable the study of molecular mechanisms and gene--environment interactions. In the next 5--0 years susceptibility genes for these disorders will be established. Describing their relationship to biological and behavioural function will be a far greater challenge. Asherson PJ Curran S Br J Psychiatry 2001 Aug;179:122-8.

Are abnormal event-related potentials specific to children with ADHD? A comparison with two clinical groups. Abstract: Children with attention deficit disorder and hyperactivity (ADHD) were compared with two other clinical groups, namely, children with autism and children with dyslexia, with respect to several peaks of the ERP. By using these other clinical groups, it was studied whether amplitude differences between children and ADHD and normal control children, which were found in an earlier study, were specific to children with ADHD. ERPs were measured in response to stimuli in an auditory and a visual oddball task. Kemner C Verbaten MN Koelega HS Camfferman G van Engeland H Percept Mot Skills 1998 Dec;87(3 Pt 1):1083-90.

Are dyslexics' visual deficits limited to measures of dorsal stream function? Abstract: We tested the hypothesis that the differences in performance between developmental dyslexics and controls on visual tasks are specific for the detection of dynamic stimuli. We found that dyslexics were less sensitive than controls to coherent motion in dynamic random dot displays. However, their sensitivity to control measures of static visual form coherence was not significantly different from that of controls. Hansen PC Stein JF Orde SR Winter JL Talcott JB Neuroreport 2001 May 25;12(7):1527-30.

Are RAN- and phonological awareness-deficits additive in children with reading disabilities? Abstract: The double-deficit hypothesis (Wolf, M. and Bowers, P.G. (1999) The double-deficit hypothesis for the developmental dyslexias. Journal of Educational Psychology, 91, 415-438) proposes that deficits in phonological processing and rapid automatized naming (RAN) are separable sources of reading dysfunction. Further, the double-deficit hypothesis predicts that the presence of deficits in both phonological processing and RAN have an additive negative influence on reading performance above and beyond that of a single deficit. Compton DL DeFries JC Olson RK Dyslexia 2001 Jul-Sep;7(3):125-49.

Are speech perception deficits associated with developmental dyslexia? Abstract: Phonological awareness and phoneme identification tasks were administered to dyslexic children and both chronological age (CA) and reading-level (RL) comparison groups. Dyslexic children showed less sharply defined categorical perception of a bath-path continuum varying voice onset time when compared to the CA but not the RL group. The dyslexic children were divided into two subgroups based on phoneme awareness. Manis FR Mcbride-Chang C Seidenberg MS Keating P Doi LM Munson B Petersen A J Exp Child Psychol 1997 Aug;66(2):211-35.

Arena, John I., comp. Building spelling skills in dyslexic children, edited by John I. Arena. Assisted by Bonnie Harrington. San Rafael, Calif, Academic Therapy Publications [c1968] Description: viii, 99 p. illus. 23 cm. ISBN: 0878790012 LC Classification: LB1574.A73 Dewey Class No.: 371.9/14

Arguing over why Johnny can't read. Roush W Science 1995 Mar 31;267(5206):1896-8.

Arkell, Helen. Dyslexia, introduction: a dyslexic's eye view / by Helen Arkell. London: Helen Arkell Dyslexia Centre, 1974. Description: [5], 23 p.; 21 cm. ISBN: 095036262X: LC Classification: LB1050.5.A74 NLM Class No.: WL340 A721d 1974 Dewey Class No.: 618.9/28/553 National Bib. No.: GB75-08217

Articulatory processes and phonologic dyslexia. Abstract: Grapheme-to-phoneme conversion (GPC) allows the pronunciation of nonword letter strings and of real words with which the literate reader has no previous experience. Although cross-modal association between visual (orthographic) and auditory (phonemic-input) representations may contribute to GPC, many cases of deep or phonologic alexia result from injury to anterior perisylvian regions. Thus, GPC may rely upon associations between orthographic and articulatory (phonemic-output) representations Detailed analysis of a patient with phonologic alexia suggests that defective knowledge of the position and motion of the articulatory apparatus might contribute to impaired transcoding from letters to sounds. Adair JC Schwartz RL Williamson DJ Raymer AM Heilman KM Neuropsychiatry Neuropsychol Behav Neurol 1999 Apr;12(2):121-7.

Ashby, Annie Barden. Dyslexia trials and triumphs: what child is he now learning, disabled or gifted? / Annie Barden Ashby. Edition Information: Rev. ed. Reston, VA: D. C. Commission on the Arts & Humanities, 1995. Description: p. cm. ISBN: 0964728109 (pbk.) LC Classification: 9506 BOOK NOT YET IN LC

Assessing reading difficulties: the validity and utility of current measures of reading skill. Abstract: Accurate assessment of reading difficulties is clearly important if appropriate support and remediation is to be provided. Many different reading tests are routinely used yet it is not clear to what extent different tests tap the same underlying skills. The nature of the relationships between different tests of reading accuracy, reading comprehension and linguistic comprehension is investigated in this paper. These findings show that different reading tests measure different aspects of the reading process and that caution should be exercised when selecting tests for the assessment of reading difficulties. Nation K Snowling M Br J Educ Psychol 1997 Sep;67 (Pt 3):359-70.

Assessment of communication impairment and the effects of resective surgery in solitary, right-sided supratentorial intracranial tumours: a prospective study. Abstract: To assess the effects of solitary, right-sided supratentorial intracranial tumours on language and communication function patients were assessed preoperatively using the Western Aphasia Battery (WAB) and Boston Naming Test (BNT). The impact of resective tumour surgery was evaluated prospectively by a comparison of test scores obtained at pre- and postoperative assessments. The WAB scores in 33 patients revealed that 21% were by definition dysphasic (i.e. Aphasia Quotient < 93.8) and 35% obtained an abnormal Language Quotient. Thomson AM Taylor R Whittle IR Br J Neurosurg 1998 Oct;12(5):423-9.

Assessment of the Dichotic Listening Test by Feldmann in children with developmental reading and spelling disorders Abstract: In Germany the dD by Feldmann is a frequently used test in child assessment. Unknown, however, is the validity of the dD in the assessment of children with specific developmental language disorders. The dD by Feldmann are pairs of three-syllable content words that are presented dichotically. In this controlled cross-sectional study 65 children took the dichotic listening test by Feldmann (dD). The experimental group comprised 34 children with developmental reading and spelling disorders de Maddalena H Watzlawick-Schumacher M Arold R Laryngorhinootologie 2001 Oct; 80(10): 610-6.

Assistive technology for dyslexia. Mercurio-Standridge A ASHA 1999 Jul-Aug;41(4):5-6.

Association of abnormal cerebellar activation with motor learning difficulties in dyslexic adults. Abstract: In addition to their impairments in literacy-related skills, dyslexic children show characteristic difficulties in phonological skill, motor skill, and balance. There is behavioural and biochemical evidence that these difficulties may be attributable to mild cerebellar dysfunction. We wanted to find out whether there was abnormal brain activation when dyslexic adults undertook tasks known normally to involve cerebellar activation. The results provided direct evidence that, for this group of dyslexic adults, the behavioural signs of cerebellar abnormality reflect underlying abnormalities in cerebellar activation. Department of Psychology, University of Sheffield, UK. r.nicolson@shef.ac.uk Nicolson RI Fawcett AJ Berry EL Jenkins IH Dean P Brooks DJ Lancet 1999 May 15;353(9165):1662-7.

Associative visual agnosia resulting from a disconnection between intact visual memory and semantic systems. Abstract: We report the case of a patient (RC) who developed a severe visual agnosia, associated to alexia without agraphia, color anomia and amnesia, following an ischemic stroke in the territory supplied by the left posterior cerebral artery. Based on his proficient performance on tests evaluating analysis of elementary visual features, formation of viewer-centered and object-centered representations of visual stimuli and discrimination between drawings representing real and unreal objects, we concluded that the critical locus of deficit was a disconnection between the normally functioning visual memory store and the semantic system. Carlesimo GA Casadio P Sabbadini M Caltagirone C Cortex 1998 Sep;34(4):563-76.

Asymmetrical visual fields distribution of attention in dyslexic children: a neuropsychological study. Abstract: Visual spatial attention was evaluated in dyslexic and normally reading children by using a flanker task. When an irrelevant distractor is presented adjacent to a target stimulus, interference is observed when the two stimuli are associated with conflicting responses. In the present study the distractor flanked the target either to the right or to the left. Results showed an asymmetric flanker effect in dyslexics, whereas it was symmetrical in normal readers. Facoetti A Turatto M Neurosci Lett 2000 Sep 1;290(3):216-8.

Athetoid quadriplegia and literacy. Abstract: To compare literacy levels in athetoid quadriplegic (AQ) patients born in the 1960s and 1970s with those born in the 1980s and 1990s. Specific and intensive reading education may be required in patients with AQ to obtain functional literacy. Beal S Zeitz H Connell T Zschorn M J Paediatr Child Health 2000 Aug;36(4):389-91.

Attention deficit hyperactivity disorder, reading disability, and personality disorders in a prison population. Abstract: Attention Deficit Hyperactivity Disorder (ADHD) has long been recognized in children, and for many the disorder persists into adulthood. There is a growing concern that the adults with ADHD who have the least favorable outcome, are among those who end up in prison. The aim of this study was to assess childhood ADHD and its persistence into adulthood among a representative sample of Norwegian prison inmates, as well as personality disorders and reading difficulties, which in previous studies have been linked to ADHD. Rasmussen K Almvik R Levander S J Am Acad Psychiatry Law 2001;29(2):186-93.

Attention factors mediating syntactic deficiency in reading-disabled children. Abstract: Syntactic context effects on the identification of spoken words, and the involvement of attention in mediating these effects, were examined in seventh-grade children with reading disabilities and children who were good readers. The subjects were asked to identify target words that were masked by white noise. All targets were final words embedded in unveiled sentences. Relative to a syntactically neutral context, the identification of targets whose morpho-syntactic structure was congruent with the context was facilitated and the identification of syntactically incongruent targets was inhibited. Deutsch A Bentin S J Exp Child Psychol 1996 Nov;63(2):386-415.

Attentional control over language lateralization in dyslexic children: deficit or delay? Abstract: Two previous verbal dichotic studies by Kershner and Morton (Neuropsychologia 28, 181-198, 1990) using the forced-attention methodology (Bryden, Strategies of Information Processing, Academic Press, London, 1978) demonstrated that the order in which the ears were monitored (LE first or RE first) determined whether learning disabled children compared to age-matched nondisabled children were more weakly or strongly lateralized. Kershner JR Graham NA Neuropsychologia 1995 Jan;33(1):39-51.

Attenuated hemispheric lateralization in dyslexia: evidence of a visual processing deficit. Abstract: There is controversial evidence that deficits in the processing of low contrast and low spatial frequency stimuli are of importance in the pathogenesis of dyslexia. Fifteen adult dyslexics and 19 controls were examined using visual evoked potentials (VEP) at varying spatial frequencies (2 and 11.33 cpd) and contrasts (0.2, 0.4, 0.6, 0.8). Our results show that the amplitude of VEPs following different spatial frequencies and contrasts did not differentiate between dyslexics and controls. Schulte-Korne G Bartling J Deimel W Remschmidt H Neuroreport 1999 Nov 26;10(17):3697-701.

Atypical cognitive disorders in a man with developmental surface dyslexia. Abstract: The neuropsychological profile of a man with a developmental surface dyslexia is presented here. This case study is of interest because J.C. exhibited a pattern of cognitive disorders rarely documented in previous data. Results showed that JC's difficulties in reading comprehension were closely related to complex memory disorders and were associated with cognitive slowness. The present observations do not support the visual memory failure hypothesis. Plaza M Picard A Weber R Marlier N Brain Cogn 2000 Jun-Aug;43(1-3):358-61.

Atypical organisation of the auditory cortex in dyslexia as revealed by MEG. Abstract: Neuroanatomical and -radiological studies have converged to suggest an atypical organisation in the temporal bank of the left-hemispheric Sylvian fissure for dyslexia. Against the background of this finding, we applied high temporal resolution magnetoencephalography (MEG) to investigate functional aspects of the left-hemispheric auditory cortex in 11 right-handed dyslexic children (aged 8-13 years) and nine matched normal subjects (aged 8-14 years). Event-related field components during a passive oddball paradigm with pure tones and consonant-vowel syllables were evaluated. Heim S Eulitz C Kaufmann J Fuchter I Pantev C Lamprecht-Dinnesen A Matulat P Scheer P Borstel M Elbert T Neuropsychologia 2000;38(13):1749-59.

Auditory attentional shifts in reading-disabled students: quantification of attentional effectiveness by the Attentional Shift Index. Abstract: A controversy has existed for some years regarding auditory attentional skills in reading-disabled children. Data have suggested highly developed attentional skills in groups of reading-disabled students, but reduced attentional shifts have been documented in equivalent groups. Attentional shifts in dichotic listening with forced or directed attention are usually inferred from a significant interaction between attentional task and ear. However, this procedure cannot be used to evaluate individual test performance, and the interaction does not give a useful measure of attentional shifts in dichotic listening meaningful for comparison with other tests of attention. Asbjornsen AE Bryden MP Neuropsychologia 1998 Feb;36(2):143-8.

Auditory backward recognition masking in children with a specific language impairment and children with a specific reading disability. Abstract: The auditory backward recognition masking (ABRM) and intensity discrimination (ID) thresholds of children with a specific language impairment and poor reading (SLI-poor readers), children with an SLI and average reading (SLI-average readers), children with a specific reading

disability and average spoken language skills (SRD-average language), and children with normal spoken and written language (controls) were estimated with "child-friendly" psychophysical tasks. McArthur GM Hogben JH J Acoust Soc Am 2001 Mar;109(3):1092-100.

Auditory ERPs during rhyme and semantic processing: effects of reading ability in college students. Abstract: Event-related potential (ERP), reaction time (RT), and response accuracy measures were obtained during the phonological and semantic categorization of spoken words in 14 undergraduates: 7 were average readers and 7 were reading-impaired. For the impaired readers, motor responses were significantly slower and less accurate than were those of the average readers in both classification tasks. ERPs obtained during rhyme processing displayed a relatively larger amplitude negativity at about 480 ms for the impaired readers as compared to the average readers, whereas semantic processing resulted in no major group differences in the ERPs at this latency. Lovrich D Cheng JC Velting DM Kazmerski V J Clin Exp Neuropsychol 1997 Jun;19(3):313-30.

Auditory event-related brain potentials in autistic children and three different control groups. Abstract: ERPs to auditory stimuli, generated during an oddball task, were obtained in a group of autistic children and three control groups (normal, ADDH, and dyslectic children, respectively). The task included the presentation of standards, deviants, and novels and had a (between-group) passive vs. active (counting) condition. It was examined whether 1) it was possible to replicate several earlier findings, 2) autistics manifest an abnormal lateralization pattern of ERPs, 3) autistics have an abnormal mismatch negativity (MMN), and 4) differences between autistics and normals are really specific to the autistic group. Kemner C Verbaten MN Cuperus JM Camfferman G van Engeland H Biol Psychiatry 1995 Aug 1;38(3):150-65.

Auditory event-related potentials in poor readers. Abstract: Although poor readers (PR) are considered the major group among reading-disabled children, there are not event-related potentials (ERP) studies reported of PR on the subject. In this study, attentional and memory processes were studied in an auditory oddball task in PR and normal controls. ERP to auditory stimuli were recorded in 19 leads of the 10/20 system, using linked earlobes as references, in 20 normal children (10 female) and 20 PR (10 female) of the same age (10-12 years old). Bernal J Harmony T Rodriguez M Reyes A Yanez G Fernandez T Galan L Silva J Fernandez- Bouzas A Rodriguez H Guerrero V Marosi E Int J Psychophysiol 2000 Apr;36(1):11-23.

Auditory event-related potentials in the study of developmental language-related disorders. Abstract: This article reviews recent auditory event-related potential (ERP) studies of developmental language disorder (DLD) and dyslexia/reading disorder (RD). The possibility of using ERPs in searching for precursors of these disorders in the early development of infants at risk is discussed. Differences in exogenous/sensory ERPs at the latency range of P1 and N1-P2 components have been reported between groups with DLD and RD and control groups. Latency differences between the groups may be related to a common timing deficit suggested by some researchers to be one of the possible underlying factors both in DLD and dyslexia Leppanen PH Lyytinen H Audiol Neurootol 1997 Sep-Oct;2(5):308-40.

Auditory evoked response data reduction by PCA: development of variables sensitive to reading disability. Abstract: Long latency auditory evoked responses (AER) were formed on 232 healthy normal and learning impaired subjects to tone pairs of 50 msec inter-stimulus interval (TA Clin Electroencephalogr 2001 Jul;32(3):168-78.

Auditory evoked responses to single tones and closely spaced tone pairs in children grouped by reading or matrices abilities. Abstract: Long latency auditory evoked responses (AER) were formed to single tones and rapid tone pairs. Using the t-statistic SPM technique, children with poorer WIAT reading scores demonstrated group difference overlying the left parietal and frontal language regions but just for AER to tone pair stimuli. Variables derived from these regions were not significantly different when the same subjects were grouped by K-BIT Matrices scores. When the same children were regrouped by Matrices scores and compared using the SPM technique, differences were now seen over the right hemisphere, especially in the parietal and frontotemporal regions, for both single and two-tone derived AERs. Duffy FH McAnulty GB Waber DP Clin Electroencephalogr 1999 Jul;30(3):84-93.

Auditory frequency discrimination in adult developmental dyslexics. Abstract: Developmental dyslexics reportedly discriminate auditory frequency poorly. A recent study found no such deficit. Unlike its predecessors, however, it employed multiple exposures per trial to the standard stimulus. To investigate whether this affects frequency discrimination in dyslexics, a traditional two-interval same-different paradigm (2I_1A_X) and a variant with six A-stimuli per trial (2I_6A_X) were used here. Frequency varied around 500 Hz; interstimulus interval (ISI) ranged between 0 and 1,000 msec. Under 2I_1A_X, dyslexics always had larger just noticeable differences (JNDs) than did controls. France SJ Rosner BS Hansen PC Calvin C Talcott JB Richardson AJ Stein JF Percept Psychophys 2002 Feb;64(2):169-79.

Auditory illusions as evidence for a role of the syllable in adult developmental dyslexics. Abstract: This study investigated whether adult developmental dyslexics differ from normal controls in early stages of spoken language processing that in turn might be related to specific reading difficulties. Subjects were required to detect prespecified targets under dichotic presentation of auditory nonword pairs.

The stimuli were made such that segment migrations were possible. The potential contribution of phonetic features, as well as that of phonemes and syllables, was investigated. de Gelder B Vroomen J Brain Lang 1996 Feb;52(2):373-85.

Auditory perceptual processing in people with reading and oral language impairments: current issues and recommendations. Abstract: A popular hypothesis holds that specific reading disability (SRD) and specific language impairment (SLI) result from an impaired ability to process rapid and brief sounds. However, the results of experiments that have tested this hypothesis are incongruous. A number of factors could explain these contradictory findings, including the questionable reliability and validity of rapid auditory processing tasks, individual differences in the auditory processing abilities of SRD and SLI populations, the age of listeners, the quality of control groups, and the relationship between verbal and non-verbal auditory processing abilities. McArthur GM Bishop DV Dyslexia 2001 Jul-Sep;7(3):150-70.

Auditory processing and dyslexia: evidence for a specific speech processing deficit. Abstract: In order to investigate the relationship between dyslexia and central auditory processing, 19 children with spelling disability and 15 controls at grades 5 and 6 were examined using a passive oddball paradigm. Mismatch negativity (MMN) was determined for tone and speech stimuli. While there were no group differences for the tone stimuli, we found a significantly attenuated MMN in the dyslexic group for the speech stimuli. Schulte-Korne G Deimel W Bartling J Remschmidt H Neuroreport 1998 Jan 26;9(2):337-40.

Auditory scene analysis in dyslexics. Abstract: It has been argued that dyslexics suffer from temporal sensory processing deficits that affect their ability to discriminate speech in quiet environments. The impact of auditory deficits on non-language aspects of perception, however, is poorly

understood. In almost every natural-listening environment, one must constantly construct scenes of the auditory world by grouping and analyzing sounds generated by multiple sources. We investigated whether dyslexics have difficulties grouping sounds. Sutter ML Petkov C Baynes K O'Connor KN Neuroreport 2000 Jun 26;11(9):1967-71.

Auditory stream segregation in dyslexic adults. Abstract: Developmental dyslexia is often associated with problems in phonological processing based on, or accompanied by, deficits in the perception of rapid auditory changes. Thirteen dyslexic adults and 18 control subjects were tested on sequences of alternating tones of high (1000 Hz) and low (400 Hz) pitch, which at short stimulus onset asynchronies (SOAs) led to perceptual separation of the sound sequence into high- and low-pitched streams. Helenius P Uutela K Hari R Brain 1999 May;122 (Pt 5):907-13.

Auditory temporal coding in dyslexia. Abstract: Developmental dyslexia is generally believed to result from impaired linguistic processing rather than from deficits in low-level sensory function. Challenging this view, we studied the perception of non-verbal acoustic stimuli and low-level auditory evoked potentials in dyslexic adults. Compared with matched controls, dyslexics were selectively impaired in tasks (frequency discrimination and binaural unmasking) which rely on decoding neural discharges phase-locked to the fine structure of the stimulus. McAnally KI Stein JF Proc R Soc Lond B Biol Sci 1996 Aug 22;263(1373):961-5.

Auditory temporal processing and lexical/nonlexical reading in developmental dyslexics. Abstract: Relationships between lexical/nonlexical reading and auditory temporal processing were examined. Poor nonlexical readers (poor nonword readers, phonologic dyslexics) had difficulty across tone tasks irrespective of speed of presentation or mode of recall. Poor lexical readers (poor irregular word readers, surface dyslexics) had difficulty recalling tones in a sequence only when they were presented rapidly. Covariate analysis supported these findings, revealing that nonlexical (nonword) reading performance is associated with general auditory performance, but lexical (irregular word) reading is particularly associated with auditory sequencing. Cestnick L Jerger J J Am Acad Audiol 2000 Oct;11(9):501-13.

Auditory temporal processing deficit in dyslexia is associated with enhanced sensitivity in the visual modality. Abstract: Developmental dyslexia has been associated with a deficit in temporal processing, but it is controversial whether the postulated deficit is pansensory or limited to the auditory modality. We present psychophysical assessment data of auditory and visual temporal processing abilities in children with dyslexia. While none of the dyslexic children displayed temporal processing abnormalities in the visual sensory modality, dyslexics with poor auditory temporal scores reached high-level visual performance. Heim S Freeman RB Jr Eulitz C Elbert T Neuroreport 2001 Mar 5;12(3):507-10.

Auditory temporal processing in disabled readers with and without oral language delay. Abstract: Inferior auditory temporal processing has been postulated as causally linked to phonological processing deficits in disabled readers with concomitant oral language delay (LDRDs), and absent in specifically disabled readers with normal oral language (SRDs). This investigation compared SRDs, LDRDs and normal readers aged 7-10 years on measures of auditory temporal processing (temporal order judgement) and phonological decoding (nonword reading). LDRDs exhibited deficits in temporal order judgement compared with normal readers, from whom SRDs did not differ significantly. Heath SM Hogben JH Clark CD J Child Psychol Psychiatry 1999 May;40(4):637-47.

Awareness of language in children who have reading difficulties: historical comparisons in a longitudinal study. Abstract: We look at the awareness of grammatical distinctions in children with reading difficulties, and at their ability to use this awareness in order to learn about the conventional spellings for morphemes like "ed" at the end of past verbs. Using longitudinal methods we show that, initially, children who are to become poor readers are actually better in this aspect of spelling and in grammatical awareness tasks than younger children of the same reading level: but they are worse than these other children in tasks that tax their knowledge of phonologically based letter-sound correspondences Bryant P Nunes T Bindman M J Child Psychol Psychiatry 1998 May;39(4):501-10.

Bakker, Dirk J. Neuropsychological treatment of dyslexia / Dirk J. Bakker; translated by Ginny Spyer. Uniform [Zijdelings. English New York: Oxford University Press, 1990. Description: xii, 94 p.: ill.; 24 cm. ISBN: 0195061322 (alk. paper) LC Classification: RC394.W6 B3513 1990 NLM Class No.: WL 340 B168z Dewey Class No.: 616.85/5306 20

Bakker, Dirk J. Temporal order in disturbed reading. Developmental and neuropsychological aspects in normal and reading-retarded children. [By] Dirk J. Bakker. Foreword by A. L. Benton. [Rotterdam] Rotterdam University Press, 1972. Description: 100 p. 23 cm. LC Classification: LC4001.M63 vol. 7 RJ496.A5 Dewey Class No.: 371.9 s 618.9/28/553 National Bib. No.: Ne72-3

Balint syndrome and associated disorders. Anamnesis--diagnosis--approaches to treatment Abstract: Balint syndrome is a combination of symptoms including simultanagnosia, a disorder of spatial and object-based attention, disturbed spatial perception and representation, and optic ataxia resulting from bilateral parieto-occipital lesions. Fixation and ocular exploration of space are severely impaired, as are reading, writing, drawing and orientation as well as movement in space. Low-level visual impairments may be associated and difficult to evaluate but are not a necessary element of Balint syndrome. Kerkhoff G Heldmann B Nervenarzt 1999 Oct;70(10):859-69.

Banks, Jacqueline Turner. Egg-drop blues / by Jacqueline Turner Banks. Boston: Houghton Mifflin, 1995. Projected Pub. Date: 9503 Description: p. cm. ISBN: 0395709318 Summary: Twelve-year-old Judge Jenkins has a low science grade because of his dyslexia, so he convinces his twin brother Jury to work with him in a science competition in order to earn extra credit. LC Classification:

Banks, Jacqueline Turner. Egg-drop blues / Jacqueline Turner Banks. Boston: Houghton Mifflin, 1995. Description: 120 p.; 22 cm. ISBN: 0395709318 Summary: Twelve-year-old Judge Jenkins has a low science grade because of his dyslexia, so he convinces his twin brother Jury to work with him in a science competition in order to earn extra credit. LC Classification: PZ7.B22593 Eg 1995 Dewey Class No.: [Fic] 20

Banova, Zakhariia. Metodichno rukovodstvo za korigirane na dislaliia i disleksichni i disgrafichni proiavi, obusloveni ot fonetiko-fonematichni narusheniia na rechta / Zakhariia Banova, Mariia Ivanova. Sofiia: Ministerstvo na narodnata prosveta, 1979. Ivanova, Mariia, joint author. LC Classification: RC394.W6 B36 National Bib. No.: Bu***

Barrie, Barbara. Adam Zigzag / Barbara Barrie. New York, N.Y.: Delacorte Press, 1994. Description: 181 p.; 21 cm. ISBN: 0385311729: Summary: Adam, who is dyslexic and has great difficulty with his homework, struggles to find the right school, resist the lure of drugs, and endure the jealousy of his older sister Caroline. LC Classification: PZ7.B275378 Ad 1994 Dewey Class No.: [Fic] 20

Basic auditory dysfunction in dyslexia as demonstrated by brain activity measurements. Abstract: Although the generality of dyslexia and its devastating effects on the individual's life are widely acknowledged, its precursors and associated neural mechanisms are poorly understood. One of the two major competing views maintains that dyslexia is based primarily on a deficit in linguistic processing, whereas the other view suggests a more general processing deficit, one involving the perception of temporal information. Here we present evidence in favor of the latter view by showing that the neural discrimination of temporal information within complex tone patterns fails in dyslexic adults Kujala T Myllyviita K Tervaniemi M Alho K Kallio J Naatanen R Psychophysiology 2000 Mar;37(2):262-6.

Basic mechanisms in cognition and language with special reference to phonological problems in dyslexia / edited by C. von Euler, I. Lundberg, and R. Llinás. Edition Information: 1st ed. Amsterdam; New York: Elsevier, 1998. Euler, Curt von, 1918- Lundberg, Ingvar. Llinás, Rodolfo R. (Rodolfo Riascos), 1934- Description: xiii, 288 p.: ill.; 24 cm. LC Classification: RJ496.A5 B37 1998 Dewey Class No.: 618.92/8553 21

Becker, Ruth, 1928- Die Lese-Rechtschreib-Schwäche aus logopädischer Sicht / Ruth Becker, unter Mitarbeit von Elke van der Meer, Ralph Weigt. Edition Information: 5, überarbeitete und erw. Aufl. Berlin: VEB Verlag Volk und Gesundheit, 1985. Meer, Elke van der. Weigt, Ralph. Description: 312 p.: ill.; 23 cm. LC Classification: RJ496.A5 B43 1985

Becker, Ruth, 1928- Die Lese-Rechtschreib-Schwäche aus logopädischer Sicht / Ruth Becker, unter Mitarbeit von R. Weigt und J. Kuhring. Edition Information: 4, überarb. Aufl. Berlin: Verlag Volk und Gesundheit, 1977. Weigt, Ralph, joint author. Kuhring, J, joint author. Description: 240 p.: ill.; 22 cm. LC Classification: RJ496.A5 B43 1977 Dewey Class No.: 618.92/8553 19 National Bib. No.: GDR

Behavioral distinctions in children with reading disabilities and/or ADHD. Abstract: To investigate behavioral distinctions between children with reading disabilities (RD) and attention-deficit hyperactivity disorder (ADHD). The results of the study indicate that children from these groups may exhibit either a "pervasive" or "situational" presentation of behavioral problems, a finding which suggests that in conducting an evaluation of ADHD it is important to obtain both parent and teacher reports of problem behaviors. Pisecco S Baker DB Silva PA Brooke M J Am Acad Child Adolesc Psychiatry 1996 Nov;35(11):1477-84.

Behaviour problems in children with dyslexia. Abstract: The association between behaviour problems and dyslexia was assessed in a population sample of 10- to 12-year-old children. Twenty-five dyslexic children and a matched control group were recruited through a screening in primary schools in the city of Bergen, Norway. For the assessment of behaviour problems the Child Behavior Checklist (CBCL), Teacher Self Report (TRF), and Youth Self Report (YSR) were filled out by parents, teachers, and children, respectively. Heiervang E Stevenson J Lund A Hugdahl K Nord J Psychiatry 2001;55(4):251-6.

Benefit of docosahexaenoic acid supplements to dark adaptation in dyslexics. Stordy BJ Lancet 1995 Aug 5;346(8971):385.

Benson, D. Frank (David Frank), 1928- Aphasia, alexia, and agraphia / D. Frank Benson. New York: Churchill Livingstone, 1979. Description: ix, 213 p.: ill.; 24 cm. ISBN: 0443080410 LC Classification: RC425.B46 NLM Class No.: W1 CL731R v. 1 WL340.5 B474a Dewey Class No.: 616.8/55 Series:

Betancourt, Jeanne. A pony in trouble / Jeanne Betancourt; illustrated by Paul Bachem. New York: Scholastic Inc, c1995. Bachem, Paul, ill. Description: 96 p.: ill.; 20 cm.ISBN: 0590485857Summary: Pam's Pony Pals try to help her find out what is making her pretty pony sick. LC Classification: PZ7.B46626 Po 1995 Dewey Class No.: [Fic] 20Other System No.: (OCoLC)31950361 NNRB (FB0784(00)) RC

Betancourt, Jeanne. My name is Brain Brian / Jeanne Betancourt. New York: Scholastic, c1993.Related Titles: My name is Brian. Description: 128 p.; 22 cm.ISBN: 0590449214:Summary: Although he is helped by his new sixth grade teacher after being diagnosed as dyslexic, Brian still has some problems with school and with people he thought were his friends. LC Classification: PZ7.B46626 My 1993 Dewey Class No.: [Fic] 20

Bilingual effects of unilingual neuropsychological treatment of dyslexic adolescents: a pilot study. Abstract: Fourteen young adolescents with specific reading disabilities received short term neuropsychological treatment--specifically left hemisphere (LH) or right hemisphere (RH) stimulation--in a clinical pilot project. The effects on single-word and passage reading were evaluated when the language of treatment was either Dutch (mother tongue) or English (foreign language). Transfer effects across the two languages were studied. Kappers EJ Dekker M J Int Neuropsychol Soc 1995 Sep;1(5):494-500.

Bimanual coordination in dyslexic adults. Abstract: Various types of dyslexia have been associated with tactile-motor coordination deficits and inefficient transfer of information between the two cerebral hemispheres. Twenty-one dyslexic adults were compared to 21 controls on the Bimanual Coordination Task, a test of tactile-motor coordination and interhemispheric collaboration. When compared to control subjects, dyslexics showed a consistent pattern of deficits in bimanual motor coordination, both with and without visual feedback. Moore LH Brown WS Markee TE Theberge DC Zvi JC Neuropsychologia 1995 Jun;33(6):781-93.

Bimodal reading: benefits of a talking computer for average and less skilled readers. Abstract: Studies have shown that when information is presented through visual and auditory channels simultaneously (i.e, bimodal presentation), speed of processing and memory recall are enhanced. The present study demonstrated the efficacy of a bimodal approach to fostering reading comprehension. Eighteen average readers (9 girls and 9 boys) and 18 less skilled readers (8 girls and 10 boys) in Grades 8 and 9 participated in the study. Students were presented with social studies and science passages via a computer. Montali J Lewandowski L J Learn Disabil 1996 May;29(3):271-9.

Biobehavioral measures of dyslexia / edited by David B. Gray, James F. Kavanagh. Parkton, Md.: York Press, c1985. Gray, David B. Kavanagh, James F. Description: xv, 328 p.: ill.; 24 cm. ISBN: 0912752106: LC Classification: RC394.W6 B56 1985 Dewey Class No.: 616.85/53 19

Blechner, Gerda. Schulversagen und Legasthenieproblematik der ausländischen Kinder in der BRD, Österreich und der Schweiz: Hintergründe, Diagnostik, Kasuistik, Lösungsformen: mit einer Anleitung zu Stützkursen und Nachhilfestunden für Gastarbeiterkinder / Gerda Blechner. Bern: P. Haupt, c1981. Description: 119 p.: ill.; 21 cm.ISBN: 3258030367 LC5158.G3 B58 1981 Dewey Class No.: 371.96/75 19

Blue, Rose. Me and Einstein: breaking through the reading barrier / by Rose Blue; illustrated by Peggy Luks. New York: Human Sciences Press, c1979. Luks, Peggy. Description: [64] p.: ill.; 22 cm.ISBN: 087705388XSummary: Having tried for years to hide the fact that he can't read, a nine-year-old boy finally discovers the reason for his problem. LC Classification: PZ7.B6248 Me Dewey Class No.: [Fic]

Blurring the image does not help disabled readers. Abstract: Previous research has found that poor readers performed a visual search task more slowly than good readers, but that this difference was virtually eliminated by blurring of the search array. Whereas blurring had little effect on the performance of the good readers, it led to a dramatic improvement in the search rate of the poor readers. The present study set out to replicate this research with groups of 10-12 yr old disabled and average readers but with methodological improvements in the procedure and the analysis. Hogben JH Pratt C Dedman K Clark CD Vision Res 1996 May;36(10):1503-7.

Bonistalli, Edo. [from old catalog] Prevenzione e trattamento della dislessia. Firenze, La nuova Italia, 1973, Description: 98, [32] p. illus. 20 cm. LC Classification: RJ496.A5 B66

Bordesoules, Roger Henry. Méthode Bordesoules: pour apprendre à lire en un temps record: méthode mnémotechnique, abréviative, antidyslexique / par Roger H. Bordesoules,... Pierre Max,...; édité par le Mouvement d'entr'aide pour le Tiers monde et la coopération. Vincennes (Centre de santé, 6, Av. Pierre-Brossolette, 94300): Mouvement d'entr'aide pour le Tiers monde et la coopération, 1975. Max, Pierre, joint author. Description: 32 p.: ill.; 21 cm. LC Classification: LB1050.5.B63 Dewey Class No.: 372.4/3National Bib. No.: F76-2612

Both coloured overlays and coloured lenses can improve reading fluency, but their optimal chromaticities differ. Abstract: Some individuals read more fluently when the text is coloured: i.e, when coloured sheets of plastic (overlays) are placed upon the page, or when coloured lenses are worn. Overlays provide a surface colour whereas lenses mimic a change in the colour of a light source. The neural mechanisms that underlie colour constancy ensure that the chromaticity of overlays and lenses is processed differently by the visual system. Lightstone A Lightstone T Wilkins A Ophthalmic Physiol Opt 1999 Jul;19(4):279-85.

Boy/girl differences in risk for reading disability: potential clues? Abstract: The authors conducted a case-control study to determine whether risk factors for reading disability (RD) differentially affect boys and girls. The study population included all children born between 1976 and 1982 in Olmsted County, Minnesota (n = 5,701). A total of 303 RD cases were identified by using intelligence quotient and achievement test scores collected from school and medical records. After excluding those who met exclusion criteria (n = 869), controls consisted of all children not identified with RD (n = 4,529). St Sauver JL Katusic SK Barbaresi WJ Colligan RC Jacobsen SJ Am J Epidemiol 2001 Nov 1;154(9):787-94.

Braams, Tom, 1959- Dyslexie: een complex taalprobleem / Tom Braams. Amsterdam: Boom, c1996. Description: 128 p.; 20 cm.ISBN: 905352276X: LC Classification: RC394.W6 B714 1996

Brain activation during reading in deep dyslexia: an MEG study. Abstract: Magnetoencephalographic (MEG) changes in cortical activity were studied in a chronic Finnish-speaking deep dyslexic patient during single-word and sentence reading. It has been hypothesized that in deep dyslexia, written word recognition and its lexical-semantic analysis are subserved by the intact right hemisphere. However, in our patient, as well as in most nonimpaired readers, lexical-semantic processing as measured by sentence-final semantic-incongruency detection was related to the left superior-temporal cortex activation. Laine M Salmelin R Helenius P Marttila R J Cogn Neurosci 2000 Jul;12(4):622-34.

Brain activation profiles in dyslexic children during non-word reading: a magnetic source imaging study. Abstract: The purpose of the study was to identify spatiotemporal brain activation profiles associated with phonological decoding in dyslexic children using magnetic source imaging. For this purpose maps of regional cerebral activation were obtained from eleven children diagnosed with dyslexia and ten children without reading problems during engagement in a pseudoword rhyme-matching task. All dyslexic children showed aberrant activation maps consisting of reduced activity in temporoparietal areas in the left hemisphere (including the posterior part of the superior temporal, angular and supramarginal gyri) and increased activity in the right homotopic region. Simos PG Breier JI Fletcher JM Foorman BR Bergman E Fishbeck K Papanicolaou AC Neurosci Lett 2000 Aug 18;290(1):61-5.

Brain activity in visual cortex predicts individual differences in reading performance. Abstract: The relationship between brain activity and reading performance was examined to test the hypothesis that dyslexia involves a deficit in a specific visual pathway known as the magnocellular (M) pathway. Functional magnetic resonance imaging was used to measure brain activity in dyslexic and control subjects in conditions designed to preferentially stimulate the M pathway. Dyslexics showed reduced activity compared with controls both in the primary visual cortex and in a secondary cortical visual area (MT+) that is believed to receive a strong M pathway input. Most importantly, significant correlations were found between individual differences in reading rate and brain activity. Demb JB Boynton GM Heeger DJ Proc Natl Acad Sci U S A 1997 Nov 25;94(24):13363-6.

Brain function and reading disabilities / edited by Lester Tarnopol and Muriel Tarnopol. Baltimore: University Park Press, c1977. Tarnopol, Lester. Tarnopol, Muriel. Description: xiii, 214 p.: ill.; 23 cm. ISBN: 0839111304 LC Classification: LB1050.5.B69 NLM Class No.: WL340 B816 Dewey Class No.: 428/.4

Brain imaging in neurobehavioral disorders. Abstract: Neuroimaging studies of neurobehavioral disorders are using new imaging modalities. In dyslexia, anatomic imaging studies demonstrate an abnormal symmetry of the planum temporale.

Functional imaging supports the hypothesis that developmental dyslexia is frequently the result of deficits in phonologic processing and that normal reading requires a patent network organization of a number of anterior and posterior brain areas. In autism, anatomic imaging studies are conflicting. Functional imaging demonstrates temporal lobe abnormalities and abnormal interaction between frontal and parietal brain areas Frank Y Pavlakis SG Pediatr Neurol 2001 Oct;25(4):278-87.

Brain imaging of reading disorders. Rumsey JM J Am Acad Child Adolesc Psychiatry 1998 Jan;37(1):12.

Brain mechanisms in normal and dyslexic readers. Abstract: Developmental dyslexics, individuals with an unexplained difficulty reading, have been shown to have deficits in phonological processing -- the awareness of the sound structure of words -- and, in some cases, a more fundamental deficit in rapid auditory processing. In addition, dyslexics show a disruption in white matter connectivity between posterior and frontal regions. These results give continued support for a neurobiological etiology of developmental dyslexia. However, more research will be required to determine the possible causal relationships between these disruptions and dyslexia. Temple E Curr Opin Neurobiol 2002 Apr;12(2):178-83.

Brain morphology in children with specific language impairment. Abstract: The planum temporale and pars triangularis have been found to be larger in the left hemisphere than the right in individuals with normal language skills. Brain morphology studies of individuals with developmental language disorders report reversed asymmetry or symmetry of the planum, although the bulk of this research has been completed on adults with dyslexia. Pars triangularis has not been studied in the developmental language impaired population. In this study, magnetic resonance imaging (MRI) was used for quantitative comparisons of the planum temporale (Wernicke's area) and pars triangularis (Broca's area) in children with specific language impairment (SLI) and children with normal language skills. Gauger LM Lombardino LJ Leonard CM J Speech Lang Hear Res 1997 Dec;40(6):1272-84.

Brain plasticity for sensory and linguistic functions: a functional imaging study using magnetoencephalography with children and young adults. Abstract: In this report, the newest of the functional imaging methods, magnetoencephalography, is described, and its use in addressing the issue of brain reorganization for basic sensory and linguistic functions is documented in a series of 10 children and young adults. These patients presented with a wide variety of conditions, ranging from tumors and focal epilepsy to reading disability. Papanicolaou AC Simos PG Breier JI Wheless JW Mancias P Baumgartner JE Maggio WW Gormley W Constantinou JE Butler II J Child Neurol 2001 Apr;16(4):241-52.

Brain potentials in developmental dyslexia: differential effects of word frequency in human subjects. Abstract: The differences of word processing between a group of adult developmental dyslexics and control subjects were examined with the event-related potential (ERP) technique. In particular, the effects of word frequency and word recognition were assessed. The subjects viewed a series of frequently and infrequently used words, most of which were repeated after some intervening items and they discriminated between first and second presentations of the words. It can be shown that in the range from 300 to 550 ms post stimulus the amplitude of the N400 component, an ERP measure of semantic processing, is reduced for high frequency words. Johannes S Mangun GR Kussmaul CL Munte TF Neurosci Lett 1995 Aug 11;195(3):183-6.

Brain structures of reading Japanese words with functional MRI Abstract: This review examines recent progress in understanding mechanisms involved in language related brain functions using functional magnetic resonance imaging (fMRI). The main focus is to detect differences in reading processes between the ideogram (Japanese kanji) and the phonogram (Indo-European language or Japanese kana). Inferior temporal (IT) areas on the language dominant side are involved in reading both characters. A plasticity model is introduced to explain the different localizations that have been ascribed to kana or kanji, respectively. Makabe T Edmister WB Jenkins BG Rosen BR Nippon Rinsho 1997 Jul;55(7):1699-705.

Bravo Valdivieso, Luis. Dislexias y retardo lector: enfoque neuropsicológico / Luis Bravo Valdivieso. Santiago, Chile: Ediciones Universidad Católica de Chile, [1984] Description: 259 p.; 19 cm. LC Classification: RC394.W6 B72 1984 Dewey Class No.: 616.85/53 20

Bravo Valdivieso, Luis. Teorías sobre la dislexia y su enfoque científico / Luis Bravo Valdivieso. Santiago de Chile: Editorial Universitaria, [1981], c1980. Description: 87 p.; 18 cm. LC Classification: RC394.W6 B73 1981 Dewey Class No.: 616.85/53 20

British Dyslexia Association. International Conference (2nd: 1991: Oxford, England) Dyslexia: integrating theory and practice: selected papers from the second International Conference of the British Dyslexia Association "Meeting the Challenge", Oxford, 1991 / edited by Margaret Snowling and Michael Thomson. London and New Jersey: Whurr Publishers, c1992. Snowling, Margaret J. Thompson, Michael L. Description: xx, 332 p.: ill.; 24 cm.ISBN: 1870332474 LC Classification: LC4710.G7 B75 1992 Dewey Class No.: 371.91/44 20

British Dyslexia Association. International Conference (3rd: 1994: Manchester, England) Reading development and dyslexia: selected papers from the Third International Conference of the British Dyslexia Association "Dyslexia--Towards a Wider Understanding," Manchester, 1994 / edited by Charles Hulme and Margaret Snowling. London: Whurr; San Diego, Calif.: Distributed in the USA by Singular Pub. Group, 1994. Hulme, Charles. Snowling, Margaret J. Description: xiii, 246 p.: ill.; 24 cm.ISBN: 1897635850 LC Classification: LB1050.5.B76 1994 Dewey Class No.: 371.9144 20National Bib. No.: GB94-31506Other System No.: (OCoLC)30438408

Broomfield, Hilary. Overcoming dyslexia: a practical handbook for the classroom / by Hilary Broomfield and Margaret Combley; consultant in dyslexia, Margaret Snowling. San Diego, Calif.: Singular Pub. Group, c1997. Combley, Margaret. Snowling, Margaret J. Description: x, 226 p.: ill.; 25 cm.ISBN: 1565938364 LC Classification: LC4709.B76 1997 Dewey Class No.: 371.91/44 21

Brown, Dale S. Learning a living: a guide to planning your career and finding a job for people with learning disabilities, attention deficit disorder, and dyslexia / Dale S. Brown.Edition Information: 1st ed. Bethesda, MD: Woodbine House, 2000. Description: xxvi, 340 p.: ill.; 28 cm.ISBN: 0933149875 (pbk.) LC Classification: HV1568.5.B76 2000 Dewey Class No.: 331.7/02/087 21

Brown, Dale, 1954- I know I can climb the mountain / written by Dale S. Brown; illustrated by Lisa Freeman. Columbus, OH: Mountain Books, c1995. Freeman, Lisa, ill. Description: 93 p.: ill.; 22 cm.ISBN: 1881650049 LC Classification: PS3552.R68542 I2 1995 Dewey Class No.: 811/.54 20

Buchanan, Ben. My year with Harry Potter: how I discovered my own magical world / Ben Buchanan. New York: Lantern Books, c2001. Description: 112 p.: ill.; 23 cm.ISBN: 1930051506 (alk. paper) LC Classification: GV1312.B84 2001 Dewey Class No.: 794/.092 B 21

Bühler-Niederberger, Doris. Legasthenie: Geschichte und Folgen einer Pathologisierung/Doris Bühler-Niederberger. Opladen: Leske + Budrich, 1991. Description: 250 p.: ill.; 21 cm.ISBN: 3810008974 LC Classification: RJ496.A5 B84 1991NLM Class No.: JJ1250 [HV 888] Dewey Class No.: 618.92/8553 20 Other System No.: (OCoLC)26673851

Building number skills in dyslexic children / edited by John I. Arena. San Rafael, Calif.: Academic Therapy Publications, 1972, 1974 printing. Arena, John I. Description: 108 p.: ill.; 23 cm. ISBN: 0878790403: LC Classification: QA11.B86 Dewey Class No.: 371.9/14

Bulletin of the Orton Society. Bulletin of the Orton Society Bull. Orton Soc. Waterbury, Conn. [etc.] Orton Society. Orton Society. Description: 31 v. ill. 23 cm. v. 1-31; 1951-81. Current Frequency: Annual Continued by: Annals of dyslexia 0736-9387 (OCoLC)8872116 (DLC) 83641415 1982 ISSN: 0474-7534 Cancel/Invalid LCCN: sn 80001740 CODEN: ORSBBT LC Classification: RJ496.A5 O78 NLM Class No.: W1 OR868 Dewey Class No.: 618.9/28/553005 Other System No.: (OCoLC)ocm01638876 Serial Record Entry: Orton Society. Bulletin. Towson, Md. sv89-4592

Bundesverband Legasthenie, Germany. Legasthenie: Bericht über d. Fachkongress 1978 / Hrsg, Bundesverb. Legasthenie e.V, Volker Ebel. Bonn: Reha-Verlag, 1979. Ebel, Volker. Description: 248 p.: ill, graphs; 21 cm.ISBN: 3882390409: LC Classification: LB1050.5.B86 1979National Bib. No.: GFR79-A49

Bursak, George J, 1913- If I can do it, so can you: triumph over dyslexia / by George J. Bursak. [S.l.]: G.J. Bursak, c1999. Description: xiii, 47 p.: ill.; 24 cm. LC Classification: RC394.W6 B87 1999 Dewey Class No.: 362.1/968553/0092 B 21

Callosal transfer in different subtypes of developmental dyslexia. Abstract: Sixteen controls (age 6-13) and 20 native Italian children with developmental dyslexia (age 7-15) received a test of callosal transfer of tactile information. Among the dyslexic children, 7 had a diagnosis of L-type, 7 of P-type and 6 of M-type dyslexia according to Bakker's classification. Both control children and children with dyslexia made a significantly larger number of errors in the crossed localization condition (implying callosal transfer of tactile information) vs. the uncrossed condition. Fabbro F Pesenti S Facoetti A Bonanomi M Libera L LorusJournalML Cortex 2001 Feb;37(1):65-73.

Callosal transfer of finger localization information in phonologically dyslexic adults. Abstract: Dyslexia, particularly phonological dyslexia, has been hypothesized to be associated with deficits in interhemispheric interactions mediated by the corpus callosum. Twenty-one dyslexic subjects were compared to 21 controls on the Finger Localization Test in order to observe patterns of tactile-motor integration and interhemispheric collaboration. When compared to control subjects, dyslexics showed consistent deficits in finger localization, particularly when more complex trials had to be completed. Moore LH Brown WS Markee TE Theberge DC Zvi JC Cortex 1996 Jun;32(2):311-22.

Can contrast sensitivity functions in dyslexia be explained by inattention rather than a magnocellular deficit? Abstract: We examined whether data demonstrating contrast sensitivity losses in dyslexia that have been interpreted as evidence for loss of magnocellular visual function could be explained by inattention. Computer simulations of observers with poor concentration yielded inflated estimates of threshold that were a constant proportion of the true threshold across spatial frequencies. Data from many, but not all, studies supporting the magnocellular deficit theory are well described by these simulations, which predicted no interaction between observer group and spatial frequency. Stuart GW McAnally KI Castles A Vision Res 2001 Nov;41(24):3205-11.

Can treatment for pure alexia improve letter-by-letter reading speed without sacrificing accuracy? Abstract: An experimental treatment study designed to improve both the accuracy and the speed of reading was administered to a patient with pure alexia and impaired letter naming. The study focused on the use of letter-by-letter reading. A two-stage approach was employed. The first stage implemented a tactile-kinesthetic strategy to improve accuracy. The second stage concentrated on speed. At the end of the treatment, patient DL was reading both trained and untrained words more accurately and with considerably greater speed than prior to treatment. Accuracy and speed of reading at the sentence level improved as well. Nitzberg Lott S Friedman RB Brain Lang 1999 May;67(3):188-201.

Carlson, Trudy. Learning disabilities: how to recognize and manage learning and behavioral problems in children / by Trudy Carlson.Edition Information: 1st ed. Duluth, Minn.: Benline Press, c1997. Description: 133 p.; 22 cm.ISBN: 0964244322 LC Classification: RJ506.H9 C37 1997 Dewey Class No.: 618.92/8589 21

Carris, Joan Davenport. Aunt Morbelia and the screaming skulls / Joan Carris; illustrated by Doug Cushman.Edition Information: 1st ed. Boston: Little, Brown, c1990. Cushman, Doug, ill. Description: 134 p.: ill.; 22 cm.ISBN: 0316129453:Summary: The peaceful life of a boy with dyslexia is interrupted when his great-aunt, who has a morbid fascination with ghosts and death omens, moves in. LC Classification: PZ7.C2347 Au 1990 Dewey Class No.: [Fic] 20

Casanova, María Antonia. La dislexia / [por] M.a Antonia Casanova Rodríguez. Salamanca: Anaya, 1976. Description: 46 p.; 22 cm.ISBN: 8420718033: LC Classification: RJ496.A5 C38 Dewey Class No.: 616.85/53 19National Bib. No.: Sp77-Jan

Case study: a virtual non-reader achieves a degree. Abstract: J, a mature age student with severe dyslexia, entered university with virtually no reading and writing. She could recognize very few words, she had difficulty with spelling simple words and her handwriting was poor. She had distinctive difficulties with numbers. Yet, she graduated successfully 3 years after entry. In this paper, the characteristics of her disabilities are discussed and the teaching programme and support systems set up to help her are described. Some theoretical and practical implications which arise from J's case are considered. Cooke A Dyslexia 2002 Apr-Jun;8(2):102-15.

Cases: when the hospital becomes alive Landi Pereira L Breda ML Riv Inferm 1995 Oct-Dec;14(4):181-3.

Category specificity in reading and writing: the case of number words. Abstract: In standard models, word meanings contribute to reading words aloud and writing them to dictation. It is known that categories of knowledge and the associated word meanings can be spared or impaired selectively, but it has not been possible to demonstrate that category-specific effects apply to reading and writing. Here we report the case of a neurodegenerative patient with selectively spared numerical abilities whose brain damage left him able to read and write only number words. Butterworth B Cappelletti M Kopelman M Nat Neurosci 2001 Aug;4(8):784-6.

Cavazzuti Pavarotti, Carla. La rieducazione del dislessico nella scuola elementare / Carla Cavazzuti Pavarotti, Franca Toni Giovanardi. Brescia: La scuola, [1974] Toni Giovanardi, Franca, joint author. Description: 173 p.: ill.; 21 cm. LC Classification: LB1050.5.C35National Bib. No.: It75-Jan

Central auditory processing disorder in school-aged children: a critical review. Abstract: The rationale to evaluate for central auditory processing disorder (CAPD) in school-aged children is based on the assumption that an auditory-specific perceptual deficit underlies many learning problems including specific reading and language disabilities. A fundamental issue in this area is whether convincing empirical evidence exists to validate this proposition. Herein, we consider the issue of modality specificity by examining the extent to which reading, language, and attention disorders in school-aged children involve perceptual dysfunctions limited to a single sensory modality. Cacace AT McFarland DJ J Speech Lang Hear Res 1998 Apr;41(2):355-73.

Central auditory processing, MRI morphometry and brain laterality: applications to dyslexia. Abstract: We review data from our laboratory related to a view of dyslexia as a biological disorder, or deficit, caused by both structural and functional brain abnormalities. The review is focused on central auditory processing in dyslexia, and the possibility that impairments in the auditory or acoustic features of the phonological code may be at the heart of the impairments seen in dyslexia. Three methodological approaches by which to investigate central auditory processing deficits are outlined: dichotic listening (DL) to consonant-vowel syllables; magnetic resonance imaging (MRI), and the use of event-related potentials (ERPs). Hugdahl K Heiervang E Nordby H Smievoll AI Steinmetz H Stevenson J Lund A Scand Audiol Suppl 1998;49:26-34.

Central transmission time in children with the delayed language development Abstract: The prolonged central transmission time (CTT) in ABR examinations in children with the delayed speech was described in 1992. Now after 4 years the examinations were repeated. The children with actually good speech revealed normalization of CTT, but in children with dyslalia and dyslexia this interpeak latencies were once

again prolonged. Pracownia Audiologiczno-Foniatryczna Centrum Medycznego Ksztalcenia Podyplomowego w Dziekanowie Lesnym. Zaleski T Kielska E Otolaryngol Pol 2000; 54(1):71-3.

Cerebral lateralisation and rate of maturation. Abstract: Multifactorial inheritance applied to brain development implies a large continuum of normal variation with deviation from the norm at the extremes of maturational rate. The greater population of neurons, greater arborization of neural networks and excessive synaptic density in early maturation imply that adaptability (plasticity) is a main advantage, as opposed to a deficit in adaptability associated with the reduced number of neurons, reduced connectivity and reduced synaptic density in late slow maturation. It is hypothesised that Planum Temporale (PT) asymmetry and hand-preference predict the rate of CNS maturation as does the cognitive profile on the Wechsler Adult Intelligence Scale (WAIS): PT leftward asymmetry, right-handedness and a left-hemisphere cognitive advantage signifies early fast maturation: PT rightward asymmetry, left-handedness and a right-hemisphere cognitive advantage signify late maturation, while PT symmetry and ambilaterality represent rates of maturation in between Saugstad LF Int J Psychophysiol 1998 Jan;28(1):37-62.

Cerebral localization of the center for reading and writing music. Abstract: The mechanisms that underlie the ability to read and write music remain largely unclear compared to those involved in reading and writing language. We had the extremely rare opportunity to study the cerebral localization of the center for reading and writing music in the case of a professional trombonist. During rehearsal immediately before a concert, he suffered a hemorrhage that was localized to the left angular gyrus, the area that has long been known as the center for the ability to read and write. Detailed tests revealed that he showed symptoms of alexia with agraphia for both musical scores and language. Department of Neurology, Showa University School of Medicine, Tokyo, Japan. Kawamura M Midorikawa A Kezuka M Neuroreport 2000 Sep 28;11(14):3299-303.

Cerebral mechanisms involved in word reading in dyslexic children: a magnetic source imaging approach. Abstract: The purpose of the present investigation was to describe spatiotemporal brain activation profiles during word reading using magnetic source imaging (MSI). Ten right-handed dyslexic children with severe phonological decoding problems and eight age-matched non-impaired readers were tested in two recognition tasks, one involving spoken and the other printed words. Dyslexic children's activation profiles during the printed word recognition task consistently featured activation of the left basal temporal cortices followed by activation of the right temporoparietal areas (including the angular gyrus). Simos PG Breier JI Fletcher JM Bergman E Papanicolaou AC Cereb Cortex 2000 Aug;10(8):809-16.

Characteristics of dyslexia in a Dutch family. Abstract: This study investigates the characteristics of 19 members of a Dutch family. Nine of them, recognized as dyslexic in their early years, are compared with six non-dyslexic members, whereas four form a non-classified category. From their personal histories, it is clear that the dyslexics had a long and troublesome educational career, while the non-dyslexics did not. However, probably because the dyslexic members had considerable intellectual resources and talents in mathematics and technical skills, most succeeded in getting degrees of a reasonably high standard and jobs that more or less matched their talents. van der Leij A de Jong PF Rijswijk-Prins H Dyslexia 2001 Jul-Sep;7(3):105-24.

Chassagny, Claude. [from old catalog] La rééducation du langage écrit; nouveau manuel pour la rééducation de la lecture et de l'orthographe. Paris, Néret [1972] Description: 449 p. illus. 22 cm. LC Classification: LB1050.5.C49

Chassagny, Claude. Pédagogie relationnelle du langage / Claude Chassagny,.... Paris: Presses universitaires de France, 1977. Description: 238 p.: ill.; 22 cm. LC Classification: LB1050.5.C485 Dewey Class No.: 448.4/2National Bib. No.: F78-2257

Chicorel abstracts to reading and learning disabilities. Portion of Abstracts to reading and learning disabilities Chicorel abstracts to reading and learning disabilities Chicorel abstr. read. learn. disabil. New York City: American Library Pub. Co, Chicorel, Marietta. Description: v.; 24 cm. Began with 1975 vol. Current Frequency: Annual ISSN: 0149-533X Cancel/Invalid LCCN: sn 79004440 LC Classification: LB1050.5.C52 NLM Class No.: Z 5814.V4 C53 Dewey Class No.: 371.9 Other System No.: (OCoLC)ocm03488225

Chicorel index to reading and learning disabilities, an annotate guide: Books. Chicorel index to reading and learning disabilities [New York] Chicorel Library Pub. Corp. Chicorel, Marietta ed. Description: v. 27 cm. 1976- ISSN: 0149-5496 Cancel/Invalid LCCN: sn 78002117 LC Classification: Z5818.L3 C55 LB1050.5 NLM Class No.: Z 5814.V4 C5305 Dewey Class No.: 016.3719 Other System No.: (OCoLC)ocm03487987

Childhood bacterial meningitis: impact of age at illness and acute medical complications on long term outcome. Abstract: This study compared postmeningitic children (N = 130) with grade and sex matched controls (N = 130) selected from target children's schools on measures of intellectual, linguistic, learning, and reading skills. Results showed that children with a history of meningitis are at greater risk for impairment in these areas, with experience of the disease prior to 12 months of age being an important risk factor. Within the postmeningitic sample presence of medical complications was associated with poorer verbal abilities.

Anderson V Bond L Catroppa C Grimwood K Keir E Nolan T J Int Neuropsychol Soc 1997 Mar;3(2):147-58.

Children with benign focal sharp waves in the EEG--developmental disorders and epilepsy. Abstract: Focal sharp waves (shw) in the childhood EEG with predominantly centrotemporal localization are a diagnostic hallmark of idiopathic partial epilepsy and have been shown to be genetically determined. Absence of neurological and neuropsychological impairment was long considered to be a prerequisite for diagnosis. For years, this diagnostic paradigm obscured the large phenotypic variability of genetically determined focal shw. Doose H Neubauer B Carlsson G Neuropediatrics 1996 Oct;27(5):227-41.

Children's language disorders from the point of view of brain research--dyslexia as an example Lyytinen H Leppanen P Duodecim 2000;116(4):449-55.

Chivers, Maria. Practical strategies for living with dyslexia / by Maria Chivers. Philadelphia, PA: Jessica Kingsley Publishers, 2000.Projected Pub. Date: 0009 Description: p. cm.ISBN: 185302905X (pbk.: alk. paper). LC Classification: RJ496.A5 C475 2000 Dewey Class No.: 618.92/8553 21

Chromosome 6p influences on different dyslexia-related cognitive processes: further confirmation. Abstract: In this study, which is a continuation and an extension of an earlier study, we enrolled two new families (N=31) and recruited more individuals from the previously ascertained families (N=56). The eight multiplex families (N=171) presented in this study were ascertained from a sample of adult probands whose childhood reading history is well documented through archival information. Six phenotypes were constructed to span a range of dyslexia-related cognitive processes. These phenotypes were (1) phonemic awareness (of spoken words); (2) phonological decoding (of printed

nonwords); (3) rapid automatized naming (of colored squares or object drawings); (4) single-word reading (orally, of printed real words); (5) vocabulary; and (6) spelling (of dictated words). Grigorenko EL Wood FB Meyer MS Pauls DL Am J Hum Genet 2000 Feb;66(2):715-23.

Chromosome Workshop: chromosomes 11, 14, and 15. Abstract: This report describes linkage data presented at the Workshop on Chromosomes 11, 14, and 15 at the Sixth World Congress of Psychiatric Genetics in Bonn, Germany, together with relevant linkage data submitted to the chair and co-chair, and it is presented in the context of the previous literature concerning these chromosomes. We have attempted to collate current linkage data to provide a guide to potentially interesting findings on chromosomes 11, 14, and 15 for the phenotypes of bipolar disorder, schizophrenia, alcoholism, autism, and spelling and reading disability. Craddock N Lendon C Am J Med Genet 1999 Jun 18;88(3):244-54.

Clark, Diana Brewster. Dyslexia: theory & practice of remedial instruction / Diana Brewster Clark. Parkton, Md.: York Press, c1988. Description: xiii, 240 p.: ill.; 24 cm.ISBN: 0912752173 0912752165 (pbk.) LC Classification: LB1050.5.C548 1988 Dewey Class No.: 371.91/44 20

Clark, Diana Brewster. Dyslexia: theory & practice of remedial instruction / Diana Brewster Clark, Joanna Kellogg Uhry.Edition Information: 2nd ed. Baltimore: York Press, c1995. Uhry, Joanna Kellogg. Description: xiv, 284 p.: ill.; 23 cm.ISBN: 0912752432 (pbk.) LC Classification: LB1050.5.C548 1995 Dewey Class No.: 371.91/44 20

Clinical application of functional magnetic resonance imaging Abstract: Three types of researches have been carried out on brain-mind relationships: 1. researches on anatomical correlates of special talents (for example, perfect pitch) or deficits (for example, dyslexia), 2. researches to examine the relationship between a given cognitive syndrome and the site of brain damage, 3. researches to localize human cognitive function in the brain in vivo using functional magnetic resonance imaging (fMRI) and positron emission tomography (PET). fMRI is a particularly important because it is noninvasive, Sugishita M No To Hattatsu 2002 Mar;34(2):111-8.

Clinical characteristics of a population of dyslexic children in Assiut, Egypt. Abstract: Two groups of pupils from special tract learning schools were randomly selected for this study. The first group (55 pupils) fulfilled the World Federation of Neurology (WFN) definition of developmental dyslexia (DD). The second group (retarded readers, RR) included 20 pupils with IQs between 80 and 90. A group of normal readers was randomly selected from the 5 school grades as a control group. This study showed that the performance IQ of the DD group was not only higher than the verbal IQ, but the DD group had superior performance IQ compared to normal readers. Farrag AF Shaker H Hamdy NA Wafaa MA Neuroepidemiology 1995;14(2):92-9. ss

Cognitive and behavioral characteristics of children with learning disabilities / edited by Joseph K. Torgesen. Austin, Tex.: PRO-ED, c1990. Torgesen, Joseph K. Donald D. Hammill Foundation. Austin Invitational Research Symposium (1988) Related Titles: [Journal of learning disabilities. Description: ix, 237 p.: ill.; 24 cm. ISBN: 0890792070 LC4704.C6 1990 Dewey Class No.: 371.9 20

Cognitive and neurophysiological evaluation of Japanese dyslexia. Abstract: Seven Japanese dyslexic boys were evaluated as to their pedagogic performance on the pupil rating scale (PRS), and psychological and neurophysiological characteristics. One of them suffered from severe English dyslexia despite that his Japanese dyslexia was feeble. PRS did not successfully reveal their reading difficulties. Psychological examination

(WISC-R and K-ABC) revealed their cognitive dysfunction, but the results were heterogeneous. The Token test was most useful for detecting their poor reading comprehension. Electroencephalogram (EEG) coherence analysis showed high inter- and intra-hemispheric values. Shiota M Koeda T Takeshita K Brain Dev 2000 Oct;22(7):421-6.

Cognitive arithmetic and problem solving: a comparison of children with specific and general mathematics difficulties. Abstract: This study examined problem-solving and number-fact skills in two subgroups of third-grade children with mathematics difficulties (MD): MD-specific (n = 12) and MD-general (n = 12). The MD-specific group had difficulties in mathematics but not in reading, and the MD-general group had difficulties in reading as well as in mathematics. A comparison group of nonimpaired children (n = 24) was included. The findings showed that on both story and number-fact problems, the MD-specific group performed worse than the nonimpaired group in timed conditions but not in untimed conditions. Jordan NC Montani TO J Learn Disabil 1997 Nov-Dec;30(6):624-34, 684.

Cognitive assessment of dyslexic students in higher education. Abstract: Previous studies have shown that the phonological deficits that characterise dyslexia persist into adulthood. There is a growing number of dyslexic students in higher education for whom sensitive diagnostic tests of their reading and reading related difficulties are required. The study highlighted the difficulties of dyslexic adults. The persisting difficulties of dyslexic students that affect their study skills need to be recognised by HE institutions Journalthat appropriate support programmes can be put in place. Hatcher J Snowling MJ Griffiths YM Br J Educ Psychol 2002 Mar;72(Pt 1):119-33.

Cognitive components of picture naming. Abstract: A substantial research literature documents the effects of diverse item attributes, task conditions, and participant characteristics on the case of picture naming. The authors review what the research has revealed about 3 generally accepted stages of naming a pictured object: object identification, name activation, and response generation. They show that dual coding theory gives a coherent and plausible account of these findings without positing amodal conceptual representations, and they identify issues and methods that may further advance the understanding of picture naming and related cognitive tasks. Johnson CJ Paivio A Clark JM Psychol Bull 1996 Jul;120(1):113-39.

Cognitive deficits in developmental disorders. Abstract: The existence of specific developmental disorders such as dyslexia and autism raises interesting issues about the structure of the normally developing mind. In these disorders distinct cognitive deficits can explain a range of behavioural impairments and have the potential to be linked to specific brain abnormalities. One possibility is that there are specific mechanisms dedicated to particular types of information processing. Frith U Scand J Psychol 1998 Sep;39(3):191-5.

Cognitive disorders: searching for the circumstances of effective treatment: introduction by the symposium organizer. Gonzalez Rothi LJ J Int Neuropsychol Soc 1998 Nov;4(6):593-4.

Cognitive intervention in unemployed individuals with reading and writing disabilities. Abstract: Sixty native-born Swedish unemployed participants with reading and writing disabilities (R&WD) participated in a 20-week educational program aimed at improving reading and writing, verbal memory, self-confidence, and flexibility of perspectives. They were tested with a comprehensive battery (interviews, questionnaires, and tests of academic achievement) before and after the intervention. Sixteen controls, matched for sex, age, education, and nonverbal IQ, participated in the pre- and posttest sessions but received only standard unemployment interventions Jensen J Lindgren M Andersson K Ingvar DH Levander S Appl Neuropsychol 2000;7(4):223-36.

Cognitive mechanisms for processing nonwords: evidence from Alzheimer's disease. Abstract: Repetition and reading of various types of pronounceable nonwords (pseudowords) was examined in patients with probable Alzheimer's disease (AD) and healthy elderly controls. Overall accuracy of performance was lower in AD patients compared to controls, but the two groups showed qualitatively similar response patterns when reading different kinds of pseudowords aloud and when repeating pseudowords composed of familiar phonological forms, analogous to those in real English words. Glosser G Friedman RB Kohn SE Sands L Grugan P Brain Lang 1998 Jun 1;63(1):32-49.

Cognitive neuropsychological analysis and neuroanatomic correlates in a case of acute anomia. Abstract: We describe an analysis of lexical processing performed in a patient with the acute onset of an isolated anomia. Based on a model of lexical processing, we evaluated hypotheses as to the source of the naming deficit. We observed impairments in oral and written picture naming and oral naming to definition with relatively intact semantic processing across input modalities, suggesting that output from the semantic system was impaired. In contrast to previous reports, we propose that this pattern represents an impairment that arises late in semantic processing prior to accessing mode-specific verbal and graphemic output lexicons. Raymer AM Foundas AL Maher LM Greenwald ML Morris M Rothi LJ Heilman KM Brain Lang 1997 Jun 1;58(1):137-56.

Cognitive neuropsychological and regional cerebral blood flow study of a developmentally dyslexic Japanese child. Kaneko M Uno A Kaga M Matsuda H Inagaki M Haruhara N J Child Neurol 1998 Sep;13(9):457-61.

Coherence in short narratives written by Spanish-speaking children with reading disabilities. Abstract: A novel analysis of coherence using a combination of three criteria (syntactic connexity, pragmatic complexity, and rhetorical well-roundedness) was applied to short narratives produced by a group of 60 Spanish-speaking children of different ages and grades with reading disabilities and compared to those produced by normal children. We posit a scale of 6 degrees of increasing coherence. Matute E Leal F Zarabozo D Appl Neuropsychol 2000;7(1):47-60.

Coherent motion detection and letter position encoding. Abstract: We identified 24 'good' and 24 'poor' coherent motion detectors from an unselected sample of young adults. The two groups were matched for reading ability, age and IQ. All subjects carried out two tasks in which optimal performance depended on accurate letter position encoding: a lexical decision task and a primed reaction time task. We found that accurate letter position encoding was predicted by performance in the motion detection task. Cornelissen PL Hansen PC Gilchrist I Cormack F Essex J Frankish C Vision Res 1998 Jul;38(14):2181-91.

College students with dyslexia: persistent linguistic deficits and foreign language learning. Abstract: The first of these two studies compared college students with dyslexia enrolled in modified Latin and Spanish classes and non-dyslexic students enrolled in regular foreign language classes on measures of foreign language aptitude, word decoding, spelling, phonological awareness and word repetition. The groups did not differ on age or grade point average. Analyses indicated that students with dyslexia performed significantly poorer on the foreign language aptitude measures as well as on both phonological tasks, reading and spelling. Downey DM Snyder LE Hill B Dyslexia 2000 Apr-Jun;6(2):101-11.

Colloque sur les difficultés et les échecs d'apprentissage de la langue écrite (1970: Paris) La dyslexie en question. Avec la collaboration de M. Abbadie [et.al.] Paris, A. Colin [1972] Abbadie, Madeleine. Centre de recherche de l'éducation spécialisée et de l'adaptation scolaire. Description: 174 p. illus. 24 cm. LC Classification: RJ498.A5 C63 1970Other System No.: (OCoLC)1748650

Colored filters and reading difficulties: a continuing controversy. Evans BJ Optom Vis Sci 1997 May; 74(5):239-40.

Colored overlays for visual perceptual deficits in children with reading disability and attention deficit/hyperactivity disorder: are they differentially effective? Abstract: The Transient Channel Deficit (TCD) model of reading disability was evaluated by examining the effects of color overlays on the reading ability of four groups of children (n = 15 each) with reading disability and comorbid conditions involving math and ADHD. These 60 children were evaluated for reading accuracy and rate on measures of word decoding and reading comprehension under three color transparency conditions (blue, red, no overlay). Results indicated that color overlays did not differentially affect the reading performance of individuals with and without reading disabilities. Iovino I Fletcher JM Breitmeyer BG Foorman BR J Clin Exp Neuropsychol 1998 Dec;20(6):791-806.

Comment on Eden et al. (1995) Cherkes-Julkowski M J Learn Disabil 1996 Jan;29(1):4-6.

Comorbidity of learning and attention disorders. Separate but equal. Abstract: Children with learning and attention disorders commonly present with symptoms of both types of disorders. In many children, this co-occurrence represents comorbid disorders that are separate but overlapping. Because of comorbidity, the presence of one disorder signals the need to evaluate for the other disorders. Evaluation and treatment approaches must address both disorders when present. Fletcher JM Shaywitz SE Shaywitz BA Pediatr Clin North Am 1999 Oct;46(5):885-97, vi.

Comorbidity of mathematics and reading deficits: evidence for a genetic etiology. Abstract: In order to assess the genetic etiology of the comorbidity of reading and mathematics difficulties, data were ascertained from two samples: (1) 102 identical and 77 same-sex fraternal twin pairs in which at least one member of each pair is reading disabled and (2) 42 identical and 23 same-sex fraternal twin pairs in which at least one member is math disabled. Composite reading and mathematics performance data from each sample were fitted to the basic multiple regression model for the analysis of selected twin data and its bivariate extension. Knopik VS Alarcon M DeFries JC Behav Genet 1997 Sep;27(5):447-53.

Comorbidity of reading and mathematics disabilities: genetic and environmental etiologies. Abstract: Although children with learning disabilities frequently manifest comorbid reading and mathematics deficits, the cause of this comorbidity is unknown. To assess the extent to which comorbidity between reading and mathematics deficits is due to genetic and environmental influences, we conducted a twin study of reading and mathematics performance. Data from 148 identical and 111 fraternal twin pairs in which at least one member of the pair had a reading disability were subjected to a cross-concordance analysis and fitted to a bivariate extension of the basic multiple regression model for the analysis of selected twin data. Light JG DeFries JC J Learn Disabil 1995 Feb;28(2):96-106.

Complex hereditary diseases with psychiatric symptoms Abstract: Family and adoption studies indicate that genetic factors play a role in the development of many psychiatric disorders. A variable number of possible interacting genes giving a predisposition to the diseases is likely. The genetic dissection has been hampered by

genetic complexity as well as by difficulties in defining the phenotypes. Genetic mapping efforts using sib pairs, twins and individual large families have revealed preliminary or tentative evidence of susceptibility loci for a number of psychiatric disorders. Wetterberg L Tidsskr Nor Laegeforen 1999 Feb 28;119(6):839-45.

Computational neuroimaging of human visual cortex. Abstract: Functional magnetic resonance imaging is a new neuroimaging method for probing the intact, alert, human brain. With this tool, brain activity that has been hidden can now be measured. Recent advances in measuring and understanding human neural responses underlying motion, color, and pattern perception are reviewed. Wandell BA Annu Rev Neurosci 1999;22:145-73.

Concentrating on weaknesses or compensating by strengths? Comparison of 2 strategies for remediation of children with comprehensive reading-spelling disorder Abstract: Our study compares the efficiency and acceptance of two different methods of treating dyslexia in children. The first method addresses the most commonly encountered deficits in sequential processing. It relies primarily upon the "Kieler Lese-Rechtschreibaufbau". The second proceeds from the child's relative resources with regard to simultaneous processing as described by Kaufman. Training materials are those prescribed by Kaufman. Normally gifted primary school third-graders were trained in two groups (n = 13 and n = 12) and achieved a mean SIF score of SW = 101 on the K-ABC. Strehlow U Haffner J Busch G Pfuller U Rellum T Zerahn-Hartung C Z Kinder Jugendpsychiatr Psychother 1999 May;27(2):103-13.

Congres over Dyslexie, Woordblindheid, Lees- en Schrijfstoornissen (1st: 1984: Katholieke Universiteit te Nijmegen) Dyslexie: verslag van het Congres over Dyslexie, Woordblindheid, Lees- en Schrijfstoornissen, gehouden aan de

Katholieke Universiteit te Nijmegen op 20 en 21 juni 1984 / onder redactie van A. van der Leij, L.M.

Connection between reading disability/dyslexia and hyperactivity Johannesen KP Ugeskr Laeger 1997 Aug 11;159(33):4999.

Connectionism, phonology, reading, and regularity in developmental dyslexia. Abstract: Tests of the "phonological deficit" account of developmental dyslexia have produced apparently inconsistent results. We show how a connectionist approach to dyslexic reading development can resolve the paradox. A "dyslexic" model of reading was created by reducing the quality of the phonological representations available to the model during learning. The model behaved similarly to dyslexic children in that it had a selectively reduced ability to process nonwords, but showed normal effects of words' spelling-to-sound regularity. Brown GD Brain Lang 1997 Sep;59(2):207-35.

Connectionist modeling of the recovery of language functions following brain damage. Abstract: This paper reviews the contribution of connectionism to our understanding of behavioral changes in language functions after brain damage. Connectionism is founded upon a neural metaphor in that connectionist networks are made up of many simple, neuron-like units. It is possible to lesion these networks and explore the effects of that damage. It is widely held that damaging connectionist networks informs our understanding of neuropsychology and cognitive psychology. To what extent then does it currently tell us, or is likely to tell us, anything about behavioral change following brain damage? Current connectionist models simulate either spontaneous recovery or the effects of retraining, and I discuss both approaches. Harley TA Brain Lang 1996 Jan;52(1):7-24.

Connections between reading disability and behavior problems: testing temporal and causal hypotheses. Abstract: In this study of children's reading and behavior problem status from Grade 2 to Grade 4 of elementary school, we tested hypotheses concerned with the temporal and causal connections between these two closely associated disorders. Children with both, either, or neither kinds of problems were followed up over 2 years. While reading disability remained stable over time, there was greater variability in behavior problem status. Our data did not support the claim that reading problems lead to the development of behavior problems. Smart D Sanson A Prior M J Abnorm Child Psychol 1996 Jun;24(3):363-83.

Connectivity of ectopic neurons in the molecular layer of the somatosensory cortex in autoimmune mice. Abstract: Approximately 50% of New Zealand Black mice (NZB/BINJ) and 80% of NXSM-D/EiJ mice prenatally develop neocortical layer I ectopias, mostly in somatosensory cortices. These cortical anomalies are similar to those seen in the brains of individuals with dyslexia. Neurofilament staining revealed a radial column of tightly packed fiber bundles in the layers underlying ectopias. This suggested that the connectivity of the ectopic neurons was aberrant. Jenner AR Galaburda AM Sherman GF Cereb Cortex 2000 Oct;10(10):1005-13.

Contrast sensitivity and coherent motion detection measured at photopic luminance levels in dyslexics and controls. Abstract: Development dyslexics perform differently from controls on a number of low level visual tasks. We carried out three experiments to explore some of these differences. Dyslexics have been found to have reduced luminance contrast sensitivity at mesopic luminance levels. We failed to replicate this finding at photopic luminance levels. We compared the (photopic) coherent motion detection thresholds of groups of child and adult dyslexics with those of age matched controls. Dyslexics were significantly less sensitive to motion. Cornelissen P Richardson A Mason A Fowler S Stein J Vision Res 1995 May;35(10):1483-94.

Contrast sensitivity differences between proficient and disabled readers using colored lenses. Abstract: Colored overlays or lenses (e.g, Irlen lenses) have been used in attempts to remediate reading difficulties. The present study included four middle-socioeconomic status (SES) adults and four middle-SES children with reading disabilities as well as an equal number of nondisabled readers of the same age groups and SES. Examined were (a) the relationship of wavelength (lens color) to visual grating performance, (b) the effect of reading disability on performance with each lens-color/luminosity-grating combination, (c) group performances on a visual detection task with the clear and chromatic lenses, and (d) peripheral retinal brightness thresholds. Spafford CS Grosser GS Donatelle JR Squillace SR Dana JP J Learn Disabil 1995 Apr;28(4):240-52.

Contrast sensitivity in dyslexia. Abstract: Contrast sensitivity was determined for dyslexic and normal readers. When testing with temporally ramped (i.e. stimuli with gradual temporal onsets and offsets) gratings of 0.6, 4.0, and 12.0 cycles/deg, we found no difference in contrast sensitivity between dyslexic readers and controls. Using 12.0 cycles/deg gratings with transient (i.e. abrupt) onsets and offsets, we found that dyslexic individuals had, compared to controls, markedly inferior contrast sensitivity at the shortest stimulus durations (i.e. 17, 34, and 102 ms Gross-Glenn K Skottun BC Glenn W Kushch A Lingua R Dunbar M Jallad B Lubs HA Levin B Rabin M et al. Vis Neurosci 1995 Jan-Feb;12(1):153-63.

Contrast sensitivity in dyslexia: deficit or artifact? Peli E Garcia-Perez MA Optom Vis Sci 1997 Dec;74(12):986-90.

Contrasting effects of letter-spacing in alexia: further evidence that different strategies generate word length effects in reading. Abstract: The reading behaviour of two alexic patients (SA and WH) is reported. Both patients are severely impaired at reading single words, and both show abnormally strong effects of word length when reading. These two symptoms are characteristic of letter-by-letter reading. Experiment 1 examined the pattern of errors when the patients read large and small words. Further experiments examined the effects of inter-letter spacing on word naming (Experiments 2a and 2b) and the identification of letters in letter strings (Experiment 3). For both patients, letter identification was better for widely spaced letters in letter strings, and this effect was most pronounced for the central letters in the strings. Price CJ Humphreys GW Q J Exp Psychol A 1995 Aug;48(3):573-97.

Converging evidence for the role of occipital regions in orthographic processing: a case of developmental surface dyslexia. Abstract: Recently, there have been several reports focusing on the neural basis for word recognition. Two different views have emerged: one emphasizing the role of the left angular gyrus in recognizing printed words, and the second view suggesting that visual word processing activates the left extrastriate cortex. This paper describes the case of EBON, a 14-year-old girl with an extensive early (most likely congenital) brain lesion in the left occipital lobe. She demonstrates a clear pattern of developmental surface dyslexia in that she is more successful at reading and spelling regular words than irregular words and makes frequent regularization errors Samuelsson S Neuropsychologia 2000;38(4):351-62.

Converging methods for understanding reading and dyslexia / edited by Raymond M. Klein and Patricia McMullen. Cambridge, Mass.: MIT Press, c1999. Klein, Raymond M. McMullen, Patricia. Description: xi, 524 p.: ill.; 24 cm. ISBN: 0262112477 (alk. paper) LC Classification: LB1050.5.C662 1999 Dewey Class No.: 371.91/44 21

Corpus callosum morphology, as measured with MRI, in dyslexic men. Abstract: To test the hypothesis of anomalous anatomy in posterior brain regions associated with language and reading, the corpus callosum was imaged in the midsagittal plane with magnetic resonance. The areas of the anterior, middle, and posterior segments were measured in 21 dyslexic men (mean age 27 yrs, SD 6) and in 19 matched controls. As predicted, the area of the posterior third of the corpus callosum, roughly equivalent to the isthmus and splenium, was larger in dyslexic men than in controls. Rumsey JM Casanova M Mannheim GB Patronas N De Vaughn N Hamburger SD Aquino T Biol Psychiatry 1996 May 1;39(9):769-75.

Cortical activation during spoken-word segmentation in nonreading-impaired and dyslexic adults. Abstract: We used magnetoencephalography to elucidate the cortical activation associated with the segmentation of spoken words in nonreading-impaired and dyslexic adults. The subjects listened to binaurally presented sentences where the sentence-ending words were either semantically appropriate or inappropriate to the preceding sentence context. Half of the inappropriate final words shared two or three initial phonemes with the highly expected semantically appropriate words. Two temporally and functionally distinct response patterns were detected in the superior temporal lobe Helenius P Salmelin R Service E Connolly JF Leinonen S Lyytinen H J Neurosci 2002 Apr 1;22(7):2936-44.

Cortical auditory signal processing in poor readers. Abstract: Magnetoencephalographic responses recorded from auditory cortex evoked by brief and rapidly successive stimuli differed between adults with poor vs. good reading abilities in four important ways. First, the response amplitude evoked by short-duration acoustic stimuli was stronger in the post-stimulus time range of 150-200 ms in poor readers than in normal readers. Second, response amplitude to rapidly successive and brief stimuli that were identical or that differed significantly in frequency were substantially weaker in poor readers compared with controls, for interstimulus intervals of 100 or 200 ms, but not for an interstimulus interval of 500 ms. Nagarajan S Mahncke H Salz T Tallal P Roberts T Merzenich MM Proc Natl Acad Sci U S A 1999 May 25;96(11):6483-8.

Cortical responses of infants with and without a genetic risk for dyslexia: II. Group effects. Abstract: Infants born to families with a background of developmental dyslexia have an increased risk of becoming dyslexic. In our previous study no major group or stimulus effects in the event-related potentials (ERPs) of at-risk and control infants were found until the age of 6 months. However, in the current study, when we made the stimulus presentation rate slower, the ERPs to the short deviant /ka/ were different from those to the long standard /kaa/ stimulus already in newborns. In addition, clear group differences in the ERPs were found. Leppanen PH Pihko E Eklund KM Lyytinen H Neuroreport 1999 Apr 6;10(5):969-73.

Cortical responses of infants with and without a genetic risk for dyslexia: I. Age effects. Abstract: We studied auditory event-related potentials (ERP) in newborns and 6-month-old infants, about half of whom had a familial risk for dyslexia. Syllables varying in vowel duration were presented in an oddball paradigm, in which ERPs to deviating stimuli are assumed to reflect automatic change detection in the brain. The ERPs of newborns had slow positive deflections typical of their age, but significant stimulus and group effects were found only by the age of 6 months. Pihko E Leppanen PH Eklund KM Cheour M Guttorm TK Lyytinen H Neuroreport 1999 Apr 6;10(5):901-5.

Could platelet activating factor play a role in developmental dyslexia? Abstract: Post-mortem studies by Galaburda and colleagues on the brains of developmental dyslexics found characteristic neuronal abnormalities: ectopias, microgyria, and fewer large-soma cells in sensory thalamus. An association between dyslexia and immune dysfunction has been proposed. We describe a mechanism which may explain these observations. Platelet-activating factor (PAF) is a pro-inflammatory lipid implicated in neurological disorders. We propose that PAF may be involved in dyslexia. Taylor KE Richardson AJ Stein JF Prostaglandins Leukot Essent Fatty Acids 2001 Mar;64(3):173-80.

Could pure alexia be due to a disconnection syndrome? Mark VW Neurology 1998 Mar;50(3):835.

Critical conceptual and methodological considerations in reading intervention research. Abstract: Research designed to identify the instructional and ecological conditions that foster the development of literacy skills in children with reading disabilities reflects a complex, multivariate enterprise. In essence, such research must be able to ultimately identify the teacher characteristics and instructional components that are critical for individual children and the interrelationships among these components. Lyon GR Moats LC J Learn Disabil 1997 Nov-Dec;30(6):578-88.

Critical periods of vulnerability for the developing nervous system: evidence from humans and animal models. Abstract: Vulnerable periods during the development of the nervous system are sensitive to environmental insults because they are dependent on the temporal and regional emergence of critical developmental processes (i.e, proliferation, migration, differentiation, synaptogenesis, myelination, and apoptosis). Evidence from numerous sources demonstrates that neural development extends from the embryonic period through adolescence. In general, the sequence of events is comparable among species, although the time scales are considerably different. Rice D Barone S Jr Environ Health Perspect 2000 Jun;108 Suppl 3:511-33.

Critical response to dyslexia, literacy and psychological assessment. (report by a working party of the division of educational and child psychology of the British psychological society). A view from the chalk face. PG - 47-52 Dyslexia Unit, School of Psychology, University of Wales, Bangor, Gwynedd LL57 2DG, UK. Cooke A Working Party of the Division of Educational and Child Psychology of the British Psychological Society. Dyslexia 2001 Jan-Mar;7(1):47-52.

Cross-modal priming evidence for phonology-to-orthography activation in visual word recognition. Abstract: Subjects were asked to indicate which item of a word/nonword pair was a word. On critical trials the nonword was a pseudohomophone of the word. RTs of dyslexics were shorter in blocks of trials in which a congruent auditory prime was simultaneously presented with the visual stimuli. RTs of normal readers were longer for high frequency words when there was auditory priming. This provides evidence that phonology can activate orthographic representations; the size and direction of the effect of auditory priming on visual lexical decision appear to be a function of the relative speeds with which sight and hearing activate orthography. Whatmough C Arguin M Bub D Brain Lang 1999 Feb 1;66(2):275-93.

Crossmodal temporal order and processing acuity in developmentally dyslexic young adults. Abstract: We investigated crossmodal temporal performance in processing rapid sequential nonlinguistic events in developmentally dyslexic young adults (ages 20-36 years) and an age- and IQ-matched control group in audiotactile, visuotactile, and audiovisual combinations. Two methods were used for estimating 84% correct temporal acuity thresholds: temporal order judgment (TOJ) and temporal processing acuity (TPA). TPA requires phase difference detection: the judgment of simultaneity/nonsimultaneity of brief stimuli in two parallel, spatially separate triplets. Laasonen M Service E Virsu V Brain Lang 2002 Mar;80(3):340-54.

Cross-modality temporal processing deficits in developmental phonological dyslexics. Abstract: Neuroanatomical evidence suggests that poor readers may have abnormal lateral (LGN) and medial (MGN) geniculate nuclei responsible for temporal processing in visual and auditory domains respectively (Livingstone & Galaburda, 1993). Although behavioral evidence does support this neuroanatomical evidence in that poor readers have performed poorly on visual and auditory tasks thought to require the utilization of the LGN and MGN, respectively, appropriate examination of the coexistence of these behavioral abnormalities in the same population of poor readers has yet to take place. Cestnick L Brain Cogn 2001 Aug;46(3):319-25.

Cross-over, completion and confabulation in unilateral spatial neglect. Abstract: Patients with left-sided neglect generally mis-bisect horizontal lines to the right of mid-position. However, with short lines they frequently cross over and place their marks to the left; a phenomenon not easily explained by current theories of neglect. It is difficult to ascertain whether patients neglect the ipsilateral segment of short lines, perceptually distort these lines, or extend these lines leftward at a representational level. Reading horizontally arrayed letter strings is an alternative task potentially capable of sorting between these hypotheses, providing this task could be demonstrated to be comparable to line bisections Chatterjee A Brain 1995 Apr; 118 (Pt 2):455-65.

Current concepts in dyslexia. Edited by Jack Hartstein. With 34 illus. Saint Louis, C. V. Mosby Co, 1971. Hartstein, Jack, 1924- Description: xii, 212 p. illus. 26 cm. ISBN: 0801620902 LC Classification: RJ496.A5 C86 Dewey Class No.: 618.92/8/553

Current directions in dyslexia research / edited by Kees. P. van den Bos... [et al.]. Lisse: Swets & Zeitlinger, c1994. Bos, Kees P. van den. Description: 286 p.: ill.; 25 cm.

ISBN: 902651297X LC Classification: RC394.W6 C87 1994 Dewey Class No.: 616.85/53 20 Other System No.: (OCoLC)30905688

Current research in search of neurobiological correlates of reading and spelling disorder Abstract: The present article provides an overview of the main approaches in the current literature on the neurobiological correlates of developmental dyslexia. The first approach is not specific enough with regard to negative results, whereas the second and third seem particularly promising. Breitenbach E Lenhard W Z Kinder Jugendpsychiatr Psychother 2001 Aug;29(3):167-77.

Current reviews of higher nervous system dysfunction / editor, Walter J. Friedlander; sponsored by the Clinical Neurology Information Center and the National Institute of Neurological Diseases and Stroke. New York: Raven Press, [1975] Friedlander, Walter J, 1919- University of Nebraska (Central administration). Medical Center. Clinical Neurology Information Center. National Institute of Neurological Diseases and Stroke. Description: ix, 195 p.; 25 cm. ISBN: 0911216782 LC Classification: RJ496.A5 C87 Dewey Class No.: 616.8/5

DAMP and dyslexia--don't listen to the fashionable slogans Gulfe A Lakartidningen 1997 Oct 22;94(43):3830.

Dark adaptation, motor skills, docosahexaenoic acid, and dyslexia. Abstract: Dyslexia is a widespread condition characterized by difficulty with learning and movement skills. It is frequently comorbid with dyspraxia (developmental coordination disorder), the chief characteristic of which is impaired movement skills, indicating that there may be some common biological basis to the conditions. Visual and central processing deficits have been found. The long-chain polyunsaturated fatty acids (LCPUFAs) are important components of retinal and brain membranes. Stordy BJ Am J Clin Nutr 2000 Jan;71(1 Suppl):323S-6S.

Deaf poor readers' pattern reversal visual evoked potentials suggest magnocellular system deficits: implications for diagnostic neuroimaging of dyslexia in deaf individuals. Abstract: Deafness and developmental dyslexia in the same individual may jointly limit the acquisition of reading skills for different underlying reasons. A diagnostic marker for dyslexia in deaf individuals must therefore detect the presence of a neurobiologically based dyslexia but be insensitive to the ordinary developmental influences of deafness on reading skill development. We propose that the functional status of the magnocellular visual system in deaf individuals is potentially such a marker. Samar VJ Parasnis I Berent GP Brain Lang 2002 Jan;80(1):21-44.

Deconstructing dyslexia. Blame it on the written word. Kher U Time 2001 Mar 26;157(12):56.

Deep dyslexia / edited by Max Coltheart, Karalyn Patterson and John C. Marshall. Edition Information: 2nd ed. London; New York: Routledge & Kegan Paul, 1987. Coltheart, Max. Description: xi, 490 p.: ill.; 22 cm. ISBN: 0710212356 Series: International library of psychology LC Classification: MLCS 91/06069 (R)

Deep dyslexia / edited by Max Coltheart, Karalyn Patterson, and John C. Marshall. London; Boston: Routledge & Kegan Paul, 1980. Coltheart, Max. Patterson, Karalyn. Marshall, John C. Description: xi, 444 p.: ill.; 22 cm. ISBN: 0710004567: LC Classification: RC394.W6 D36 Dewey Class No.: 616.85/53 19 National Bib. No.: GB***

Deep dyslexia in the two languages of an Arabic/French bilingual patient. Abstract: We present a single case study of an Arabic/French bilingual patient, ZT, who, at the age of 32, suffered a cerebral vascular accident that resulted in a massive infarct in the left peri-sylvian region. ZT's reading displays the characteristics of the deep dyslexia syndrome in both languages, that is, production of semantic, visual, and morphological errors, and concreteness effect in reading aloud and impossibility of reading nonwords. In the first part of this paper, using a three-route model of reading, we account for the patient's performance by positing functional lesions, which affect the non-lexical, the semantic lexical and the non-semantic lexical routes of reading Beland R Mimouni Z Cognition 2001 Dec;82(2):77-126.

Deep dyslexia is right-hemisphere reading. Abstract: Two views exist concerning the proper interpretation of the form of acquired dyslexia known as deep dyslexia: (a) that it represents reading by a multiply damaged left hemisphere reading system; (b) that it represents reading which relies extensively on right-hemisphere orthographic and semantic processing. Price, Howard, Patterson, Warburton, Friston, and Frackowiak (1998) have recently reported a brain-imaging study whose results, they claim, "preclude an explanation of deep dyslexia in terms of purely right-hemisphere word processing." Coltheart M Brain Lang 2000 Feb 1;71(2):299-309.

Deep dyslexic phenomena in a letter-by-letter reader. Abstract: Numerous accounts of pure alexia have suggested that prelexical impairment precludes rapid access to orthographic information in patients with the disorder. We report a patient with features of both pure and partially recovered deep dyslexia in whom we demonstrate prelexical deficits in maintaining a reliable abstract representation of the right side of letter arrays, as well as in modulating a "spotlight" of visual attention Buxbaum LJ Coslett HB Brain Lang 1996 Jul;54(1):136-67.

Deficient antisaccades in the social-emotional processing disorder. Abstract: We investigated whether adolescents and adults with the developmental social-emotional processing disorder (SEPD) exhibit deficits in visual attention, as measured by eye movements, when compared with dyslexic and normal control subjects. On the antisaccade task, subjects with SEPD made more errors than either control group and were the only group to show a decrease in performance accuracy compared with prosaccade. Manoach DS Weintraub S Daffner KR Scinto LF Neuroreport 1997 Mar 3;8(4):901-5.

Deficient inhibition as a marker for familial ADHD. Abstract: The authors investigated whether deficient inhibitory control, as measured by the stop-signal paradigm, delineates a familial subgroup of attention deficit hyperactivity disorder (ADHD). Deficient inhibition delineates a familial subtype of ADHD. Psychosocial and neurobiological factors did not account for inclusion in the good inhibition group and did not act conjointly with inhibition to increase the risk for ADHD in the poor inhibition group. This study demonstrates that cognitive measures such as a laboratory measure of inhibition can serve as phenotype markers for genetic analyses. Crosbie J Schachar R Am J Psychiatry 2001 Nov;158(11):1884-90.

Deficit of temporal auditory processing in dyslexic adults. Abstract: Dyslexia is a common disorder with largely unknown pathophysiology. We tested ten dyslexic adults and 20 control subjects with trains of binaural clicks that led to illusory sound movements at short click intervals. In controls, the illusion disappeared at intervals exceeding 90-120 ms while in the dyslexics it persisted up to intervals of 250-500 ms. Dyslexic adults thus seem to have a deficit in the processing of rapid sound sequences, which is manifested in significant delays in their conscious auditory percepts. Hari R Kiesila P Neurosci Lett 1996 Feb 23;205(2):138-40.

Deficit of visual contour integration in dyslexia. Abstract: The visual processing of text occurs spontaneously in most readers. Dyslexic persons, however, often report both somatic symptoms and perceptual distortions when trying to read. It is possible that the perceptual distortions experienced by those with dyslexia reflect a disturbance in the basic mechanisms supporting perceptual organization at the early stages of visual processing. Integration of information over extended areas of visual space can be measured psychophysically in a task that requires the detection of a path defined by aligned, spatially narrow-band elements on a dense field of otherwise similar elements that are randomly oriented and positioned. In the present study a contour integration task was used to investigate such perceptual organization in dyslexia In the present study the authors have described a visual deficit in a global integration task in dyslexia. The pattern of deficits reported suggest that abnormal cooperative associations may be present in dyslexia that are indicative of poor perceptual integration. Simmers AJ Bex PJ Invest Ophthalmol Vis Sci 2001 Oct; 42(11):2737-42.

Deficits in auditory temporal and spectral resolution in language-impaired children. Abstract: Between 3 and 6 per cent of children who are otherwise unimpaired have extreme difficulties producing and understanding spoken language. This disorder is typically labelled specific language impairment. Children diagnosed with specific language impairment often have accompanying reading difficulties (dyslexia), but not all children with reading difficulties have specific language impairment. Some researchers claim that language impairment arises from failures specific to language or cognitive processing. Wright BA Lombardino LJ King WM Puranik CS Leonard CM Merzenich MM Nature 1997 May 8;387(6629):176-8.

Deficits in long-term memory are not characteristic of ADHD. Attention Deficit Hyperactivity Disorder. Abstract: To separate the influence of inattentiveness from memory, we examined savings scores on material previously learned in 53 children with Attention Deficit Hyperactivity Disorder (ADHD), 63 with a reading disability (RD), 63 with both

ADHD and RD combined, and 112 controls. Children with reading disabilities were impaired in their ability to remember previously-learned material unless it was repeated over four trials, whereas children with only ADHD performed as well as the controls for material presented only once. Kaplan BJ Dewey D Crawford SG Fisher GC J Clin Exp Neuropsychol 1998 Aug;20(4):518-28.

Deficits of motion transparency perception in adult developmental dyslexics with normal unidirectional motion sensitivity. Abstract: We assessed motion integration ability in seven adult developmental dyslexics using unidirectional and bidirectional (transparent) random dot kinematograms (RDKs) that varied in the number of frames. All adult dyslexics performed as well as normally reading age-matched controls with unidirectional RDKs, regardless of frame number. However, using orthogonal motion transparent stimuli, deficits were obvious in six dyslexics and depended on frame number. Whereas controls needed on average only 4.4 frames (144 ms) to identify both directions correctly on 75% of presentations, dyslexics needed on average 14.6 frames (483 ms) to achieve this level of performance Hill GT Raymond JE Vision Res 2002 Apr;42(9):1195-203.

Defining and classifying learning disabilities and attention-deficit/hyperactivity disorder. Abstract: This paper provides an overview of current conceptualizations of learning disabilities and ADHD, a conceptual framework critical for defining and classifying each disorder and for distinguishing each disorder from the other and from other, less common problems of childhood. At a most basic level, reading disability or dyslexia (the most common and best defined of the learning disabilities) and ADHD represent two distinct disorders that may frequently cooccur in the same unfortunate child but that can be clearly distinguished from one another. Shaywitz BA Fletcher JM Shaywitz SE J Child Neurol 1995 Jan;10 Suppl 1:S50-7.

Defining dyslexia. Duane DD Mayo Clin Proc 2001 Nov;76(11):1075-7.

Defining dyslexia. Levelt WJ Science 2001 May 18;292(5520):1300-1.

Definition and treatment of dyslexia: a report by the Committee on Dyslexia of the Health Council of The Netherlands. Abstract: A committee of the Health Council of the Netherlands prepared a report on the definition and treatment of dyslexia at the request of the Minister of Health, Welfare, and Sport (see Note). The Health Council, as charged by the Health Act, is to inform the government on the state of science with respect to public health issues. The Council is entirely funded by the government but otherwise completely independent (an independence guaranteed by law). Gersons-Wolfensberger DC Ruijssenaars WA J Learn Disabil 1997 Mar-Apr;30(2):209-13.

Delayed P300 during Sternberg and color discrimination tasks in poor readers. Abstract: The P300 ERP component was studied in poor and normal readers, using Sternberg and color discrimination (Spaceships) tasks. During the first one, subjects must decide if a probe item belongs or not to a set of digits previously presented. In the second one, the participants must shoot violet spaceships with one key and other than violet spaceships with another key. There were no significant differences between groups with respect to reaction times, but a larger proportion of errors was observed in poor readers. Silva-Pereyra J Fernandez T Harmony T Bernal J Galan L Diaz-Comas L Fernandez-Bouzas A Yanez G Rivera-Gaxiola M Rodriguez M Marosi E Int J Psychophysiol 2001 Feb;40(1):17-32.

Des enfants hors du lire / sous la direction de Christiane Préneron, Claire Meljac et Serge Netchine; avec la collaboration de Maïté Auzanneau... [et al.]. Paris: Bayard: INSERM: CTNERHI, c1994. Préneron, Christiane. Meljac, Claire. Netchine, Serge. Description: 457 p.: ill.; 21 cm.

ISBN: 2227005688 (Bayard): 2855985994 (INSERM) 2877100871 (CTNERHI) LC Classification: LB1050.5.E54 1994 Dewey Class No.: 371.91/44/0944 20

Detection and explanation of sentence ambiguity are unaffected by hippocampal lesions but are impaired by larger temporal lobe lesions. Abstract: We address the recent suggestion that the "hippocampal system" is important for understanding ambiguities in language (MacKay et al, J Cogn Neurosci 1998;10:377-394). Seven amnesic patients and 11 controls first decided whether a sentence was ambiguous and then tried to explain the ambiguity. Three amnesic patients with damage limited to the hippocampal formation and one amnesic patient with primarily diencephalic damage performed like the controls in all respects. Schmolck H Stefanacci L Squire LR Hippocampus 2000;10(6):759-70.

Development of a magnocellular function in good and poor primary school-age readers. Abstract: Abnormal functioning of the transient visual pathway (the M-pathway) has been implicated in specific reading disability (SRD). The aim of this study is to examine the contrast thresholds for flicker-defined form discrimination in primary school children, and to compare its development with reading and mentation development as a means of identifying children at risk of SRD. It appears that there is a developmental improvement in perceptual capacity for tasks attributed to magnocellular function, which plateaus at the age of about 8 to 10 years. However, despite the reported reduction of magnocellular function in specific reading disabled children, no significant difference in contrast threshold for flicker-defined letter discrimination was found between good and poor readers. Barnard N Crewther SG Crewther DP Optom Vis Sci 1998 Jan;75(1):62-8.

Development of the magnocellular VEP in children: implications for reading disability. Crewther SG Crewther DP

Klistorner A Kiely PM Electroencephalogr Clin Neurophysiol Suppl 1999;49:123-8.

Developmental and acquired dyslexia: neuropsychological and neurolinguistic perspectives / edited by Che Kan Leong and R. Malatesha Joshi. Dordrecht; Boston: Kluwer Academic, c1995. Leong, Che Kan. Joshi, R. Malatesha. Related Titles: [Reading disabilities. Description: x, 290 p.: ill.; 25 cm. ISBN: 0792331664 (alk. paper) LC Classification: RC394.W6 D44 1995 NLM Class No.: W1 NE342DG v. 9 1995 WM 475 D4888 1995 Dewey Class No.: 616.85/53 20

Developmental deep dyslexia in Japanese: a case study. Abstract: This report demonstrates the existence of developmental deep dyslexia involving Japanese orthography. When asked to read (or name) isolated kanji, T.S, a sixth grader with a normal IQ and no speech impairment, produced a number of visual, selection, and semantic errors. It is suggested that these errors arise from an interaction between phonological coding impairment and the relative sparing of direct visual processing, which are taken to be characteristic of developmental deep dyslexia. Yamada J Brain Lang 1995 Dec;51(3):444-57.

Developmental dyscalculia and brain laterality. Abstract: The correlation between arithmetic dysfunction and brain laterality was studied in 25 children with developmental dyscalculia (DD). The children were tested on a standardized arithmetic battery and underwent a neurological and neuro-psychological evaluation. A diagnosis of left hemisphere dysfunction (n = 13) was based on right side soft neurological signs, performance IQ (PIQ) > verbal IQ (VIQ), dyslexia and intact visuo-spatial functions. The criteria for right hemisphere dysfunction (n = 12) were left body signs, VIQ > PIQ, impaired visuo-spatial functions and normal language skills Shalev RS Manor O Amir N Wertman-Elad R Gross-Tsur V Cortex 1995 Jun;31(2):357-65.

Developmental dyscalculia behavioral and attentional aspects: a research note. Abstract: Behavioral characteristics of 140 children with developmental dyscalculia (DC) were evaluated using the Child Behavior Checklist. DC children demonstrated more behavior problems than normal children but significantly fewer problems than children psychiatrically referred. DC children had significantly more attentional problems although they had normal levels of anxiety/depression. Significantly higher scores on all syndrome scales were found for DC children who had attentional problems in the clinical range. Shalev RS Auerbach J Gross-Tsur V J Child Psychol Psychiatry 1995 Oct;36(7):1261-8.

Developmental dyscalculia. Abstract: Developmental dyscalculia is a specific learning disability affecting the acquisition of arithmetic skills in an otherwise-normal child. Although poor teaching, environmental deprivation, and low intelligence have been implicated in the etiology of developmental dyscalculia, current data indicate that this learning disability is a brain-based disorder with a familial-genetic predisposition. The neurologic substrate of developmental dyscalculia is thought to involve both hemispheres, particularly the left parietotemporal areas. Shalev RS Gross-Tsur V Pediatr Neurol 2001 May;24(5):337-42.

Developmental dyscalculia: prevalence and demographic features. Abstract: One hundred and forty-three 11-year-old children with development dyscalculia, from a cohort of 3029 students, were studied to determine demographic features and prevalence of this primary cognitive disorder. They were evaluated for gender, IQ, linguistic and perceptual skills, symptoms of attention-deficit hyperactivity disorder (ADHD), socio-economic status and associated learned disabilities. The IQs of the 140 children (75 girls and 65 boys) retained in the study group (three were excluded because of low IQs) ranged from 80 to 129 (mean 98.2,

SD 9.9). 26 per cent of the children had symptoms of ADHD, and 17 per cent had dyslexia. Manor O Shalev RS Dev Med Child Neurol 1996 Jan;38(1):25-33.

Developmental dyscalculia: prevalence and prognosis. Abstract: The prevalence of developmental dyscalculia (DC) in the school population ranges from 3-6 %, a frequency similar to that of developmental dyslexia and ADHD. These studies fulfilled the criteria for an adequate prevalence study, i.e, were population based, using standardized measures to evaluate arithmetic function. Although the variation in prevalence is within a narrow range, the differences are probably due to which definition of dyscalculia was used, the age the diagnosis was made and the instrument chosen to test for DC. Shalev RS Auerbach J Manor O Gross-Tsur V Eur Child Adolesc Psychiatry 2000;9 Suppl 2:II58-64.

Developmental dyslexia and dysgraphia--a case report Abstract: We reported a 7-year-old, right-handed boy whose reading and writing of kana and kanji were impaired. He showed a severe deficit in visuo-spatial perception skills. Nevertheless, his ability to read and write kana characters was facilitated by means of the Japanese Syllabaries. It is generally considered that the Syllabary involve two kinds of language modalities: auditory-verbal and visuo-verbal language systems. In spite of his intact auditory-verbal language system, his visuo-verbal language skills involved in writing kanji were severely impaired. Kaneko M Uno A Kaga M Inagaki M Haruhara N No To Hattatsu 1997 May;29(3):249-53.

Developmental dyslexia and learning disorders: diagnosis and treatment / volume editors, D. Bakker... [et al.]. Basel; New York: Karger, 1987. Bakker, Dirk J. Description: 166 p, 1 p. of plates: ill. (some col.); 25 cm. ISBN: 3805545851: LC Classification: RJ496.A5 D48 1987 NLM Class No.: W1 CH661T v. 5 WM 475 D489 1986 Dewey Class No.: 618.92/8553 19

Developmental dyslexia: a motor-articulatory feedback hypothesis. Abstract: Reading is mediated by parallel and widely distributed modular systems. There are, therefore, multiple loci in these systems where dysfunction may lead to developmental dyslexia. However, most normal children learn to read using the alphabetic system. Learning to use this system requires awareness that words are comprised of a system of speech sounds (phonological awareness) and the knowledge of how to convert letters (graphemes) into these speech sounds (phonemes). Most dyslexic children have deficient phonological awareness and have difficulty converting graphemes into phonemes. Heilman KM Voeller K Alexander AW Ann Neurol 1996 Mar;39(3):407-12.

Developmental dyslexia: an update on genes, brains, and environments. Abstract: The science of reading and developmental dyslexia has experienced spectacular advances during the last few years. Five aspects of this research are discussed in the article. (1) The holistic phenomenon of reading is complex. Many lower-level psychological processes (e.g, phonemic awareness, phonological decoding, ability to process stimuli rapidly and automatize this process, memory, ability to recognize words) contribute to a single act of reading. Conceptualizing the complex process of reading through its partly overlapping but partly independent components--which contribute to, but do not fully explain, the holistic process of reading--provides an excellent model for understanding complex hierarchies of higher mental functions Grigorenko EL J Child Psychol Psychiatry 2001 Jan;42(1):91-125.

Developmental dyslexia: atypical cortical asymmetries and functional significance. Abstract: Using brain magnetic resonance imaging, we measured in 16 young developmental dyslexic adults and 14 age-matched controls cortical asymmetries of posterior language-related areas, including Planum temporale and parietal operculum cortical ribbon, and of the inferior frontal region related in the left hemisphere to speech processing. In addition, we assessed the sulcal morphology of the inferior frontal gyrus in both groups according to a qualitative method. Robichon F Levrier O Farnarier P Habib M Eur J Neurol 2000 Jan;7(1):35-46.

Developmental dyslexia: contribution of modern neuropsychology Abstract: In France about 1 million children are thought to present learning disabilities for reading that in most cases correspond to developmental dyslexias. These are specific and constitutional deficits that prevent rapid and automatic reading abilities from developing, in spite of a normal intelligence and normal visual and auditory acuity. Demonet JF Habib M Rev Neurol (Paris) 2001 Sep;157(8-9 Pt 1):847-53.

Developmental dyslexia: neural, cognitive, and genetic mechanisms / edited by Christopher H. Chase, Glenn D. Rosen, and Gordon F. Sherman. Baltimore, Md.: York Press, c1996. Chase, Christopher H. Rosen, Glenn D. Sherman, Gordon F. Description: ix, 277 p.: ill.; 23 cm. ISBN: 0912752394 LC Classification: RJ496.A5 D486 1996 Dewey Class No.: 616.85/53 20

Developmental dyslexia: passive visual stimulation provides no evidence for a magnocellular processing defect. Abstract: Livingstone et al. [Livingstone, M. S, Rosen, G. D, Drislane, F. W. and Galaburda, A. M. Physiological and anatomical evidence for a magnocellular defect in developmental dyslexia. Proceedings of the National Academy of Science U.S.A. 88, 7943-7947, 1991] presented evidence for a defect of the magnocellular visual processing stream in developmental dyslexia. Johannes S Kussmaul CL Munte TF Mangun GR Neuropsychologia 1996 Nov;34(11):1123-7.

Developmental dyslexia: re-evaluation of the corpus callosum in male adults. Abstract:

Using a new method based upon the measurement of four angles, we analyzed the corpus callosum of 23 adult male dyslexics and 25 age-matched controls on MRI sagittal scans. Two out of the four angles measured showed significant differences between the groups that are consistent with previous findings concerning the size of the corpus callosum in dyslexics. In particular, posterior regions are concerned, displaying a lowered corpus callosum in dyslexics. Robichon F Bouchard P Demonet J Habib M Eur Neurol 2000;43(4):233-7.

Developmental dyslexia: the cerebellar deficit hypothesis. Abstract: Surprisingly, the problems faced by many dyslexic children are by no means confined to reading and spelling. There appears to be a general impairment in the ability to perform skills automatically, an ability thought to be dependent upon the cerebellum. Specific behavioural and neuroimaging tests reviewed here indicate that dyslexia is indeed associated with cerebellar impairment in about 80% of cases. Nicolson RI Fawcett AJ Dean P Trends Neurosci 2001 Sep;24(9):508-11.

'Developmental dysmusia (developmental musical dyslexia)'. Gordon N Dev Med Child Neurol 2000 Mar;42(3):214-5.

Developmental learning disorders: clues to their diagnosis and management. Capin DM Pediatr Rev 1996 Aug;17(8):284-90.

Developmental neuropathology and impact of perinatal brain damage. III: gray matter lesions of the neocortex. Abstract: The evolving neuropathology of primarily undamaged cortical regions adjacent to the injured site has been studied in 36 infants who survived a variety of perinatally acquired encephalopathies (microgyrias, ulegyrias, multicystic encephalopathies, porencephalies, and hydranencephalies) and later died of unrelated causes. Their survival times range from hours, days, weeks, or months, to several years. Ten of these children developed epilepsy, 2 developed cerebral palsy, and several were neurologically and mentally impaired. Marin-Padilla M J Neuropathol Exp Neurol 1999 May;58(5):407-29.

Developmental surface dyslexia is not associated with deficits in the transient visual system. Abstract: Deficits of the transient visual system have been reported in unselected groups of dyslexics. The aim of this study was to examine whether this finding holds when subjects with a specific type of developmental reading disorder (surface dyslexia) are considered. Ten Italian children were examined. They all presented the characteristic markers of surface dyslexia: slow and laborious reading with errors in tasks which cannot be solved with a grapheme-phoneme conversion (i.e, homophones). Spinelli D Angelelli P De Luca M Di Pace E Judica A Zoccolotti P Neuroreport 1997 May 27;8(8):1807-12.

Diagnosis of dyslexia is often very much delayed. A retrospective study of 102 pupils Fohrer U Johnsen UB Lakartidningen 1998 Mar 4;95(10):1024-6.

Diagnosis of reading and spelling disorder Abstract: The ICD-10 calls for the use of tables that account for the correlation between intelligence and spelling or reading, respectively (regression model) in the diagnosis of dyslexia. In this paper we discuss the consequences that arise from this recommendation with respect to the interpretation of psychometric tests. In addition, a table is presented that contains the data required to make diagnostic decisions based on the regression model. Schulte-Korne G Deimel W Remschmidt H Z Kinder Jugendpsychiatr Psychother 2001 May;29(2):113-6.

Diagnostic defaitism worsens the pressure on patients with dyslexia! Gulfe A Lakartidningen 1997 Oct 29;94(44):3954.

Diagnostic testing methods for skill assessment in reading, writing, and arithmetic. A critical review Abstract: The diagnosis of a specific developmental disorder of reading, writing and arithmetic can be made based upon individually applied standardized methods for testing scholastic achievement and IQ. To make the choice of suitable methods easier for the administrator of the test, a critical survey of German-language methods for assessing skills in reading, writing and arithmetic is presented.: There is a need for new constructions, respectively a need to update published scholastic achievement tests. Hemminger U Roth E Schneck S Jans T Warnke A Z Kinder Jugendpsychiatr Psychother 2000 Aug;28(3):188-201.

Dichotic listening CV lateralization and developmental dyslexia. Abstract: The present study was carried out on a sample of 125 right-handed boys who are described as follows: 50 boys with dyslexia, 50 controls of a similar age, and 25 controls according to reading level. Using an objective procedure based on regression, we selected three subgroups from among the poor readers: children with difficulties in the lexical pathway (surface dyslexics), children with difficulties in the sublexical pathway (phonological dyslexics), and children with problems in both pathways (mixed dyslexics). Martinez JA Sanchez E J Clin Exp Neuropsychol 1999 Aug;21(4):519-34.

Dichotic listening to temporal tonal stimuli by good and poor readers. Abstract: The hypothesis that reading disability is associated with impairment in the lateralization of temporal stimuli was tested by presenting 123 good- and poor-reading boys (Grades 4 through 6) with dichotic sets of temporal and nontemporal tonal stimuli for recognition. Reading ability was assessed by measuring proficiency in reading consonants, vowels, words, sentences and short stories. On the tone test, good readers showed a right-ear advantage in reporting the temporal stimuli, and a left-ear advantage in reporting the nontemporal stimuli. Harel S Nachson I Percept Mot Skills 1997 Apr;84(2):467-73.

Dichotic pitch: a new stimulus distinguishes normal and dyslexic auditory function. Abstract: Two patterns of appropriately filtered acoustic white noise can be binaurally fused by the human auditory system to extract pitch and location information that is not available to either ear alone. This phenomenon is called dichotic pitch. Here we present a new method for generating more effective and useful dichotic pitch stimuli. These novel stimuli allow the psychophysical assessment of dichotic pitch detection thresholds. Dougherty RF Cynader MS Bjornson BH Edgell D Giaschi DE Neuroreport 1998 Sep 14;9(13):3001-5.

Differences in visuospatial judgement in reading-disabled and normal children. Abstract: Both visual and verbal impairments have been reported in two independent streams of research into the etiology of dyslexia or reading-disability. To address the question of the presence of either abnormality in reading-disabled children, visuospatial and phonological ability were assessed and contrasted in 39 Normal and 26 Reading-disabled children. To assess whether these deficits are unique to dyslexia, scores were compared to those of a group of 12 Poor Readers ("garden-variety" backward readers with low IQs. Eden GF Stein JF Wood HM Wood FB Percept Mot Skills 1996 Feb;82(1):155-77.

Different neural circuits subserve reading before and after therapy for acquired dyslexia. Abstract: Rehabilitative measures for stroke are not generally based on basic neurobiological principles, despite evidence from animal models that certain anatomical and pharmacological changes correlate with recovery. In this report, we use functional magnetic resonance imaging (fMRI) to study in vivo human brain reorganization in a right handed patient with an acquired reading disorder from stroke. With phonological dyslexia, her whole-word (lexical) reading approach included inability to read nonwords and poor reading of function words. Small SL Flores DK Noll DC Brain Lang 1998 Apr;62(2):298-308.

Differential categorization of words by learning disabled, gifted, and nonexceptional students. Abstract: This research was done to answer whether learning disabled students attend to different word features than nonexceptional and gifted students and whether there is a difference by grade. Word sorts of meaningful and nonsense words were used to estimate differences between 145 first- and fifth-grade learning disabled, nonexceptional, and gifted groups. Analyses indicated that 54 learning disabled students were more likely to provide no response or to give simpler responses than 61 nonexceptional or 30 gifted peers. Siegel J Cook R Gerard J Percept Mot Skills 1995 Aug;81(1):243-50.

Differential effects of orthographic transparency on dyslexia: word reading difficulty for common English words. Abstract: Orthographic transparency is increasingly being recognised as an important factor in determining the manifestation of dyslexic tendencies in individuals. Recent evidence has shown that normal English-speaking children have reading deficits in the range associated with same age dyslexic German-speaking children for less frequently used words, and English orthography has been identified as a contributing factor. Spencer (Reading (1999) 33(2), 72-77; Journal of Research in Reading (1999) 22(3), 283-292) has proposed a predictive model for English children's reading and spelling deficits, based on orthographic features. Spencer K Dyslexia 2001 Oct-Dec;7(4):217-28.

Differentiation between dyslexia and ocular causes of reading disorders Abstract: Dyslexia is defined as a reading and/or writing disability persisting after exclusion of organic causes. Studies show that ocular disorders, especially small refraction errors, hypoaccommodation and symptomatic heterophoria, are often not detected or treated in cases of reading and/or writing problems which were otherwise diagnosed as dyslexia. Our results underline the importance of the correction of even small refraction and/or motility errors in the presence of reading and writing difficulties. Motsch S Muhlendyck H Ophthalmologe 2001 Jul;98(7):660-4.

Difficulties in reading the optotype Abstract: The paper presents in its first part the actual knowledge about the literal paralexias taking into consideration that the main method to examine the visual acuity includes the literal gnosia that has a symbolic character. The literal paralexias represents a normal cerebral phenomenon at the limit of the visual acuity. The typology of the paralexias is being studied by the morphological entiry of the letter and by the degree of being aware of them. After these methods we can divide the subjects in 3 types. Zolog A Zolog I Oftalmologia 1998;42(1):39-40.

Diffusion tensor imaging: concepts and applications. Abstract: The success of diffusion magnetic resonance imaging (MRI) is deeply rooted in the powerful concept that during their random, diffusion-driven displacements molecules probe tissue structure at a microscopic scale well beyond the usual image resolution. As diffusion is truly a three-dimensional process, molecular mobility in tissues may be anisotropic, as in brain white matter. With diffusion tensor imaging (DTI), diffusion anisotropy effects can be fully extracted, characterized, and exploited, providing even more exquisite details on tissue microstructure. Le Bihan D Mangin JF Poupon C Clark CA Pappata S Molko N Chabriat H J Magn Reson Imaging 2001 Apr;13(4):534-46.

Digit span and other WISC-R scores in the diagnosis of dyslexia in children. Abstract: The examination of subtest scores on the Wechsler Intelligence Scale is needed to provide confirmatory evidence for various subtest categorizations as there is no consensus about what patterns might be diagnostically useful. The present study supports the use of the ACID/AVID profiles (Arithmetic, Coding or Vocabulary, Information, and Digit Span) as elements in the diagnosis of dyslexia. WISC-R scores from 44 subjects were analyzed for specific subtest patterns of scores which might separate dyslexic individuals from the WISC-R standardization group. Vargo FE Grosser GS Spafford CS Percept Mot Skills 1995 Jun;80(3 Pt 2):1219-29.

Disability and the ADA: learning impairment as a disability. Winner BJ J Law Med Ethics 2000 Winter;28(4):410-1.

Discourse level writing in dyslexics--methods, results, and implications for diagnosis. Abstract: In this paper, we investigate some aspects of the written language production process in dyslexic writers. A group of adult dyslexic writers are compared with a control group and a group of congenitally deaf writers. We present analyses of the actions of both constructing and editing linguistic units during on-line writing. The results suggest that in order to understand the organization of how linguistic units are constructed in writing, we need to take both cognitive and socio-communicative factors into account. Wengelin A Stromqvist S Logoped Phoniatr Vocol 2000;25(1):22-8.

Disrupted neural responses to phonological and orthographic processing in dyslexic children: an fMRI study. Abstract: Developmental dyslexia, characterized by difficulty in reading, has been associated with phonological and orthographic processing deficits. fMRI was performed on dyslexic and normal-reading children (8-12 years old) during phonological and orthographic tasks of rhyming and matching visually presented letter pairs. During letter rhyming, both normal and dyslexic reading children had activity in left frontal brain regions, whereas only normal-reading children had activity in left temporo-parietal cortex. During letter matching, normal-reading children showed activity throughout extrastriate cortex, especially in occipito-parietal regions, whereas dyslexic children had little

activity in extrastriate cortex during this task. Temple E Poldrack RA Salidis J Deutsch GK Tallal P Merzenich MM Gabrieli JD Neuroreport 2001 Feb 12,;12(2):299-307.

Disruption of residual reading capacity in a pure alexic patient after a mirror-image right-hemispheric lesion. Abstract: A 74-year-old woman became a letter-by-letter reader after the occurrence of a left occipito-temporal hematoma. Seven months later, she suffered a second, mirror-image hematoma in the right hemisphere. After this second lesion, her residual reading capacity deteriorated dramatically in terms of both accuracy and reading latencies for words and isolated letters. Our findings support the hypothesis that the right hemisphere contributes to the residual reading capacities of pure alexic patients. Bartolomeo P Bachoud-Levi AC Degos JD Boller F Neurology 1998 Jan;50(1):286-8.

Disruption of the neural response to rapid acoustic stimuli in dyslexia: evidence from functional MRI. Abstract: The biological basis for developmental dyslexia remains unknown. Research has suggested that a fundamental deficit in dyslexia is the inability to process sensory input that enters the nervous system rapidly and that deficits in processing rapid acoustic information are associated with impaired reading. Functional magnetic resonance imaging (fMRI) was used to identify the brain basis of rapid acoustic processing in normal readers and to discover the status of that response in dyslexic readers. Temple E Poldrack RA Protopapas A Nagarajan S Salz T Tallal P Merzenich MM Gabrieli JD Proc Natl Acad Sci U S A 2000 Dec 5;97(25):13907-12.

Dissociation in the recovery from neglect dyslexia and visuospatial unilateral neglect: a case report. Abstract: The recovery of the ability to read of a patient affected by persistent visuospatial neglect suggests the functional independence of the two phenomena. Neglect dyslexia seems to be an example of a dissociation between an implicit and explicit knowledge of the characteristics of the stimulus. Cantoni C Piccirilli M Ital J Neurol Sci 1997 Feb;18(1):41-3.

Dissociation of normal feature analysis and deficient processing of letter-strings in dyslexic adults. Abstract: Neuroimaging studies have revealed that the functional organization of reading differs between developmentally dyslexic and non-impaired individuals. However, it is not clear how early in the reading process the differences between fluent and dyslexic readers start to emerge. We studied cortical activity of ten dyslexic adults using magnetoencephalography (MEG), as they silently read words or viewed symbol-strings which were clearly visible or degraded with Gaussian noise. Helenius P Tarkiainen A Cornelissen P Hansen PC Salmelin R Cereb Cortex 1999 Jul-Aug;9(5):476-83.

Dissociation of reading strategies: letter-by-letter reading in the native language and normal reading in the learned language. A case study. Abstract: In letter-by-letter reading, which is typically observed in Dejerine's (1892) "pure alexia," oral reading seems to be mediated by the naming of the constituent letters of the printed sequence: reading time rises abnormally as a function of the number of letters of the target item. We describe a patient with fluent aphasia who showed the unusual pattern of letter-by-letter reading together with surface dyslexia in her native language (French) and apparently normal reading in the second, learned language (English). Kremin H Chomel-Guillaume S Ferrand I Bakchine S Brain Cogn 2000 Jun-Aug;43(1-3):282-6.

Dissociations between reading responses and semantic priming effects in a dyslexic patient. Abstract: We report a patient (Y.Y.) with senile dementia of the Alzheimer's type. The patient read aloud some words composed of two or three kanji characters with errors applying typical pronunciations of each character

and defined them in keeping with the mispronunciation if the pronunciation represented another real word. The results of single-word semantic priming in a lexical decision task, however, suggested normal recognition processes for these kanji-words, despite the patient's reading errors. Nakamura H Nakanishi M Hamanaka T Nakaaki S Furukawa T Masui T Cortex 1997 Dec;33(4):753-61.

Distribution in normal subjects of performance in Token test: a basic study for the diagnosis of learning disabilities Abstract: For the diagnosis of specific reading disorder (SRD) we studied the distribution in 187 elementary school children of the scores of Token test. Token test was performed under two conditions: listening and reading by presenting the same sentences. The diagnosis required a normal score under the listening condition, an abnormally low score under the reading condition and significantly large discrepancy between them. This test is valid and convenient for the diagnosis of SRD. Koeda T Terakawa S Shiota M No To Hattatsu 2000 Jan;32(1):25-8.

Disturbed visual processing contributes to impaired reading in Alzheimer's disease. Abstract: The relationship between visual processing dysfunction and oral reading impairment was investigated in 17 patients with probable or possible Alzheimer's disease (AD). When dementia severity was controlled, a significant relationship was found between single word oral reading impairments and difficulties discriminating words written in different fonts and photographs of objects in different orientations, which are all functions believed to be dependent on the integrity of left ventral temporal-occipital visual association regions Glosser G Baker KM de Vries JJ Alavi A Grossman M Clark CM Neuropsychologia 2002;40(7):902-9.

Do visual neurophysiological tests reflect magnocellular deficit in dyslexic children? Abstract: To address the question of a possible magnocellular visual deficit in children with reading problems (dyslexia), we examined pattern ERG and VEP responses to stimulation with checks of 24', 49' and 180' in size and of 5%, 42% and 100% contrast level. Neurophysiological difference between children with reading problems and those without them was found confined to VEP which showed a significant prolongation of P100 wave in dyslexic children at highest contrast (100%) and smallest checks (24'). Pattern ERG was normal. Brecelj J Strucl M Raic V Pflugers Arch 1996;431(6 Suppl 2):R299-300.

Do visual problems cause dyslexia? Evans BJ Ophthalmic Physiol Opt 1999 Jul;19(4):277-8.

Dodds, Patricia S. Beyond the rainbow: a guide for parents of children with dyslexia and other disabilities / written by Patricia S. Dodds, Nancy T. Robeson, Paula Z. Rosteet; edited by June M. Turer. Baytown, Tex. (P.O. Box 1753, Baytown 77522): Educational Interventions, c1991. Robeson, Nancy T. Rosteet, Paula Z. Turer, June M. Description: 123 p.: ill.; 21 cm. Classification: LC4709.D63 1991 Dewey Class No.: 371.91/44 20

Does dyslexia develop from learning the alphabet in the wrong hemisphere? A cognitive neuroscience analysis. Abstract: A new perspective is described which views developmental dyslexia as the outcome of learning to write the alphabet in the nondominant (right) hemisphere. The letter-level and whole-word subtypes of dyslexia are seen as differing responses adopted to cope with this predicament. Striking similarities between dyslexics and callosotomy patients in the allocation of covert attention to lateralized stimuli provide direction for integrating a diversity of dyslexic research within this framework. Mather DS Brain Lang 2001 Mar;76(3):282-316.

Does intelligence make a difference? Spelling and phonological readiness in specific and nonspecific reading/spelling disabilities Abstract: In an investigation involving, 1800 second-to-fourth graders, the children were divided into three groups according to their reading and spelling achievement and the results of a nonverbal intelligence test: children with average achievement in oral reading and spelling, and those with poor achievements in both which were either discrepant or non-discrepant to their good-to-average scores on the intelligence test Klicpera C Klicpera BG Z Kinder Jugendpsychiatr Psychother 2001 Feb;29(1):37-49.

Does recognizing orally spelled words depend on reading? An investigation into a case of better written than oral spelling. Abstract: In this study we describe an investigation into the residual spelling skills of a patient (BRK) with a deep dysgraphia. His written spelling was significantly superior to his oral spelling and he had grave difficulties in recognizing orally spelled words. In addition, his impairment in recognizing orally spelled words was qualitatively very similar to his difficulties in oral spelling. In contrast, he could read and repeat the stimuli he could no longer spell. Cipolotti L Warrington EK Neuropsychologia 1996 May;34(5):427-40.

Does the Conners' Continuous Performance Test aid in ADHD diagnosis? Abstract: The performance of clinic-referred children aged 6-11 (N = 100) was examined using the Conners' Continuous Performance Test (CPT) and measures of auditory attention (Auditory Continuous Performance Test; ACPT), phonological awareness, visual processing speed, and visual-motor competence. The Conners' CPT overall index was unrelated to measures of visual processing speed or visual-motor competence. Although the Conners' CPT converged with the ACPT, the latter demonstrated age and order effects. McGee RA Clark SE Symons DK J Abnorm Child Psychol 2000 Oct;28(5):415-24.

Does training change the brain? Rosenberger PB Rottenberg DA Neurology 2002 Apr 23;58(8):1139-40.

Donnelly, Karen. Coping with dyslexia / Karen Donnelly. Portion of Dyslexia Edition Information: 1st ed. New York: Rosen Pub. Group, 2000. Description: 121 p.; 24 cm. ISBN: 0823928500 (lib. bdg.) LC Classification: RJ496.A5 D66 2000 Dewey Class No.: 616.85/53 21

Draper, Sharon M. (Sharon Mills) Double Dutch / by Sharon M. Draper. New York: Atheneum Books for Young Readers, 2002. Projected Pub. Date: 0204 Description: p. cm. ISBN: 0689842309 Summary: Three eighth-grade friends, preparing for the International Double Dutch Championship jump rope competition in their home town of Cincinnati, Ohio, cope with Randy's missing father, Delia's inability to read, and Yo Yo's encounter with the class bullies. LC Classification: PZ7.D78325 Do 2002 Dewey Class No.: [Fic] 21

Drawing performance in children with special learning difficulties. Abstract: The present study examined drawings on 5 tasks of 45 dyslexic and 45 nondyslexic children aged 6-9 years old. Children who show low performance in written language and phonological awareness are expected to get low scores on drawing tasks which require similar skills such as comprehension of difference, coordination of parts in an organized whole, spatial movement, classification or distinction of figures. The present hypotheses were constructed accordingly. Analysis showed that the drawings of the dyslexic participants presented inadequate planning, difficulties in the depiction of contrast, size-scaling and canonicality, lack of details, and stereotypic depiction. Mati-Zissi H Zafiropoulou M Bonoti F Percept Mot Skills 1998 Oct;87(2):487-97.

DRC: a dual route cascaded model of visual word recognition and reading aloud. Abstract: This article describes the Dual Route Cascaded (DRC) model, a computational model of visual word recognition and reading aloud. The DRC is a computational realization of the dual-route theory of reading, and is the only computational model of reading that can perform the 2 tasks most commonly used to study reading: lexical decision and reading aloud. For both tasks, the authors show that a wide variety of variables that influence human latencies influence the DRC model's latencies in exactly the same way. Coltheart M Rastle K Perry C Langdon R Ziegler J Psychol Rev 2001 Jan;108(1):204-56.

Dual-route and connectionist models: a step towards a combined model. Abstract: Current models of word recognition are mainly constructed within the frameworks of either dual-route or connectionist theories. The most important test of a word recognition model is how it succeeds in accounting for various reading behaviors. In the present paper dual-route and connectionist word recognition models are briefly described and evaluated. As a further development of these models, a combined framework is proposed. An amalgamation of the two main types of models might give a more satisfactory account of various phenomena within word recognition. Bjaalid IK Hoien T Lundberg I Scand J Psychol 1997 Mar;38(1):73-82.

Dynamic assessment and instructional strategies for learners who struggle to learn a foreign language. Abstract: In this paper the authors discuss how the concept of dynamic (cognitive) assessment and instruction might relate to the assessment and instruction of at-risk foreign/second language learners. They describe its relevance to a diagnostic/prescriptive approach to instruction for teaching a foreign language to students with identified dyslexia and other at-risk students. They explain how to assess learners' knowledge of the native/foreign/second language through questions and guided discovery. Schneider E Ganschow L Dyslexia 2000 Jan-Mar;6(1):72-82.

Dynamic visual perception of dyslexic children. Abstract: This study describes the capacity of children to detect fast changes of a small visual pattern. Three visual detection tasks for a group of normally reading (N = 140) and another group of dyslexic children (N = 366) in the age range of 7 to 16 years have been used. All three tasks require the detection of the fast changing orientation of a small pattern before it disappears. In one task, stationary fixation was required, because the orientation changes took place always at the same location antisaccade task, a parallel development of the performance of both Fischer B Hartnegg K Mokler A Perception 2000;29(5):523-30.

Dynamics of blood flow velocity in middle cerebral arteries in dyslexic persons Abstract: The aim of our study was to investigate the blood flow in middle cerebral arteries during the different forms of cognitive activity in dyslectic persons. Two group of subjects were tested. The first group consisted of 10 students with school difficulties, diagnosed neuropsychologically as having a particular form of dyslexia, i.e. dysgraphy or dysorthography. 6 of them were right lateralized and 4--left lateralized. Fersten E Luczywek E Zabolotny W Szelag E Czernicki Z Neurol Neurochir Pol 1999 Sep-Oct;33(5):1099-108.

Dyscalculia and dyslexia after right hemisphere injury in infancy. Abstract: To use the findings from neuropsychological evaluation and functional magnetic resonance imaging (fMRI) to assess interhemispheric reorganization of function after early unilateral brain injury. Interhemispheric reorganization of function may be bidirectional rather than a feature unique to the left hemisphere substrate for language. Levin HS Scheller J Rickard T Grafman J Martinkowski K Winslow M Mirvis S Arch Neurol 1996 Jan;53(1):88-96.

Dyslexia - samuel t. orton and his legacy [edited by] Marcia K. Henry. Edition Information: 1st ed. Baltimore, MD: International Dyslexia Association, 1999. Projected Pub. Date: 9910 Henry, Marcia

K. Brickley, Susan G. Description: p. cm. ISBN: 0892140208

Dyslexia after "one hundred years of solitude" Gadoth N Harefuah 1998 Mar 1;134(5):365-6.

Dyslexia among Swedish prison inmates in relation to neuropsychology and personality. Abstract: Several investigations have reported high frequencies of reading and writing disabilities in criminal populations. The aims of the present study were to assess the frequency of dyslexia among Swedish prison inmates and to relate dyslexia to other indices of neuropsychological functions. Sixty-three prison inmates with Swedish as their native language, age 19 to 57 years, were examined by interviews, tests of academic achievement, and neuropsychological assessment. Jensen J Lindgren M Meurling AW Ingvar DH Levander S J Int Neuropsychol Soc 1999 Jul;5(5):452-61.

Dyslexia and bilingual children--does recent research assist identification? Abstract: This paper analyses some of the recent research into dyslexia in relation to monolingual and bilingual children. It focuses on the phonological approach to the identification of dyslexia. It reviews the literature on those aspects of phonological development which allow dyslexic children to be identified at increasingly younger ages. The literature on the phonological development of children who speak English as an additional language, and who are bilingual or multilingual, is then reviewed to compare the possibilities for identification of these children in comparison with those for monolingual children. Durkin C Dyslexia 2000 Oct-Dec;6(4):248-67.

Dyslexia and corpus callosum morphology. Abstract: There is evolving evidence that developmental dyslexia is associated with anomalous cerebral morphology in the bilateral frontal and left temporoparietal regions. This study examined the morphology of the corpus callosum, as possible deviations in other important structures are poorly understood in this behaviorally diagnosed syndrome Subtle neurodevelopmental variation in the morphology of the corpus callosum may be associated with the difficulty that dyslexic children experience in reading and on tasks involving interhemispheric transfer. Hynd GW Hall J Novey ES Eliopulos D Black K Gonzalez JJ Edmonds JE Riccio C Cohen M Arch Neurol 1995 Jan;52(1):32-8.

Dyslexia and criminal behavior. Prout C Tex Med 2000 Jun;96(6):76.

Dyslexia and development: neurobiological aspects of extra-ordinary brains / edited by Albert M. Galaburda. Cambridge, Mass.: Harvard University Press, 1993. Galaburda, Albert M, 1948- Description: xxi, 378 p.: ill.; 24 cm. ISBN: 0674219406 (alk. paper) LC Classification: RC394.W6 D953 1993 NLM Class No.: WL 340.6 D998 Dewey Class No.: 616.85/53 20

Dyslexia and developmental verbal dyspraxia. McCormick M Dyslexia 2000 Jul-Sep;6(3):210-4.

Dyslexia and dyspraxia: commentary. Nicolson R Dyslexia 2000 Jul-Sep;6(3):203-4.

Dyslexia and familial high blood pressure: an observational pilot study. Abstract: Developmental dyslexia is a neurodevelopmental learning disability characterised by unexpectedly poor reading and unknown aetiology. One hypothesis proposes excessive platelet activating factor, a potent vasodilator, as a contributor, implying that there should be a negative association between dyslexia and high blood pressure (HBP). Since both conditions have a partial genetic basis, this association may be apparent at the familial level HBP+ family history is associated with better performance on reading. The prediction of a negative association between dyslexic status and familial high blood pressure is therefore confirmed. Taylor K Stein J Arch Dis Child 2002 Jan;86(1):30-3.

Dyslexia and literacy: an introduction to theory and practice / [edited by] Gavin Reid and Janice Wearmouth. Chichester, West Sussex, UK; New York: J. Wiley & Sons, 2002. Projected Pub. Date: 0208 Reid, Gavin, 1950- Wearmouth, Janice. Description: p. cm. ISBN: 0471486337 (cased) 0471486345 (pbk.: alk. paper) LC Classification: LB1050.5.D92 2002 Dewey Class No.: 372.43 21

Dyslexia and mathematics / edited by T.R. and E. Miles. London; New York: Routledge, 1992. Miles, T. R. (Thomas Richard) Miles, Elaine. Description: xiii, 127 p.: ill.; 23 cm. ISBN: 0415064805 0415049873 (pbk.) LC Classification: QA11.D97 1991 Dewey Class No.: 371.91/44 20

Dyslexia and self-control. An ego psychoanalytic perspective. Abstract: Dyslexia and the self-control problems that frequently accompany it are viewed from an ego psychoanalytic perspective. Dyslexia is conceptualized as resulting from an ego deficit in language processing; this deficit is seen as contributing to the ADHD-type symptoms often seen in dyslexic children. Lacking certain crucial components of linguistic competence, the dyslexic child is therefore lacking a basic tool of impulse control. As a result, this child may exhibit a type of language deficit based impulsivity that has dynamic characteristics which are diagnostically significant. Migden S Psychoanal Study Child 1998;53:282-99.

Dyslexia and the centre-of-gravity effect. Abstract: When human observers are presented with a double target display, a saccadic eye movement is triggered to an intermediate position close to the 'centre-of-gravity' of the configuration. This study examined the saccadic eye movements of dyslexic and normal readers in response to displays of single and double targets. Eye movement analyses revealed no differences in the spatial position of saccadic eye movements of dyslexic and normal readers in response to single targets presented at 5 degrees or 10 degrees. However, when presented with two targets simultaneously at 5 degrees AND 10 degrees, in contrast to normal readers who generated saccades to an intermediate position between the two targets (towards the 'centre-of gravity'), dyslexics generated saccades that landed close to the near target eccentricity. These findings suggest that dyslexia is associated with a deficit in the processing of global spatial information for the control of saccadic eye movements. Mental Health and Neural Systems Research Unit, Department of Psychology, Lancaster University, Lancaster Exp Brain Res 2001 Mar;137(1):122-6.

Dyslexia and the learning of a foreign language in school: where are we going? Abstract: The difficulties which many dyslexic students encounter in the learning of the English language often extend to the learning of a foreign language in school. Although this problem has been acknowledged for some time, and although the learning of a modern foreign language is a core element in the Scottish curriculum, there has been little research into how modern languages can be presented to offer the best learning opportunities to dyslexic students. Crombie MA Dyslexia 2000 Apr-Jun;6(2):112-23.

Dyslexia and the new science of reading. Kantrowitz B Underwood A Newsweek 1999 Nov 22;134(21):72-8.

Dyslexia and visual-spatial talents: compensation vs deficit model. Abstract: There are both theoretical and empirical reasons to support the hypothesis that dyslexia is associated with enhancement of right-hemisphere, visual-spatial skills. However, the neurological evidence is neutral with respect to whether dyslexic visual-spatial abilities should be superior (a compensation model) or inferior (a deficit model). In three studies we tested the hypothesis that dyslexia is associated with superior visual-spatial skills. Winner E von Karolyi C Malinsky D French L Seliger C Ross E Weber C Brain Lang 2001 Feb;76(2):81-110.

Dyslexia as a disfunction in successive processing Abstract: We present a study on reading and writing difficulties after normal instruction during a year. Verifying if these patients showed a specific pattern of PASS (Planning, Attention, Sequential and Simultaneous) cognitive processing; if so, it allows us a rapid diagnosis and a useful cognitive remediation according to the PASS theory of intelligence. A kind of dyslexia may be defined by disfunction in PASS successive processing. Perez-Alvarez F Timoneda-Gallart C Rev Neurol 2000 Apr 1-15;30(7):614-9.

Dyslexia in adults is associated with clinical signs of fatty acid deficiency. Abstract: Developmental dyslexia is a complex syndrome whose exact cause remains unknown. It has been suggested that a problem with fatty acid metabolism may play a role, particularly in relation to the visual symptoms exhibited by many dyslexics. We explored this possibility using two self-report questionnaires, designed on the basis of clinical experience, to assess (1) clinical signs of fatty acid deficiency; and (2) symptoms associated with dyslexia in known dyslexic and non-dyslexic subjects. Taylor KE Higgins CJ Calvin CM Hall JA Easton T McDaid AM Richardson AJ Prostaglandins Leukot Essent Fatty Acids 2000 Jul-Aug;63(1-2):75-8.

Dyslexia in children: multidisciplinary perspectives / edited by Angela Fawcett, Rod Nicolson. New York: Harvester Wheatsheaf, 1994. Fawcett, Angela. Nicolson, Rod. Description: xxiii, 248 p.: ill.; 22 cm. ISBN: 0745016367 (pbk.) 0133428583 (pbk.) LC Classification: RJ496.A5 D955 1994 Dewey Class No.: 618.92/8553 20

Dyslexia in Hebrew. Cole M Lerner AJ J Neurol Neurosurg Psychiatry 2000 Apr;68(4):537-8.

Dyslexia in practice: a guide for teachers / edited by Janet Townend and Martin Turner. New York: Kluwer Academic/Plenum Publishers, c2000.

Townend, Janet. Turner, Martin, 1948-
Description: xx, 349 p.: ill.; 24 cm. ISBN:
0306462516 (hard) 0306462524 (pbk.)
Classification: LC4710.G7 D94 2000
Dewey Class No.: 371.91/44 21 Other
System No.: (DLC) 99043454

Dyslexia may show a different face in different
languages. Abstract: Since research into
dyslexic difficulties has been conducted
predominately among those whose first
language is English, assumptions may
have been made about the nature of
dyslexia which are dependent on the
complex features of that language. This
paper considers first a sample of
'transparent' languages without those
particular inconsistencies of phoneme-
grapheme correspondence: they seem to
produce fewer children with problems but
nevertheless do present some different
inconsistencies of their own. Miles E
Dyslexia 2000 Jul-Sep;6(3):193-201.

Dyslexia research and its applications to
education / edited by George Th. Pavlidis
and T.R. Miles. Chichester [West Sussex];
New York: J. Wiley, c1981. Pavlidis,
George Th. Miles, T. R. (Thomas Richard)
Description: xxi, 307 p.: ill.; 24 cm. ISBN:
0471278416   LC   Classification:
LB1050.5.D95 1981 Dewey Class No.:
371.91/4 19

Dyslexia   Schafer   WD   Klin   Monatsbl
Augenheilkd 1997 Oct;211(4):215-6.

Dyslexia screening measures and bilingualism.
Abstract: A series of measures used in a
number of dyslexia screening tests was
administered to groups of 7-8-year old
English monolinguals and Sylheti/English
bilinguals. Within these groups a subgroup
of children was distinguished by poor
spelling and reading in the absence of
general ability, sensory, emotional or
behavioural problems, i.e. specific literacy
difficulties   (SpLD).   General   ability
(assessed   by   Raven's   matrices),
chronological age, male/female ratio and
mono/bilingualism   were   controlled
between SpLD and control groups. Everatt

J Smythe I Adams E Ocampo D Dyslexia
2000 Jan-Mar;6(1):42-56.

Dyslexia-- successful inclusion in the
secondary school / edited by Lindsay Peer
and Gavin Reid; foreword by David
Blunkett. London: D. Fulton Publishers,
2001. Peer, Lindsay. Reid, Gavin, 1950-
British Dyslexia Association. Description:
x, 278 p.: ill.; 25 cm. ISBN: 1853467421
(pbk.) LC Classification: LC4710.G7 D99
2001 Dewey Class No.: 371.91/44 21
Other   System   No.:
(UkLWHE)b000095010

Dyslexia   Symposium,   Melbourne,   1968.
Dyslexia symposium; proceedings, edited
and compiled by R. N. Harrison and Freda
Hooper. [Melbourne] Australian College
of Speech Therapists [1968?] Harrison, R.
N, ed. Hooper, Freda, ed. Australian
College of Speech Therapists. Description:
232 p. diagrs, tables. 21 cm. LC
Classification: LB1050.D93 1968 Dewey
Class No.: 428.4/2 National Bib. No.:
Aus69-571

Dyslexia, ADDH (Attention Deficit Disorder)
and   Asperger   syndrome.   Healthy
individuals are declared sick in a
diagnosis-oriented society Elinder L
Lakartidningen 1997 Sep 24;94(39):3391-
3; discussion 3393-4.

Dyslexia, development and the cerebellum.
Nicolson R Fawcett AJ Dean P Trends
Neurosci 2001 Sep;24(9):515-6.

Dyslexia, fluency, and the brain / edited by
Maryanne Wolf. Timonium, Md.: York
Press, 2001. Wolf, Maryanne. Description:
xxv, 423 p.: ill.; 23 cm. ISBN:
0912752602   LC   Classification:
RC394.W6 D958 2001 Dewey Class No.:
616.85/53 21

Dyslexia, gender, and brain imaging. Abstract:
Future brain imaging studies of dyslexia
should have a sufficient number of males
and females to detect possible gender
differences   in   the   neurological
underpinning of this disorder. Detailed
knowledge about such differences may

clarify our understanding of the structural and functional impairments which lead to the phonological deficits that characterize dyslexia. Functional brain imaging studies have shown that males and females exhibit different patterns of brain activation during phonological processing Lambe EK Neuropsychologia 1999 May;37(5):521-36.

Dyslexia, interdisciplinary approaches to reading disabilities / Herman K. Goldberg, Gilbert B. Schiffman, Michael Bender; with a foreword by Leo Kanner. New York: Grune & Stratton, c1983. Goldberg, Herman K. Schiffman, Gilbert B. Bender, Michael, 1943- Description: xiii, 217 p.; 24 cm. ISBN: 0808914847: LC Classification: RJ496.A5 D97 1983 NLM Class No.: WL 340 G618d Dewey Class No.: 616.85/53 19

Dyslexia, neurolinguistic ability, and anatomical variation of the planum temporale. Abstract: This article addresses the relationship between patterns of planum temporale symmetry/asymmetry and dyslexia and neurolinguistic abilities. Considerable research indicates that dyslexic individuals typically do not display the predominant pattern of leftward planum temporale asymmetry. Variable findings on the structural basis of symmetry are due partially to measurement issues, which are examined in some detail in this critical review. Morgan AE Hynd GW Neuropsychol Rev 1998 Jun;8(2):79-93.

Dyslexia, speech and language: a practitioner's handbook / [edited by] Margaret Snowling and Joy Stackhouse. San Diego, CA: Singular Pub. Group, 1996. Snowling, Margaret J. Stackhouse, Joy. Description: ix, 267 p.: ill.; 24 cm. ISBN: 1897635486 LC Classification: LC4710.G7 D97 1996 Other System No.: (OCoLC)35300516

Dyslexia. Bases of reading. Reading-writing disorder. Ocular reading disorder Trauzettel-Klosinski S Schafer WD Klosinski G Ophthalmologe 2002 Mar;99(3):208-27; quiz 228-9.

Dyslexia. Diller LH N Engl J Med 1998 Jun 18;338(25):1853.

Dyslexia. Manilla GT N Engl J Med 1998 Jun 18;338(25):1852-3; discussion 1853.

Dyslexia. Marshall JC N Engl J Med 1998 Jun 18;338(25):1852; discussion 1853.

Dyslexia. Melhus H N Engl J Med 1998 Jun 18;338(25):1853.

Dyslexia. Reading between the laminae. Abstract: Reading is one of the most complex tasks in which vision is involved. Our understanding of the visual system is contributing to the analysis of dyslexia, a reading disorder which may reflect abnormal visual processes. Walsh V Curr Biol 1995 Nov 1;5(11):1216-7.

Dyslexia. Shaywitz SE N Engl J Med 1998 Jan 29;338(5):307-12.

Dyslexia. Shaywitz SE Sci Am 1996 Nov;275(5):98-104.

Dyslexia. Talk of two theories. Ramus F Nature 2001 Jul 26;412(6845):393-5.

Dyslexia: a developmental language disorder. Abstract: The acquisition of literacy in an alphabetic script such as English makes heavy demands on linguistic skills. The relation between spoken and written language however, is far from straightforward. This article reviews the research that suggests that phonological processing skills are crucial in the translation of symbols to sounds, and the development of rapid and automatic decoding skills. It examines research that indicates that children whose phonological processing skills are compromised in some way, are at-risk of experiencing difficulties in the acquisition of literacy; it supports the suggestion that dyslexia can be viewed as lying on the continuum of developmental language disorders Simpson S Child Care Health Dev 2000 Sep;26(5):355-80.

Dyslexia: a hundred years on. Snowling MJ BMJ 1996 Nov 2;313(7065):1096-7.

Dyslexia: a multidisciplinary approach / editors, Patience Thomson, Peter Gilchrist. New York: Chapman & Hall, 1996. Description: p. cm. ISBN: 1565934385 (pbk.) LC Classification: 9611 BOOK NOT YET IN LC

Dyslexia: a neuroscientific approach to clinical evaluation / edited by Frank H. Duffy, Norman Geschwind. Edition Information: 1st ed. Boston: Little, Brown, c1985. Duffy, Frank H. Geschwind, Norman. Description: xii, 223 p, [3] p. of plates: ill. (some col.); 25 cm. ISBN: 0316194549 LC Classification: RJ496.A5 D94 1985 Dewey Class No.: 616.85/53 19

Dyslexia: a validation of the concept at two age levels. Abstract: The 144 participants were administered tasks with a demonstrated relationship to reading. Both older students (8 to 10 years old) and younger students (6 to 7 years old) included three groups of poor readers (matched on word reading but differing in the discrepancy from expected reading level) and age-matched average readers. Older poor readers had a control group of reading-matched younger subjects. The study provided no support for the concept of dyslexia at age 6 to 7 years. Among older participants there was support for the concept of dyslexia as a phonological deficit and of nondiscrepant garden-variety poor reading as a developmental lag. Badian NA J Learn Disabil 1996 Jan;29(1):102-12.

Dyslexia: actual status of our neurological and neuropsychological knowledge Abstract: Developmental dyslexia is a neurological syndrome of unknown origin. Historical, conceptual, etiological, epidemiological aspects of developmental dyslexia are reviewed in a neuropsychological perspective. This article reviews the known neuroanatomic, neuropathologic, and diagnostic basis of developmental dyslexia. Dislexic typology, with specific deficits in language, the visual domain or both, is discussed. Developmental dyslexia may be associated with several neuropsychological deficits. Estevez-Gonzalez A Garcia-Sanchez C Rev Neurol 1996 Jan;24(125):31-9.

Dyslexia: advances in theory and practice / edited by Ingvar Lundberg, Finn Egil Tønnessen & Ingolv Austad. Dordrecht; Boston, Mass: Kluwer Academic, c1999. Lundberg, Ingvar. Tønnessen, Finn Egil. Austad, Ingolv. Description: viii, 291 p.: ill.; 25 cm. ISBN: 0792358376 (hardcover: alk. paper) LC Classification: RC394.D9525 1999 Dewey Class No.: 616.85/53 21

Dyslexia: biology, cognition, and intervention / edited by Charles Hulme and Margaret Snowling. San Diego, Calif.: Singular Pub. Group, c1997. Hulme, Charles. Snowling, Margaret J. Description: xiii, 288 p.: ill.; 24 cm. ISBN: 1565938925 LC Classification: RC394.W6 D955 1997 Dewey Class No.: 616.85/53 21

Dyslexia: cultural diversity and biological unity. Abstract: The recognition of dyslexia as a neurodevelopmental disorder has been hampered by the belief that it is not a specific diagnostic entity because it has variable and culture-specific manifestations. In line with this belief, we found that Italian dyslexics, using a shallow orthography which facilitates reading, performed better on reading tasks than did English and French dyslexics. However, all dyslexics were equally impaired relative to their controls on reading and phonological tasks. Paulesu E Demonet JF Fazio F McCrory E Chanoine V Brunswick N Cappa SF Cossu G Habib M Frith CD Frith U Science 2001 Mar 16;291(5511):2165-7.

Dyslexia: empowering parents to become their child's educational advocate. Linday J Dev Behav Pediatr 1995 Oct;16(5):359-61.

Dyslexia: impact on the family. Elyachar A J Child Neurol 1995 Jan;10 Suppl 1:S110-1.

Dyslexia: its neuropsychological classification and treatment Bakker DJ Zh Nevropatol Psikhiatr Im S S Korsakova 1996;96(2):72-8.

Dyslexia: its neuropsychology and treatment / edited by George Th. Pavlidis and Dennis F. Fisher. Chichester; New York: Wiley, c1986. Pavlidis, George Th. Fisher, Dennis F. Orton Dyslexia Society. International Academy for Research in Learning Disabilities. World Congress on Dyslexia (2nd: 1983: Chalkidik‾e, Greece) Description: xx, 316 p.: ill.; 24 cm. ISBN: 0471908754: LC Classification: RC394.W6 D96 1986 NLM Class No.: WM 475 D9983 1983 Dewey Class No.: 616.85/53 19

Dyslexia: neuronal, cognitive, & linguistic aspects: proceedings of an international symposium held at the Wenner-Gren Center, Stockholm, June 3-4, 1980 / edited by Yngve Zotterman. Edition Information: 1st ed. Oxford; New York: Pergamon Press, 1982. Zotterman, Yngve. Sweden. Utbildningsdepartementet. Statens medicinska forskningsråd (Sweden) Wenner-Grenska samfundet. Description: xix, 172 p.: ill.; 26 cm. ISBN: 0080268633: Classification: RC394.W6 D97 1982 NLM Class No.: W 3 WE429 v. 35 1980 WM 475 D9984 1980 Dewey Class No.: 616.85/53 19

Dyslexia: oral and written language disorder. A new look at old links. Abstract: It is now generally accepted that written language attainment is directly associated with oral language ability, and that deficits in oral language will be reflected in written language. This paper examines the links that exist between these two modes of communication from a historical perspective, as well as from current research. The concept and terminology of dyslexia - written language disability - are explored. The impact of deficits in phonology, vocabulary, semantics and syntax on the acquisition of written language is discussed. Supple MD Folia Phoniatr Logop 2000 Jan-Jun;52(1-3):7-13.

Dyslexia: the link with visual deficits. Abstract: Some research reports suggest that visual anomalies may have a causative role in dyslexia, and on this basis certain forms of therapy have been proposed. Recently, we have published the initial results of a matched group study which found dyslexia to be associated with binocular instability, reduced amplitude of accommodation, and reduced contrast sensitivity for both low spatial frequencies and uniform field flicker. Evans BJ Drasdo N Richards IL Ophthalmic Physiol Opt 1996 Jan;16(1):3-10.

Dyslexia: verbal impairments in the absence of magnocellular impairments. Abstract: Sensitivity to dynamic visual and auditory stimuli was assessed in dyslexic children (Grade 7) who at school entrance had suffered from the well-established double-deficit of impaired phonological sensitivity and deficient rapid naming performance. A visual magnocellular deficit was assessed by the coherent motion detection task of the Oxford group. An auditory magnocellular deficit was assessed by the illusory sound movement perception task of Hari and Kiesila. Kronbichler M Hutzler F Wimmer H Neuroreport 2002 Apr 16;13(5):617-20.

Dyslexia-specific brain activation profile becomes normal following successful remedial training. Abstract: To examine changes in the spatiotemporal brain activation profiles associated with successful completion of an intensive intervention program in individual dyslexic children. These findings suggest that the deficit in functional brain organization underlying dyslexia can be reversed after sufficiently intense intervention lasting as little as 2 months, and are consistent with current proposals that reading difficulties in many children represent a variation of normal development that can be altered by intensive intervention. Simos PG Fletcher JM Bergman E Breier JI Foorman BR Castillo EM Davis RN Fitzgerald M Papanicolaou AC Neurology 2002 Apr 23;58(8):1203-13.

Dyslexic and category-specific aphasic impairments in a self-organizing feature map model of the lexicon. Abstract:

DISLEX is an artificial neural network model of the mental lexicon. It was built to test computationally whether the lexicon could consist of separate feature maps for the different lexical modalities and the lexical semantics, connected with ordered pathways. In the model, the orthographic, phonological, and semantic feature maps and the associations between them are formed in an unsupervised process, based on cooccurrence of the lexical symbol and its meaning. After the model is organized, various damage to the lexical system can be simulated, resulting in dyslexic and category-specific aphasic impairments similar to those observed in human patients. Mikkulainen R Brain Lang 1997 Sep;59(2):334-66.

Dyslexic children have abnormal brain lactate response to reading-related language tasks. Abstract: Children with dyslexia have difficulty learning to recognize written words owing to subtle deficits in oral language related to processing sounds and accessing words automatically. The purpose of this study was to compare regional changes in brain lactate between dyslexic children and control subjects during oral language activation Dyslexic and control children differ in brain lactate metabolism when performing language tasks, but do not differ in nonlanguage auditory Richards TL Dager SR Corina D Serafini S Heide AC Steury K Strauss W Hayes CE Abbott RD Craft S Shaw D Posse S Berninger VW AJNR Am J Neuroradiol 1999 Sep;20(8):1393-8.

Dysphasia and dyslexia in the light of PASS theory Abstract: The PASS theory of intelligence understands the cognitive function as an information process or program that can be differentiated in planning, attention, successive and simultaneous. Every process is linked to an anatomical region: planning to frontal cortex, attention to frontal cortex and subcortical structures, successive to frontal cortex and non-frontal cortex and simultaneous to non-frontal cortex. Effective remediation is possible when a PASS pattern is known. Dysphasia and

dyslexia show a typical PASS pattern that allows an appropriate remedial training as a neurocognitive approach. The PASS diagnosis is a psychogenetic diagnosis which is different from the usual diagnosis based on semiology or results obtained with tests that explore non-PASS cognitive function. Perez-Alvarez F Timoneda C Rev Neurol 1999 Apr 1-15;28(7):688-93.

Early dentine lead levels and educational outcomes at 18 years. Abstract: The associations between early dentine lead levels measured at the age of 6-8 years and educational outcomes measured at 18 years were examined in a birth cohort of 1265 New Zealand children. Analyses showed significant (p <.005) dose/response relationships between early dentine lead levels and later outcomes: at age 18 children with early elevated lead levels had poorer reading abilities, had more often left school early, had more often left school without qualifications, and had lower levels of success in school examinations. Fergusson DM Horwood LJ Lynskey MT J Child Psychol Psychiatry 1997 May;38(4):471-8.

Early reading development in children at family risk for dyslexia. Abstract: In a 3-year longitudinal study, middle- to upper-middle-class preschool children at high family risk (HR group, N = 67) and low family risk (LR group, N = 57) for dyslexia (or reading disability, RD), were evaluated yearly from before kindergarten to the end of second grade. Both phonological processing and literacy skills were tested at each of four time points. Consistent with the well-known familiarity of RD, 34% of the HR group compared with 6% of the LR group became RD. Pennington BF Lefly DL Child Dev 2001 May-Jun;72(3):816-33.

Early reading difficulties and later conduct problems. Abstract: The relationships between early reading difficulties and later conduct problems were examined in a birth cohort of New Zealand children studied from the point of school entry to the age of 16. Children with early reading difficulties had increased rates of conduct problems up to the age of 16 years. These associations depended on context, being more evident for boys and tending to reduce with increasing age. Fergusson DM Lynskey MT J Child Psychol Psychiatry 1997 Nov;38(8):899-907.

Early reading for low-SES minority language children: an attempt to 'catch them before they fall'. Abstract: Minority language and low socioeconomic status (SES) students are at high risk for language and learning disabilities. In an attempt to 'catch them before they fall', an early reading project was initiated in four kindergarten classes, in a low-SES bilingual school (English/French as a second language), where minority language children form a majority. The project included: (1) teaching reading and writing to kindergarten students, and outcome research: individual pre- and post-treatment assessment using a computer software to measure phonological processing and decoding skills; (2) reading testing of grade 1 students, graduates of traditional kindergartens with no explicit reading instruction programs Hus Y Folia Phoniatr Logop 2001 May-Jun;53(3):173-82.

Early screening for dyslexia--a collaborative pilot project. Abstract: An ongoing collaborative project, currently being piloted in 12 Wiltshire primary schools, is described. The aim is to provide a means of identifying potentially dyslexic children by the end of Key Stage 1 (Year 2) with a view to early intervention. The causal links identified by research between phonological skills and literacy development are taken as the theoretical basis of an initial screening procedure, and an intervention package is implemented for identified children. Ball S Becker T Boys M Davies S Noton H Int J Lang Commun Disord 2001;36 Suppl:75-9.

Early speech development, articulation and reading ability up to the age of 9. Abstract: Speech development, the occurrence of articulatory errors, speech therapy received and literacy were evaluated in children at preschool and school age. Data were obtained with questionnaires sent to the parents and teachers of 1,708 second-grade children in 119 school classes selected by multistage random sampling among Finnish-speaking schools throughout the country. Completed questionnaires were received from 1,531 parents (89.6%) and 1,601 teachers (93.7%). Early speech development was slower among the boys than among the girls. Luotonen M Folia Phoniatr Logop 1995;47(6):310-7.

Eclamptogenic Gerstmann's syndrome in combination with cortical agnosia and cortical diplopia. Abstract: Cortical blindness is defined as a loss of vision due to bilateral retrogeniculate lesions (geniculocalcarine blindness). Gerstmann's syndrome is a combination of disorientation for left and right, finger agnosia, and profound agraphia, alexia, and acalculia. It is due to a lesion in the left angular gyrus, situated at the confluence of the temporal, parietal, and occipital lobes. We report on a patient who suffered from severe underdiagnosed eclampsia and who developed bilateral extensive medial temporal, parietal, and calcarine ischemic infarctions during an eclamptic fit. Kasmann B Ruprecht KW Ger J Ophthalmol 1995 Jul;4(4):234-8.

Educational support for nursing and midwifery students with dyslexia. Abstract: This article sets out to begin the process of discussing and investigating the support of nursing students and midwives with dyslexia. Although concentrating on academic support, there are implications for practitioners who support students on clinical placements. Wright D Nurs Stand 2000 Jun 28-Jul 4;14(41):35-41.

Edwards, Janice. The scars of Dyslexia: eight case studies in emotional reactions / Janice Edwards. London; New York: Cassell, c1994. Description: 182 p.: ill.; 25 cm. ISBN: 0304329460 (hc) 0304329444 (pbk.). LC Classification: LC4709.5.E39 1994 Dewey Class No.: 371.91/44 20

EEG power spectra of adolescent poor readers.
Abstract: EEG power spectra were studied in two poor-reading adolescent groups (dysphonetic and phonetic) as the students viewed strings of letters and easy words (seven categories). The students ranged in age from 12 to 16 years; 29 were male, 9 were female. Bilateral results are reported from frontal, parietal, and occipital regions. Significant Group x Hemisphere effects were found in the alpha and beta bands, with the phonetic group showing right greater than left asymmetry. Ackerman PT McPherson WB Oglesby DM Dykman RA J Learn Disabil 1998 Jan-Feb;31(1):83-90.

Effect of luminance on visual evoked potential amplitudes in normal and disabled readers. Abstract: Considerable evidence exists that some reading-disabled children have disordered visual processing, specifically in the fast processing magnocellular (M) pathway. The presence of a weaker VEP response in reading-disabled children suggests a deficit early in visual processing. The significant difference in VEP amplitudes between the two reading groups provides an objective measure of a deficit in the M pathway that has been implicated in this condition. Whether serial VEP recordings might help to assess the effects of optometric therapy by providing an independent index of therapeutic efficiency is of special interest. Brannan JR Solan HA Ficarra AP Ong E Optom Vis Sci 1998 Apr;75(4):279-83.

Effect of oculomotor and other visual skills on reading performance: a literature review. Abstract: The diagnosis and management of many oculomotor anomalies is within the domain of optometry. Thus, a thorough understanding of these systems and their relation to reading performance is vital. Efficient reading requires accurate eye movements and continuous integration of the information obtained from each fixation by the brain. A relation between oculomotor efficiency and reading skill has been shown in the literature. Frequently, these visual difficulties can be treated successfully with vision therapy.

Kulp MT Schmidt PP Optom Vis Sci 1996 Apr;73(4):283-92.

Effect of time and frequency manipulation on syllable perception in developmental dyslexics. Abstract: Many people with developmental dyslexia have difficulty perceiving stop consonant contrasts as effectively as other people and it has been suggested that this may be due to perceptual limitations of a temporal nature. Accordingly, we predicted that perception of such stimuli by listeners with dyslexia might be improved by stretching them in time-equivalent to speaking slowly. Conversely, their perception of the same stimuli ought to be made even worse by compressing them in time-equivalent to speaking quickly. McAnally KI Hansen PC Cornelissen PL Stein JF J Speech Lang Hear Res 1997 Aug;40(4):912-24.

Effects and significance of specific spelling problems in young adults--empirical studies in an epidemiologic patient sample Abstract: With reference to an epidemiological sample of adolescents and young adults the impact of different models on the number of children classified as having specific spelling problems is investigated. Because of the high impact of spelling ability for educational success, dyslexic children need help by early intervention. Furthermore scholastic promotion is necessary to enable a school carer appropriate to the intellectual possibilities of the child. Haffner J Zerahn-Hartung C Pfuller U Parzer P Strehlow U Resch F Z Kinder Jugendpsychiatr Psychother 1998 May;26(2):124-35.

Effects of a phonologically driven treatment for dyslexia on lactate levels measured by proton MR spectroscopic imaging. Abstract: Dyslexia is a language disorder in which reading ability is compromised because of poor phonologic skills. The purpose of this study was to measure the effect of a phonologically driven treatment for dyslexia on brain lactate response to language stimulation as measured by proton MR spectroscopic imaging.

Richards TL Corina D Serafini S Steury K Echelard DR Dager SR Marro K Abbott RD Maravilla KR Berninger VW AJNR Am J Neuroradiol 2000 May;21(5):916-22.

Effects of a red background on magnocellular functioning in average and specifically disabled readers. Abstract: Two experiments were conducted using metacontrast masking to examine responses in the magno system of adults, average reading adolescents and adolescents with specific reading disability. In Experiment 1 the effects of a red background field on the metacontrast functions of adult subjects were investigated. Results showed that a red, compared to a photometrically matched white background field, significantly attenuated metacontrast magnitude, supporting the interpretation of metacontrast as due to magno system suppression of parvo system responses. Edwards VT Hogben JH Clark CD Pratt C Vision Res 1996 Apr;36(7):1037-45.

Effects of accelerated reading rate on processing words' syntactic functions by normal and dyslexic readers: event related potentials evidence. Abstract: In the present study, the authors examined differences in brain activity, as measured by amplitudes and latencies of event related potentials (ERP) components, in Hebrew-speaking adult dyslexic and normal readers when processing sentence components with different grammatical functions. Participants were 20 dyslexic and 20 normally reading male college students aged 18-27 years. The authors examined the processing of normal word strings in word-by-word reading of sentences having subject-verb-object (SVO) syntactic structure in self- and fast-paced conditions Breznitz Z Leikin M J Genet Psychol 2001 Sep;162(3):276-96.

Effects of replicating primary-reflex movements on specific reading difficulties in children: a randomised, double-blind, controlled trial. Abstract: Children with specific reading difficulties have problems that extend beyond the range of underlying language-related deficits (eg, they have difficulties with balance and motor control). We investigated the role of persistent primary reflexes (which are closely linked in the earliest months of life to the balance system) in disrupting the development of reading skills This study provides further evidence of a link between reading difficulties and control of movement in children. In particular, our study highlights how the educational functioning of children may be linked to interference from an early neurodevelopmental system (the primary-reflex system). A new approach to the treatment of children with reading difficulties is proposed involving assessment of underlying neurological functioning, and appropriate remediation. McPhillips M Hepper PG Mulhern G Lancet 2000 Feb 12;355(9203):537-41.

Effects of response and trial repetition on sight-word training for students with learning disabilities. Abstract: Alternating treatments designs were used to compare the effects of trial repetition (one response within five trials per word) versus response repetition (five response repetitions within one trial per word) on sight-word acquisition for 3 elementary students diagnosed with specific learning disabilities in reading. Although both interventions occasioned the same number of accurate responses per word during training, the trial-repetition condition, which involved complete antecedent-response-feedback sequences, resulted in more words mastered for all 3 students. Belfiore PJ Skinner CH Ferkis MA J Appl Behav Anal 1995 Fall;28(3):347-8.

Effects of visual training on saccade control in dyslexia. Abstract: This study reports the effects of daily practice of three visual tasks on the saccadic performance of 85 dyslexic children in the age range of 8 to 15 years. The children were selected from among other dyslexics because they showed deficits in their eye-movement control, especially in fixation stability and/or voluntary saccade control. Their eye movements were measured in an overlap prosaccade and a gap antisaccade task before and after the training. Fischer B Hartnegg K Perception 2000;29(5):531-42.

Egocentric mental rotation in Hungarian dyslexic children. PG - 3-11Abstract: A mental rotation task was given to 27 dyslexic children (mean age 9 years, 2 months) and to 28 non-dyslexic children (mean age 8 years, 8 months). Pictures of right and left hands were shown at angles of 0, 50, 90 and 180 degrees, and the subjects were required to indicate whether what was shown was a right hand or a left hand. It was found that, in this task, the dyslexics did not show the normal pattern of response times at different angles, and also, that they made more errors than the controls. It is argued that this result is compatible with hypothesis that, in typical cases of dyslexia, there is a malfunctioning in the posterior parietal area. Neuropsychology Laboratory, University Medical School Pecs, Institute of Behavioural Sciences, Szigeti u. 12, H-7623, Pecs, Hungary. Karadi K Kovacs B Szepesi T Szabo I Kallai J Dyslexia 2001 Jan-Mar;7(1):3-11.

Eisenson, Jon, 1907- Really now, why can't our Johnnies read? / Jon Eisenson. Palo Alto, Calif.: Pacific Books, c1989. Description: 160 p.: ill.; 24 cm. ISBN: 0870152580: LC Classification: LC151.E57 1989 Dewey Class No.: 372.4/145 19

Elbeck, Alice. [from old catalog] Dyslexi og mundtligt formuleringsniveau. København: GMT, 1974. Description: 160 p.; 22 cm. LC Classification: LB1050.5.E99

Electro-oculographic recordings reveal reading deficiencies in learning disabled children. Abstract: This study was undertaken in order to learn the functional differences in reading tasks between two groups of children: those identified as learning disabled and a group of control children. During the earliest stages of learning to read, children adopt a logographic strategy, in which letter order is ignored and phonologic factors are secondary. The children later move into an alphabetic and then to an orthographic reading stage. Reading strategies can be studied by electro-oculographic (EOG) recordings during text reading. Poblano A Cordoba de Caballero B Castillo I Cortes V Arch Med Res 1996 Winter;27(4):509-12.

Electrophysiological testing of dyslexia. Abstract: We enlarged our previous study (Kubova Z. et al. Physiol Res 1995;44:87-89) giving an evidence about magnocellular pathway involvement (delayed motion-onset visual evoked potentials (M-VEPs)) in 70% of dyslexic children. In the new group presented here, only 48% of 25 dyslexics displayed prolonged latencies of cortical responses to motion stimuli. However, there was no correlation of this defect with the used quantification of the reading skills (reading quotients). No significant EEG frequency spectrum changes were found. 10 subjects from the former group, who were re-examined 4 years after the previous study at the mean age of 14 years, exhibited significant shortening of the M-VEP latencies compared to the original values Kuba M Szanyi J Gayer D Kremlacek J Kubova Z Acta Medica (Hradec Kralove) 2001;44(4):131-4.

Empirical research on language teaching and language acquisition / edited by R. Grotjahn, E. Hopkins. Bochum [Germany]: Studienverlag Brockmeyer, 1980. Grotjahn, Rüdiger. Hopkins, E. (Edwin) Description: iv, 231 p.: ill.; 21 cm. ISBN: 3883391441 (pbk.) LC Classification: P51.E475 1980

Enhancing the phonological processing skills of children with specific reading disability. Abstract: The present study evaluated the benefits of phonological processing skills training for children with persistent reading difficulties. Children aged between 9-14 years, identified as having a specific reading disability, participated in the study. In a series of three experiments, pedagogical issues related to length of training time, model of intervention and severity of readers' phonological processing skills deficit prior to intervention, were explored. Gillon G Dodd B Eur J Disord Commun 1997;32(2 Spec No):67-90.

Enterocolitis in children with developmental disorders. Abstract: Intestinal pathology, i.e, ileocolonic lymphoid nodular hyperplasia (LNH) and mucosal inflammation, has been described in children with developmental disorders. This study describes some of the endoscopic and pathological characteristics in a group of children with developmental disorders (affected children) that are associated with behavioral regression and bowel symptoms, and compares them with pediatric controls. A new variant of inflammatory bowel disease is present in this group of children with developmental disorders. Wakefield AJ Anthony A Murch SH Thomson M Montgomery SM Davies S O'Leary JJ Berelowitz M Walker-Smith JA Am J Gastroenterol 2000 Sep;95(9):2285-95.

ERP differences among subtypes of pervasive developmental disorders. Abstract: Children with multiple complex developmental disorder (MCDD) have been distinguished from autistic children on the basis of chart reviews. It was questioned whether it is possible to find other, e.g, event-related potential (ERP), evidence for this assertion.: ERP parameters indicate that autistic and MCDD children might differ in underlying pathology and might therefore, better be regarded as two separate diagnostic entities. Kemner C van der Gaag RJ Verbaten M van Engeland H Biol Psychiatry 1999 Sep 15;46(6):781-9.

Errors in a nonlinear graphic-semantic mapping task resulting from lesions in Boltzmann machine: is it relevant to dyslexia? Abstract: One of the most fascinating aspects of brain research is the subject of language. As in many other cases, the malfunctions that occur in different persons for various reasons give us insight on the mechanisms that support our ability to talk, read and listen. Following the work of Plaut and associates, we deal with the dyslexia disorder, which is the overall name for a large number of reading disorders. A Boltzmann machine neural network scheme was trained to implement the nonlinear mapping task of graphic representation into semantic representation, which may model the brain sections responsible for the translation of a written word into meanings and syllables. Geva AB Shtram L Policker S J Int Neuropsychol Soc 2000 Jul;6(5):620-6.

Estienne-Dejong, Françoise. La part des mots, les mots à part: chantiers d'écriture / Françoise Dejong-Estienne. Louvain-la-Neuve: Cabay, 1985. Related Titles: Part des mots. Description: 318 p.: ill.; 24 cm. ISBN: 2870772874: . LC Classification: PQ1109.5.C5 E75 1985

Estienne-Dejong, Françoise. Langage et dysorthographie. Paris, Éditions universitaires [1973] Description: 2 v. illus. 24 cm. LC Classification: RJ496.A4 E85 NLM Class No.: WL340 E81La 1973 Dewey Class No.: 618.92/855 19 National Bib. No.: F***

Etiology of individual differences in reading performance: a test of sex limitation. Abstract: To test the hypothesis that the etiology of individual differences in reading performance differs in males and females, reading performance data from twin pairs tested in the Colorado Learning Disabilities Research Center were fitted to structural equation models of sex limitation. The sample included 513 pairs of twins in which at least one member of each pair has a positive school history of reading problems [228 monozygotic (MZ), 176 same-sex dizygotic (DZ), and 109 opposite-sex DZ pairs] and 302 matched control pairs [148 MZ, 98 same-sex DZ, and 56 opposite-sex DZ pairs]. Alarcon M DeFries JC Fulker DW Behav Genet 1995 Jan;25(1):17-23.

Etiology of neuroanatomical correlates of reading disability. Abstract: The heritable nature of reading disability has been well documented (DeFries & Alarcon, 1996), and possible abnormalities of brain structures have been associated with the disorder (Filipek, 1995). However, the etiology of individual differences in morphological brain measures has not been examined extensively. The purpose of this study was to apply behavioral genetic methods to assess the etiology of individual differences in neuroanatomical structures. Measures of reading performance, cognitive ability, and magnetic resonance imaging scans were obtained from 25 monozygotic (MZ) and 23 same-sex dizygotic (DZ) twin pairs with reading disability, and 9 MZ and 9 DZ control twin pairs participating in the Colorado Learning Disabilities Research Center. Alarcon M Pennington BF Filipek PA DeFries JC Dev Neuropsychol 2000;17(3):339-60.

Etiology of reading difficulties and rapid naming: the Colorado Twin Study of Reading Disability. Abstract: Children with reading deficits perform more slowly than normally-achieving readers on speed of processing measures, such as rapid naming (RN). Although rapid naming is a well-established correlate of reading performance and both are heritable, few studies have attempted to assess the cause of their covariation. Measures of rapid naming (numbers, colors, objects, and letters subtests), phonological decoding, orthographic choice, and a composite variable (DISCR) derived from the reading recognition, reading comprehension, and spelling subtests of the Peabody Individual Achievement Test were obtained from a total of 550 twin pairs with a positive school history of reading problems Davis CJ Gayan J Knopik VS Smith SD Cardon LR Pennington BF Olson RK DeFries JC Behav Genet 2001 Nov;31(6):625-35.

Evans, Martha M. Dyslexia: an annotated bibliography / Martha M. Evans. Westport, Conn.: Greenwood Press, 1982. Description: xxvi, 644 p.; 24 cm. ISBN: 0313213445 (lib. bdg.) LC Classification: Z6671.52.D97 E9 1982 RJ496.A5 Dewey Class No.: 016.61892/8553 19

Event related potentials in adults diagnosed as reading disabled in childhood. Abstract: The purpose of this study was to identify electrophysiological correlates of reading disability (RD) in adults with psychometrically documented childhood reading histories. Specific a-priori hypotheses for these correlates were generated from the findings of Harter, Anllo-Vento, Wood & Schroeder (1988a); Harter, Diering & Wood (1988b). The subjects were 32 males with normal intelligence and no history of attention deficit disorder or current major psychopathology. Event related potentials were recorded over O1, O2, C3', C4', F3, and F4 to letter stimuli using an intralocation selective attention paradigm. Naylor CE Wood FB Harter MR Int J Neurosci 1995;80(1-4):339-52.

Event-related brain potentials elicited by rhyming and non-rhyming pictures differentiate subgroups of reading disabled adolescents. Abstract: Event-related brain potentials were recorded while disabled adolescent subjects read and judged whether two sequentially presented pictures had names that rhymed. Subjects with relatively good phonetic skills displayed an N400 priming effect, i.e, a significant reduction in the amplitude of the negative peak, occurring approximately 400 msec post-stimulus, for pictures with names that rhymed with preceding pictures as compared with pictures that had names that did not rhyme with the prime. No such effect was evident for subjects with relatively poor phonetic skills. McPherson WB Ackerman PT Oglesby DM Dykman RA Integr Physiol Behav Sci 1996 Jan-Mar;31(1):3-17.

Event-related brain potentials elicited during phonological processing differentiate subgroups of reading disabled adolescents. Abstract: Visual and auditory rhyme judgment tasks were administered to adolescent dyslexics and normal readers while event-related brain potentials were recorded. Reading disabled subjects were split into two groups based on a median split of scores on a visual non-word decoding test. The better decoders were called Phonetics and the poorer decoders were referred to as Dysphonetics. Single syllable, real word stimuli were used, and both rhyming and non-rhyming targets had a 50% chance for matching orthography. McPherson WB Ackerman PT Holcomb PJ Dykman RA Brain Lang 1998 Apr;62(2):163-85.

Evidence for a susceptibility locus on chromosome 6q influencing phonological coding dyslexia. Abstract: A linkage study of 96 dyslexia families containing at least two affected siblings (totaling 877 individuals) has found evidence for a dyslexia susceptibility gene on chromosome 6q11.2-q12 (assigned the name DYX4). Using a qualitative phonological coding dyslexia (PCD) phenotype (affected, unaffected, or uncertain diagnoses), two-point parametric analyses found highly suggestive evidence for linkage between PCD and markers D6S254, D6S965, D6S280, and D6S251 (LOD(max) scores = 2.4 to 2.8) across an 11 cM region. Petryshen TL Kaplan BJ Fu Liu M de French NS Tobias R Hughes ML Field LL Am J Med Genet 2001 Aug 8;105(6):507-17.

Evidence for an articulatory awareness deficit in adult dyslexics. Abstract: Dyslexia is widely considered to be associated with impaired performance on phonological awareness tasks. However, it is likely that orthographic knowledge influences performance on these tasks. In this study, adult dyslexics, for whom reading is no longer a major problem, were compared to a control group on a measure of articulatory awareness, a task which is not confounded with orthography. The dyslexic group showed deficits on the task in comparison to the control group. Griffiths S Frith U Dyslexia 2002 Jan-Mar;8(1):14-21.

Evidence for implicit sequence learning in dyslexia. Abstract: Nicolson and Fawcett (Cognition 1990; 35: 159-182) have suggested that a deficit in the automatization of skill learning could account for the general impairments found in dyslexia. Much of the evidence for their claims has been collected via a dual task paradigm, which might allow for alternative explanations of the data. The present study examines automatic skill learning in a single task paradigm and extends previous studies by independently examining the contribution of stimulus-based and response-based learning. Kell SW Griffiths S Frith U Dyslexia 2002 Jan-Mar;8(1):43-52.

Evidence for linkage of spelling disability to chromosome 15. Schulte-Korne G Grimm T Nothen MM Muller-Myhsok B Cichon S Vogt IR Propping P Remschmidt H Am J Hum Genet 1998 Jul;63(1):279-82.

Evidence from imaging on the relationship between brain structure and developmental language disorders. Abstract: This article discusses findings using various imaging techniques regarding the neurological underpinnings of developmental language and learning disorders. Evidence from magnetic resonance imaging, functional magnetic resonance imaging, single photon emission spectroscopy, and positron emission tomography implicates the left perisylvian regions in the processing of phonemes and auditory information, as had been predicted from lesion data and from neurobiological theory. Semrud-Clikeman M Semin Pediatr Neurol 1997 Jun;4(2):117-24.

Evillen, Anna. Books for dyslexic children: a parent's guide with teachers' supplement. Edition Information: Revised [ed.]; additional list by Betty Root. Laleham, North Surrey Dyslexic Society, 1973. Root, Betty. Dyslexia Institute. North Surrey Dyslexic Society. Description: 19 p. 33 cm. ISBN: 0903992000 LC Classification: Z5814.C52 E84 1973 NLM Class No.: Z5814.C52 E93b 1973 Dewey

Class No.: 016.3719/14 National Bib. No.: GB73-17195

Evolution of a form of pure alexia without agraphia in a child sustaining occipital lobe infarction at 2 1/2 years. Abstract: The progress of cognitive visual dysfunction over an 8-year period of a child who sustained bilateral occipital-lobe infarctions at the age of 2 1/2 years is described. She survived with normal intelligence and went on to attend mainstream school. She manifested many features of cognitive visual impairment and, in particular, developed a form of pure alexia without agraphia. She achieved some letter-by-letter reading but no sight vocabulary development, including to her own name. She learned to write imaginatively employing phonetically true spelling but cannot read what she has written. O'Hare AE Dutton GN Green D Coull R Dev Med Child Neurol 1998 Jun;40(6):417-20.

Executive functions in dyslexia. Abstract: This study focused on executive functions in dyslexia. A group of 43 heavily-affected young dyslexics, divided into two groups based on the results of a receptive language test, and 20 non-dyslexic controls, were tested with a Dichotic Listening Test, the Stroop Color Word Test and the Wisconsin Card Sorting Test. The dyslexic subjects demonstrated significant impairment on all tasks, but with different patterns of impairment according to the subgrouping. The subgroups were equally impaired on the Dichotic Listening Test, but differed on the Stroop and the Wisconsin Tests Helland T Asbjornsen A Neuropsychol Dev Cogn Sect C Child Neuropsychol 2000 Mar;6(1):37-48.

Experimental study of response latency of visual search processes and premotor decision latency in dyslexic and non-dyslexic children. Model of linear regression: derived parametric estimates Abstract: For some time the question of a visual impairment in dyslexic children has been a source of controversy in the literature. Depending on the method used, the findings point either to receptor or neural impairment or to a visual deficit in information processing. The question remains of whether these findings mask retardation in the motor planning and execution of a response. cannot assume there will be a manifest visuomotor impairment in all dyslexic children when the stimulus is presented at the center and periphery of the field of vision. However, if such an impairment is present it is highly likely that the findings contain a mixture of retardation of pre-motor and visual decision latency. This would have substantial consequences for therapy, as visuomotor perception training would not be indicated in all instances. Some dyslexic children, both boys and girls, achieve completely "normal" results. Bitschnau W Z Kinder Jugendpsychiatr Psychother 1997 May;25(2):82-94.

Explicit and implicit processing of words and pseudowords by adult developmental dyslexics: A search for Wernicke's Wortschatz? Abstract: Two groups of male university students who had been diagnosed as dyslexic when younger, and two groups of control subjects of similar age and IQ to the dyslexics, were scanned whilst reading aloud and during a task where reading was implicit. The dyslexics performed less well than their peers on a range of literacy tasks and were strikingly impaired on phonological tasks. In the reading aloud experiment, simple words and pseudowords were presented at a slow pace Journalthat reading accuracy was equal for dyslexics and controls Brunswick N McCrory E Price CJ Frith CD Frith U Brain 1999 Oct;122 (Pt 10):1901-17.

Exploring the cognitive phenotype of autism: weak "central coherence" in parents and siblings of children with autism: II. Real-life skills and preferences. Abstract: Information on everyday life activities and preferences in both social and nonsocial domains was obtained from parents and children who had taken part in an experimental study of central coherence.

Comparisons were made between parents who had a son with autism, parents with a dyslexic son, and families without a history of developmental disorder, as well as the male siblings in these families. Data on everyday preferences and abilities were elicited by means of an experimental questionnaire. Significant group differences in social and nonsocial preferences were found, suggesting that some parents showed similarities with their son with autism, in preference for nonsocial activities and ability in detail-focused processing. Briskman J Happe F Frith U J Child Psychol Psychiatry 2001 Mar;42(3):309-16.

Exploring the cognitive phenotype of autism: weak "central coherence" in parents and siblings of children with autism: I. Experimental tests. Abstract: Previous twin and family studies have indicated that there are strong genetic influences in the etiology of autism, and provide support for the notion of a broader phenotype in first-degree relatives. The present study explored this phenotype in terms of one current cognitive theory of autism. Parents and brothers of boys with autism, boys with dyslexia, and normal boys were given tests of "central coherence", on which children with autism perform unusually well due to an information-processing bias favouring part/detail processing over processing of wholes/meaning. Happe F Briskman J Frith U J Child Psychol Psychiatry 2001 Mar;42(3):299-307.

Extension of a recent therapy for dyslexia. Abstract: Recently, peculiarities of visual perception were found in dyslexic patients. Therefore, we investigated visual acuity, reading and spelling capabilities, as well as peripheral letter recognition in 54 children with reading and/or spelling problems. Subsequently, the children and their parents trained at home for approximately 0.5 h daily during 2-3 months. Training consisted of reading through a small aperture and of visuomotor coordination tasks. Fahle M Luberichs J Ger J Ophthalmol 1995 Nov;4(6):350-4.

Eye fixation patterns among dyslexic and normal readers: effects of word length and word frequency. Abstract: Eye fixation patterns of 21 dyslexic and 21 younger, nondyslexic readers were compared when they read aloud 2 texts. The study examined whether word-frequency and word-length effects previously found for skilled adult readers would generalize equally to younger dyslexic and nondyslexic readers. Significantly longer gaze durations and reinspection times were found for low-frequency and long words than for high-frequency and short words. The effects showed up in the number of fixations on the target words. Hyona J Olson RK J Exp Psychol Learn Mem Cogn 1995 Nov;21(6):1430-40.

Eye movement efficiency in normal and reading disabled elementary school children: effects of varying luminance and wavelength. Abstract: This investigation examines the question of whether decreasing wavelength of light and/or reducing luminance benefits oculomotor efficiency in normal and reading disabled (RD) children. This investigation confirms a link between wavelength of light and eye movement efficiency in reading. Blue filters resulted in a significant improvement in the number of fixations and regressions and rate of reading in RD children. The outcome broadens the concept of transient system deficit established in previous research to include the effect on oculomotor efficiency. The educational implications of Solan HA Ficarra A Brannan JR Rucker F J Am Optom Assoc 1998 Jul;69(7):455-64.

Eye movement patterns in hemianopic dyslexia. Abstract: Homonymous parafoveal field loss impairs reading at the visual-sensory level. To elucidate the role of parafoveal visual field in reading, reading eye movements were recorded, by means of an infra-red registration technique, in 50 patients with homonymous hemianopia and visual field sparing ranging from 1 degree to 5 degrees; for comparison, a group of 25 normal subjects was studied. The degree of reading impairment in patients was found to depend on the extent of visual field sparing. Zihl J Brain 1995 Aug;118 (Pt 4):891-912.

Eye movement patterns in linguistic and non-linguistic tasks in developmental surface dyslexia. Abstract: Ten subjects who could be reliably assessed as surface dyslexics were selected on the basis of a large test battery. Eye movements in non-linguistic and linguistic tasks were studied in these subjects. Stability of fixation on a stationary stimulus was examined. Performance of dyslexics was no different from that of an age-matched control group. Similarly, no difference was observed between the two groups when they were requested to saccade to a rightward or leftward target. On the other hand, while reading short passages, dyslexics showed an altered pattern of eye movements with more frequent and smaller rightward saccades as well as longer fixation times. De Luca M Di Pace E Judica A Spinell D Zoccolotti P Neuropsychologia 1999 Nov;37(12):1407-20.

Eye movement patterns in reading as a function of visual field defects and contrast sensitivity loss. Abstract: Saccadic eye movements during reading were examined as a function of the side of visual field cut and the impairment of visual contrast sensitivity Five patients with various visual field defects were compared to five age-matched controls. Patients with right visual field defect showed an increase in the number of rightward saccades and a decrease in their amplitude, and patients with left visual field defects showed a pattern more similar to that of the control subjects. De Luca M Spinelli D Zoccolotti P Cortex 1996 Sep;32(3):491-502.

Eye movements and verbal reports in neglect patients during a letter reading task. Abstract: To study different typolologies from visuo-verbal behavior concerning the arrest and the treatment of visual information in patients with spatial hemineglect. Our results confirmed the heterogeneity of the mechanisms of neglect and suggest that rehabilitation procedures adapted to each profile might be useful. Beis JM Andre JM Datie AM Brugerolle B NeuroRehabilitation 2002;17(2):145-51.

Eye movements in reading / edited by Jan Ygge and Gunnar Lennerstrand. Edition Information: 1st ed. Oxford, OX, U.K.; Tarrytown, N.Y, U.S.A.: Pergamon, 1994. Ygge, Jan. Lennerstrand, Gunnar. Description: xiv, 374 p.: ill.; 24 cm. ISBN: 0080425097: LC Classification: QP477.5.E952 1994 Dewey Class No.: 612.8/46 20

Eye movements in reading and information processing: 20 years of research. Abstract: Recent studies of eye movements in reading and other information processing tasks, such as music reading, typing, visual search, and scene perception, are reviewed. The major emphasis of the review is on reading as a specific example of cognitive processing. Basic topics discussed with respect to reading are (a) the characteristics of eye movements, (b) the perceptual span, (c) integration of information across saccades, (d) eye movement control, and (e) individual differences (including dyslexia). Rayner K Psychol Bull 1998 Nov;124(3):372-422.

Eyeblink conditioning indicates cerebellar abnormality in dyslexia. Abstract: There is increasing evidence that cerebellar deficit may be a causal factor in dyslexia. The cerebellum is considered to be the major structure involved in classical conditioning of the eyeblink response. In a direct test of cerebellar function in learning, 13 dyslexic participants (mean age 19.5 years) and 13 control participants matched for age and IQ undertook an eyeblink conditioning experiment in which for 60 acquisition trials an 800-ms auditory tone (conditioned stimulus, CS) was presented. On 70% of the trials an 80-ms corneal airpuff (unconditioned stimulus, US) was presented 720 ms after the tone onset. Nicolson RI Daum I Schugens MM Fawcett AJ Schulz A Exp Brain Res 2002 Mar;143(1):42-50.

Eye-hand preference dissociation in obsessive-compulsive disorder and dyslexia. Abstract: Dyslexia may be a development disturbance in which there are alterations in visual-spatial and visual-motor processing, while obsessive-compulsive disorder (OCD) is a psychiatric disease in which there are alterations in memory, executive function, and visual-spatial processing. Our hypothesis is that these disturbances may be, at least partially, the result of a crossed eye and hand preference. In the present study 16 controls, 20 OCD (DSM-IV criteria) and 13 dyslexic adults (Brazilian Dyslexia Association criteria) were included. Siviero MO Rysovas EO Juliano Y Del Porto JA Bertolucci PH Arq Neuropsiquiatr 2002 Jun;60(2-A):242-5.

Facets of dyslexia and its remediation / edited by Sarah F. Wright, Rudolf Groner. Amsterdam; New York: North-Holland, 1993. Wright, Sarah F. Groner, Rudolf. Description: xxiii, 646 p.: ill.; 25 cm. ISBN: 0444899499 (alk. paper) LC Classification: RC394.W6 F33 1993 NLM Class No.: W1 ST937I v.3 1993 WM 475 F138 1993 Dewey Class No.: 616.85/53 20

Factors that influence phoneme-grapheme correspondence learning. Abstract: The present study examined (a) the relative impact visual and phonetic factors have on learning phoneme grapheme correspondences, and (b) the relationship between measures of visual and phonological processing and children's ability to learn novel phoneme-grapheme correspondence pairs. Participants were 20 children with reading disabilities (RD), 10 normally achieving children matched for mental age (MA), and 10 children matched for reading age (RA). Mauer DM Kamhi AG J Learn Disabil 1996 May;29(3):259-70.

Failure of blue-tinted lenses to change reading scores of dyslexic individuals. Abstract: This study was designed to address a perceived major flaw in past studies investigating tinted lenses and dyslexia; i.e, the lack of a direct, scientifically validated means of diagnosing the type and severity of dyslexia. Using DDT classification, subjects were found to have mostly dysphoneidetic (mixed pattern) dyslexia. Among this population of dyslexic students, tinted lenses appeared to provide no beneficial effect. We offer an explanation based on neuro-anatomical relationships between the visual system and reading centers in the brain. The hypothesis states that the transient system defect may be an epiphenomenon, which can coincidentally occur in cases of reading disability. Christenson GN Griffin JR Taylor M Optometry 2001 Oct;72(10):627-33.

Faludy, Tanya, 1957- A little edge of darkness: a boy's triumph over dyslexia / Tanya and Alexander Faludy. London; Bristol, Pa.: Jessica Kingsley Publishers, 1996. Faludy, Alexander, 1983- Description: x, 175 p.: ill.; 22 cm. ISBN: 1853023574 (alk. paper) LC Classification: LC4710.G7 F35 1996 Dewey Class No.: 371.91/44 20

Familial aggregation of dyslexia phenotypes. Abstract: There is evidence for genetic contributions to reading disability, but the phenotypic heterogeneity associated with the clinical diagnosis may make identification of the underlying genetic basis difficult. In order to elucidate distinct phenotypic features that may be contributing to the genotypic heterogeneity, we assessed the familial aggregation patterns of Verbal IQ and 24 phenotypic measures associated with dyslexia in 102 nuclear families ascertained through probands in grades 1 through 6 who met the criteria for this disorder Raskind WH Hsu L Berninger VW Thomson JB Wijsman EM Behav Genet 2000 Sep;30(5):385-96.

Familial aggregation of spelling disability. Abstract: This study examined the familial aggregation of spelling disability in a sample of 32 German school-aged children and their relatives. The influence of two different diagnostic criteria (low-achievement criterion, and regression-based IQ-discrepancy criterion) on the rate of affectedness was investigated. Results revealed that 52.3-61.9% of the sibs and 26-34% of the parents were spelling disabled. Little evidence was found for an influence of the diagnostic criterion on the rate of affectedness. Schulte-Korne G Deimel W Muller K Gutenbrunner C Remschmidt H J Child Psychol Psychiatry 1996 Oct;37(7):817-22.

Familial dyslexia associated with cavum vergae. Abstract: Three members of one family, diagnosed as dyslexic, are described. All of them have variations of midline cavity: cavum vergae or cavum septum pellucidum, diagnosed by neuroradiological examination. In contrast, the non dyslexic members of the same family have no neuroanatomical congenital variations. We raise the possibility of a functional correlation between the dyslexia and the anatomical findings in the affected members of this family. Lampl Y Barak Y Gilad R Eshel Y Sarova-Pinhas I Clin Neurol Neurosurg 1997 May;99(2):142-7.

Family patterns of developmental dyslexia, part II: behavioral phenotypes. Abstract: The motor control of bimanual coordination and motor speech was compared between first degree relatives from families with at least 2 dyslexic family members, and families where probands were the only affected family members. Half of affected relatives had motor coordination deficits; and they came from families in which probands showed impaired motor coordination. By contrast, affected relatives without motor deficits came from dyslexia families where probands did not have motor deficits Wolff PH Melngailis I Obregon M Bedrosian M Am J Med Genet 1995 Dec 18;60(6):494-505.

Family patterns of developmental dyslexia. Part III: Spelling errors as behavioral phenotype. Abstract: The major trends in current research on developmental dyslexia assume that impaired phonological processing is the core deficit

in this disorder. Our earlier studies indicated that half of all dyslexic persons have significant deficits of bimanual motor coordination, and that impaired temporal resolution in motor action may identify a vertically transmitted behavioral phenotype in familial dyslexia. This report examines the relationship between spelling errors as a measure of impaired phonological processing and motor coordination deficits in the same dyslexia families. Wolff PH Melngailis I Kotwica K Am J Med Genet 1996 Jul 26;67(4):378-86.

Family-based association mapping provides evidence for a gene for reading disability on chromosome 15q. Abstract: Family-based association mapping was used to follow up reports of linkage between reading disability (RD) and a genomic region on chromosome 15q. Using a two-stage approach, we ascertained 101 (stage 1) and 77 (stage 2) parent-proband trios, in which RD was characterized rigorously. In stage 1, a set of eight microsatellite markers spanning the region of putative linkage was used and a highly significant association was detected between RD and a three-marker haplotype (D15S994 D15S214 D15S146: P and empirical P < 0.001 Morris DW Robinson L Turic D Duke M Webb V Milham C Hopkin E Pound K Fernando S Easton M Hamshere M Williams N McGuffin P Stevenson J Krawczak M Owen MJ O'Donovan MC Williams J Hum Mol Genet 2000 Mar 22;9(5):843-8.

Fatty acid deficiency signs predict the severity of reading and related difficulties in dyslexic children. Abstract: It has been proposed that developmental dyslexia may be associated with relative deficiencies in certain highly unsaturated fatty acids (HUFA). In children with attention-deficit/hyperactivity disorder, minor physical signs of fatty acid deficiency have been shown to correlate with blood biochemical measures of HUFA deficiency. These clinical signs of fatty acid deficiency were therefore examined in 97 dyslexic children in relation to reading and related skills, and possible sex differences were explored.Children with high fatty acid deficiency ratings showed poorer reading (P<0.02) and lower general ability (P<0.04) than children with few such clinical signs Richardson AJ Calvin CM Clisby C Schoenheimer DR Montgomery P Hall JA Hebb G Westwood E Talcott JB Stein JF Prostaglandins Leukot Essent Fatty Acids 2000 Jul-Aug;63(1-2):69-74.

Fatty acid metabolism in neurodevelopmental disorder: a new perspective on associations between attention-deficit/hyperactivity disorder, dyslexia, dyspraxia and the autistic spectrum. Abstract: There is increasing evidence that abnormalities of fatty acid and membrane phospholipid metabolism play a part in a wide range of neurodevelopmental and psychiatric disorders. This proposal is discussed here in relation to attention-deficit/hyperactivity disorder (ADHD), dyslexia, developmental coordination disorder (dyspraxia) and the autistic spectrum. These are among the most common neurodevelopmental disorders of childhood, with significant implications for society as well as for those directly affected. Richardson AJ Ross MA Prostaglandins Leukot Essent Fatty Acids 2000 Jul-Aug;63(1-2):1-9.

Fernández Baroja, Fernanda. [from old catalog] La dislexia: Madrid: Ciencias de la Educación Preescolar y Especial, 1974. Llopis Paret, Ana Maria, [from old catalog] joint author. Pablo de Riesgo, Carmen, [from old catalog] joint author. Description: 165 p.: ill.; 24 cm. LC Classification: LB1050.5.F45

Fernández Baroja, Fernanda. La dislexia: cuaderno de recuperación / [Fernanda Fernández Baroja, Ana María Llopis Paret, Carmen Pablo de Riesgo]. [Madrid: C.E.P.E, 1974?- Llopis Paret, Ana María, joint author. Pablo de Riesgo, Carmen, joint author. Description: v.: ill.; 17 cm. LC Classification: LB1050.5.F44 National Bib. No.: Sp***

Fily, Dominique. Faut-il enseigner la lecture? / Dominique Fily. Paris: Syros, c1997. Description: 158 p.: ill.; cm. ISBN: 2841465012 LC Classification: LB1050.F45 1997 Other System No.: (FrPJT)JTL00008462

Fine mapping of the chromosome 2p12-16 dyslexia susceptibility locus: quantitative association analysis and positional candidate genes SEMA4F and OTX1. Abstract: A locus on chromosome 2p12-16 has been implicated in dyslexia susceptibility by two independent linkage studies, including our own study of 119 nuclear twin-based families, each with at least one reading-disabled child. Nonetheless, no variant of any gene has been reported to show association with dyslexia, and no consistent clinical evidence exists to identify candidate genes with any strong a priori logic. We used 21 microsatellite markers spanning 2p12-16 to refine our 1-LOD unit linkage support interval to 12cM between D2S337 and D2S286. Francks C Fisher SE Olson RK Pennington BF Smith SD DeFries JC Monaco AP Psychiatr Genet 2002 Mar;12(1):35-41.

Finnish compound structure: experiments with a morphologically impaired patient. Abstract: The present study addresses two major aspects of compound processing, namely the issues of access code and structural effects (headedness), with an extensively studied deep dyslexic patient, HH, who has previously been shown to suffer from morphological impairment. In oral reading of compounds, HH preserves their morphological structure and, at the same time, shows additional processing load in increased errors compared to monomorphemic and derived words. Our data suggest that semantically transparent Finnish compounds are decomposed into their constituents at the level of lexical access. Makisalo J Niemi J Laine M Brain Lang 1999 Jun 1-15;68(1-2):249-53.

Fitzgibbon, Gary. Adult dyslexia: a guide for the workplace / Gary Fitzgibbon and Brian O'Connor. Chichester: Wiley, c2002.

O'Connor, Brian. Description: x, 172 p.; 25 cm. ISBN: 0470847255 (alk. paper) 0471487120 (PBK.) LC Classification: RC394.W6 F54 2002 National Bib. No.: GBA2-Y1836 Other System No.: (OCoLC)ocm49350632

Fitzhugh-Bell, Kathleen B. Dyslexia in Indianapolis: studies of needs and resources / Kathleen B. Fitzhugh-Bell, principal investigator. Indianapolis, Ind.: Dyslexia Institute of Indiana, c1993. Dyslexia Institute of Indiana. Description: 1 v. (various foliations); 28 cm. LC Classification: RJ496.A5 F58 1993 Dewey Class No.: 618.92/8553/00977252 20

fMRI auditory language differences between dyslexic and able reading children. Abstract: During fMRI, dyslexic and control boys completed auditory language tasks (judging whether pairs of real and/or pseudo words rhymed or were real words) in 30 s 'on' conditions alternating with a 30 s 'off' condition (judging whether tone pairs were same). During phonological judgment, dyslexics had more activity than controls in right than left inferior temporal gyrus and in left precentral gyrus. During lexical judgment, dyslexics were less active than controls in bilateral middle frontal gyrus and more active than controls in left orbital frontal cortex. Corina DP Richards TL Serafini S Richards AL Steury K Abbott RD Echelard DR Maravilla KR Berninger VW Neuroreport 2001 May 8;12(6):1195-201.

fMRI during word processing in dyslexic and normal reading children. Abstract: The present study addresses phonological processing in children with developmental dyslexia. Following the hypothesis of a core deficit of assembled phonology in dyslexia a set of hierarchically structured tasks was applied that specifically control for different kinds of phonological coding (assembled versus addressed phonological strategies). Seventeen developmental dyslexics and 17 normal reading children were scanned during four different tasks: (1) passive viewing of letter strings (control condition), (2) passive reading of non-words, (3) passive reading of legal words, and (4) a task requiring phonological transformation. Georgiewa P Rzanny R Hopf JM Knab R Glauche V Kaiser WA Blanz B Neuroreport 1999 Nov 8;10(16):3459-65.

Focal hypersynchronous activity in the EEG of children with specific developmental deficits: is there a clinical relevance? Abstract: Focal hypersynchronous activity in children with specific developmental deficits: Are there any clinical implications? To determine the frequency of focal hypersynchronous activity (HSA) in the EEGs of a child and adolescent psychiatry client population we evaluated 762 patients between 3 and 15 years old. Children with neurological problems, including epilepsy, craniocerebral trauma and psychotic disorders, and children on medication were excluded, as well as those with general developmental delays or abnormal EEG findings (except focal HSA). Pott W Remschmidt H Z Kinder Jugendpsychiatr Psychother 1996 Dec;24(4):272-81.

Foundations of reading acquisition and dyslexia: implications for early intervention / edited by Benita A. Blachman. Mahwah, N.J.: L. Erlbaum Associates, 1997. Blachman, Benita A. Description: xxii, 463 p.: ill.; 24 cm. ISBN: 080582362X (cloth: alk. paper) 0805823638 (pbk.: alk. paper) LC Classification: LB1050.2.F69 1997 Dewey Class No.: 428.4 21

Foxhall, G. J. Dyslexia: congenital word-blindness, compiled by G. J. Foxhall. Adelaide, State Library of South Australia, 1969. Description: 22 p. 26 cm. LC Classification: Z1009.S73 no. 122 Dewey Class No.: 011 s 016.6168/553 National Bib. No.: Aus70-648

Fractal analysis of eye movements during reading. Abstract: We present a new method for the analysis of reading eye movements based on the methods of nonlinear dynamics. In this preliminary study, the eye movements of normal and abnormal readers were analyzed for evidence of chaotic, nonlinear dynamical behavior. Both power spectral density analysis and fractal dimension determination showed evidence of nonlinearity as manifest in chaotic behavior. The computed fractal dimension of the system's presumed attractor seemed directly related to qualitative assessment of reading ability. Representative subjects did not differ in a similar analysis of pursuit movements. Schmeisser ET McDonough JM Bond M Hislop PD Epstein AD Optom Vis Sci 2001 Nov;78(11):805-14.

Freinet, Célestin. La Santé mentale de l'enfant: les maladies scolaires, la dyslexie, la délinquance / Célestin Freinet. Paris: F. Maspero, 1978. Description: 153 p.: facsims.; 18 cm. ISBN: 270710986X: LC Classification: LB3081.F73 Dewey Class No.: 371.9/2 National Bib. No.: F78-8569

Frequency acuity and binaural masking release in dyslexic listeners. Hill NI Bailey PJ Griffiths YM Snowling MJ J Acoust Soc Am 1999 Dec;106(6):L53-8.

Frequency and consistency effects in a pure surface dyslexic patient. Abstract: Data are presented from a neurological patient (M.P.) with an acquired deficit for naming words with atypical spelling-sound correspondences. In Experiment 1, the degree of consistency within neighborhoods of orthographically similar words had a parallel impact on M.P.'s pronunciations of regular and irregular words and nonwords. This result is more compatible with models in which the same basic procedure, sensitive in a graded fashion to both frequency and consistency, computes pronunciations for all types of letter strings than it is with models postulating separate lexical and nonlexical mechanisms. Patterson K Behrmann M J Exp Psychol Hum Percept Perform 1997 Aug;23(4):1217-31.

Frequency of reading disability caused by ocular problems in 9- and 10-year-old children in a small town. Abstract: Of the 89 children examined, 16 (18%) had reading problems and only 3/16 had no detectable ophthalmologic explanation. Hypoaccommodation was the most common cause of reading problems (in 6 of 16). In most of the cases it had not been diagnosed before. In all of these children the reading ability improved markedly with the proper refractive correction, bifocals or prisms. Motsch S Muhlendyck H Strabismus 2000 Dec;8(4):283-5.

From "logographic" to normal reading: the case of a deaf beginning reader. Abstract: Visual word recognition of a profoundly deaf girl (AH) with developmental reading disorders was explored using an experimental technique that measures performance as a function of eye fixation within a word. AH's fixation-dependent word recognition profile revealed that she was inferring the identity of words using a "logographic" reading strategy (i. e, using salient visual features). Following this observation a special training program that enhances the understanding of grapheme-phoneme relations was applied. Aghababian V Nazir TA Lancon C Tardy M Brain Lang 2001 Aug;78(2):212-23.

From attentional gating in macaque primary visual cortex to dyslexia in humans. Abstract: Selective attention is an important aspect of brain function that we need in coping with the immense and constant barrage of sensory information. One model of attention (Feature Integration Theory) that suggests an early selection of spatial locations of objects via an attentional spotlight would solve the 'binding problem' (that is how do different attributes of each object get correctly bound together?). Our experiments have demonstrated modulation of specific locations of interest at the level of the primary visual cortex both in visual discrimination and memory tasks, where the actual locations of the targets was important in being able to perform the task Vidyasagar TR Prog Brain Res 2001;134:297-312.

From inside prison. Cox J Dyslexia 2001 Apr-Jun;7(2):97-102.

From language to reading and dyslexia. PG - 37-46Abstract: This paper reviews evidence in support of the phonological deficit hypothesis of dyslexia. Findings from two experimental studies suggest that the phonological deficits of dyslexic children and adults cannot be explained in terms of impairments in low-level auditory mechanisms, but reflect higher-level language weaknesses. A study of individual differences in the pattern of reading skills in dyslexic children rejects the notion of 'sub-types'. Instead, the findings suggest that the variation seen in reading processes can be accounted for by differences in the severity of individual children's phonological deficits, modified by compensatory factors including visual memory, perceptual speed and print exposure. Children at genetic risk who go on to be dyslexic come to the task of reading with poorly specified phonological representations in the context of a more general delay in oral language development. Their prognosis (and that of their unaffected siblings) depends upon the balance of strengths and difficulties they show, with better language skills being a protective factor. Taken together, these findings suggest that current challenges to the phonological deficit theory can be met. Department of Psychology, University of York, Heslington, York, YO24 1AX UK. mjs19@york.ac.uk Snowling MJ Dyslexia 2001 Jan-Mar;7(1):37-46.

From reading to neurons / edited by Albert M. Galaburda. Cambridge, Mass.: MIT Press, c1989. Galaburda, Albert M, 1948- Landau, Emily. Fisher-Landau Foundation. Description: xxii, 545 p.: ill.; 24 cm. ISBN: 0262071150 LC Classification: RC394.W6 F76 1989 NLM Class No.: WL 340.6 F931 1987 Dewey Class No.: 616.85/53 19

Frontal processing and auditory perception. Abstract: Disordered processing of the pattern in sound over time has been observed in a number of clinical disorders, including developmental dyslexia. This study addresses the brain mechanisms required for the perception of such a pattern. We report the systematic evaluation of temporal perception in a patient with a single intact right auditory cortex and a large right frontal lobe lesion. A striking dissociated deficit was demonstrated in the perception of temporal pattern at the level of tens or hundreds of milliseconds. Griffiths TD Penhune V Peretz I Dean JL Patterson RD Green GG Neuroreport 2000 Apr 7;11(5):919-22.

Fucks, Wolfgang. Merkmalserfassung bei legasthenen Schülern: Anleitung zu Diagnoseverfahren u. Therapiekontrolle / Wolfgang Fucks, Peter Gräff. Weinheim; Basel: Beltz, 1976. Gräff, Peter, joint author. Description: 80 p.: graphs; 19 cm. ISBN: 340762008X: LC Classification: LB1050.5.F8 National Bib. No.: GFR76-A

Functional connectivity of the angular gyrus in normal reading and dyslexia. Abstract: The classic neurologic model for reading, based on studies of patients with acquired alexia, hypothesizes functional linkages between the angular gyrus in the left hemisphere and visual association areas in the occipital and temporal lobes. The angular gyrus is thought to have functional links with posterior language areas (e.g, Wernicke's area), because it is presumed to be involved in mapping visually presented inputs onto linguistic representations. Using positron emission tomography, we demonstrate in normal men that regional cerebral blood flow in the left angular gyrus shows strong within-task, across-subjects correlations (i.e, functional connectivity) with regional cerebral blood flow in extrastriate occipital and temporal lobe regions during single word reading. Horwitz B Donohue BC Proc Natl Acad Sci U S A 1998 Jul 21;95(15):8939-44.

Functional disruption in the organization of the brain for reading in dyslexia. Abstract: Learning to read requires an awareness that spoken words can be decomposed into the phonologic constituents that the alphabetic characters represent. Such phonologic awareness is characteristically lacking in dyslexic readers who, therefore, have difficulty mapping the alphabetic characters onto the spoken word. To find the location and extent of the functional disruption in neural systems that underlies this impairment, we used functional magnetic resonance imaging to compare brain activation patterns in dyslexic and nonimpaired subjects as they performed tasks that made progressively greater demands on phonologic analysis. Shaywitz SE Shaywitz BA Pugh KR Fulbright RK Constable RT Mencl WE Shankweiler DP Liberman AM Skudlarski P Fletcher JM Katz L Marchione KE Lacadie C Gatenby C Gore JC Proc Natl Acad Sci U S A 1998 Mar 3;95(5):2636-41.

Functional magnetic resonance imaging of early visual pathways in dyslexia. Abstract: We measured brain activity, perceptual thresholds, and reading performance in a group of dyslexic and normal readers to test the hypothesis that dyslexia is associated with an abnormality in the magnocellular (M) pathway of the early visual system. Functional magnetic resonance imaging (fMRI) was used to measure brain activity in conditions designed to preferentially stimulate the M pathway. Demb JB Boynton GM Heeger DJ J Neurosci 1998 Sep 1;18(17):6939-51.

Functional magnetic resonance imaging: clinical applications and potential. Abstract: Demonstration that contrast in magnetic resonance images can be generated based on differences in blood oxygenation has led to an explosion of interest in so-called functional magnetic resonance imaging (FMRI). FMRI can be used to map increases in blood flow that accompany local synaptic activity in the brain. The technique has proved remarkably sensitive and has been used to map a broad range of cognitive, motor and sensory processes in the brain entirely non-invasively. Matthews PM Clare S Adcock J J Inherit Metab Dis 1999 Jun;22(4):337-52.

Functional neuroimaging studies of reading and reading disability (developmental dyslexia). Abstract: Converging evidence from a number of neuroimaging studies, including our own, suggest that fluent word identification in reading is related to the functional integrity of two consolidated left hemisphere (LH) posterior systems: a dorsal (temporo-parietal) circuit and a ventral (occipito-temporal) circuit. This posterior system is functionally disrupted in developmental dyslexia. Reading disabled readers, relative to nonimpaired readers, demonstrate heightened reliance on both inferior frontal and right hemisphere posterior regions, presumably in compensation for the LH posterior difficulties. Pugh KR Mencl WE Jenner AR Katz L Frost SJ Lee JR Shaywitz SE Shaywitz BA Ment Retard Dev Disabil Res Rev 2000;6(3):207-13.

Further evidence that reading ability is not preserved in Alzheimer's disease. Abstract: Pre-morbid intelligence level is routinely assessed in Alzheimer's disease using the National Adult Reading Test (NART). This practice is based on the assumption that pronunciation of irregular words remains unaffected by the disease process. Recent reports have suggested that reading ability may become compromised in moderately demented subjects. NART performance is compromised in moderate Alzheimer disease, and the measure provides a serious underestimate of pre-morbid IQ in patients with an MMSE of 13 or less. O'Carroll RE Prentice N Murray C van Beck M Ebmeier KP Goodwin GM Br J Psychiatry 1995 Nov;167(5):659-62.

Gehret, Jeanne. Learning disabilities and the don't give-up kid / by Jeanne Gehret; illustrations by Sandra Ann DePauw; [foreword by Kathryn Cappella]. Fairport, N.Y.: Verbal Images Press, c1990. DePauw, Sandra Ann, ill. Related Titles: Don't give-up kid. Description: [32] p.: ill.; 21 cm. ISBN: 0962513601 (pbk.) Summary: Alex, a child with dyslexia, learns about his and other learning problems and what is done to solve them. LC Classification: LC4704.G44 1990 Other System No.: (OCoLC)21547758

Generalization of early metalinguistic skills in a phonological decoding study with first-graders at risk for reading failure. Abstract: This training study was designed to examine the effects of training letter-sound correspondences and phonemic decoding (segmenting and blending skills) on the decoding skills of three first-grade children identified to be at risk for reading failure. This training study was to examine the degree to which the subjects could readily learn decoding skills necessary for early reading and to determine the degree to which phonemic decoding training on CVC syllable structures generalize to untrained syllable structures. Rivers KO Lombardino LJ Int J Lang Commun Disord 1998 Oct-Dec;33(4):369-91.

Genetic analysis of dyslexia and other complex behavioral phenotypes. Abstract: In this review, we discuss recent data on the genetics of developmental dyslexia and consider broader issues involved in the search for genes influencing complex behavioral phenotypes. These issues include 1) the need for a sophisticated analysis of the phenotype and the need for interdisciplinary collaboration between geneticists and cognitive neuroscientists, 2) the likelihood of genetic heterogeneity and non-Mendelian inheritance and the necessity for linkage methods to deal with these issues, and 3) how association analyses complement linkage analyses. Pennington BF Smith SD Curr Opin Pediatr 1997 Dec;9(6):636-41.

Genetic factors contributing to learning and language delays and disabilities. Abstract: Reading disability shows substantial genetic influence, and it is in this area of early-onset cognitive delays that genetic research has made the most progress. Reading disability provides the first success story for identifying replicable quantitative trait locus linkage for behavioral disorders. Language and communication disorders show substantial

genetic influence, as does general cognitive ability (intelligence), which plays a role in most cognitive disabilities. Plomin R Child Adolesc Psychiatr Clin N Am 2001 Apr;10(2):259-77, viii.

Genetic influences on language impairment and literacy problems in children: same or different? Abstract: Data from two twin studies are examined to assess genetic and environmental influences on literacy, and the etiological relationship between language and literacy. Study 1 used children from 86 families previously recruited for a study of the genetics of specific language impairment (see Bishop, North, & Donlan, 1995), who completed tests of single-word reading and spelling. Literacy problems in this sample were common, were strongly heritable, and showed a close genetic relationship with poor nonword repetition. Bishop DV J Child Psychol Psychiatry 2001 Feb;42(2):189-98.

Genetic linkage analysis with dyslexia: evidence for linkage of spelling disability to chromosome 15. Abstract: Dyslexia (reading and spelling disability) is one of the most frequently diagnosed disorders in childhood. Twin studies of dyslexia have indicated that deficits in spelling are substantially heritable and that the heritability of spelling deficits is higher than the heritability of reading deficits. We conducted a linkage study for spelling disability in seven multiplex families from Germany. Following previously reported linkage findings of components of dyslexia to chromosome 6p21-p22 and 15q21, we genotyped 26 microsatellite markers covering all of chromosome 6, and 13 microsatellite markers covering all of chromosome 15. Nothen MM Schulte-Korne G Grimm T Cichon S Vogt IR Muller-Myhsok B Propping P Remschmidt H Eur Child Adolesc Psychiatry 1999;8 Suppl 3:56-9.

Genetic susceptibility to neurodevelopmental disorders. Abstract: A large body of evidence suggests that genetic factors influence liability to many common neurodevelopmental disorders. Examples include Tourette syndrome, attention-deficit hyperactivity disorder, autism, and dyslexia. Characterization of the genetic component of susceptibility to these conditions at a molecular level should improve classification, elucidate fundamental neurobiologic mechanisms of disease, and suggest novel approaches to treatment. Susceptibility loci for complex traits could be identified by detecting linkage to a well-mapped genetic marker or by detecting association with a putative high-risk allele at a candidate locus. Ryan SG J Child Neurol 1999 Mar;14(3):187-95.

Genetics of learning disabilities. Pennington BF J Child Neurol 1995 Jan;10 Suppl 1:S69-77.

Genomic mapping of chromosomal region 2p15-p21 (D2S378-D2S391): integration of Genemap'98 within a framework of yeast and bacterial artificial chromosomes. Abstract: The region of chromosome 2 encompassed by the polymorphic markers D2S378 (centromeric) and D2S391 (telomeric) spans an approximately 10-cM distance in cytogenetic bands 2p15-p21. This area is frequently involved in cytogenetic alterations in human cancers. It harbors the genes for several genetic disorders, including Type I hereditary nonpolyposis colorectal cancer (HNPCC), familial male precocious puberty (FMPP), Carney complex (CNC), Doyne's honeycomb retinal dystrophy (DHRD), and one form of familial dyslexia (DYX-3). Kirschner LS Taymans SE Pack S Pak E Pike BL Chandrasekharappa SC Zhuang Z Stratakis CA Genomics 1999 Nov 15;62(1):21-33.

Get real: clinical testing of patients' reading abilities. Abstract: Education of cancer patients is complicated by a number of factors including timing, understanding of medical terms, and anxiety-induced inattention. The concern about patient education has led to the common practice of providing brochures about cancer, responses to cancer, treatment, and management of side effects. This material is often written at reading levels that do not match the reading ability of the patient. Research has indicated that the stated educational level is not equivalent to reading level. Foltz A Sullivan J Cancer Nurs 1998 Jun;21(3):162-6.

Gilroy, Dorothy E. Dyslexia at college / D.E. Gilroy and T.R. Miles; with contributions from C.R. Wilsher... [et al.]. Edition Information: 2nd ed. London; New York: Routledge, 1996. Miles, T. R. (Thomas Richard) Description: xii, 260 p.; 24 cm. ISBN: 0415127785 LC Classification: LB1050.5.G53 1996 Dewey Class No.: 371.91/44 20

Giordano, Luis. Los fundamentos de la dislexia escolar: el grado para alumnos disléxicos, los fundamentos para su organización y funcionamiento, medios para prevenir la dislexia escolar desde el jardín de infantes, trescientos ejercicios para la reeducación de los alumnos disléxicos / Luis Giordano y Luis Héctor Giordano. Buenos Aires: Ediciones I.A.R, 1973 [i.e. 1974] Giordano, Luis Héctor, joint author. Description: 324 p.: ill.; 20 cm. LC Classification: LB1050.5.G54

Gjessing, Hans-Jørgen. Lese- og skrivevanster: dyslexi: problemorientering, analyse og diagnose, behandling og undervisning / Hans-Jørgen Gjessing. Bergen: Universitetsforl, c1977. Description: 254 p.: diagrs.; 23 cm. ISBN: 8200016927: LC Classification: LB1050.5.G57 National Bib. No.: N77-Sept.

Goldberg, Herman K. Dyslexia: problems of reading disabilities, by Herman K. Goldberg and Gilbert B. Schiffman. New York, Grune & Stratton [1972] Schiffman, Gilbert B, joint author. Description: xiii, 194 p. illus. 23 cm. ISBN: 0808907840 LC Classification: RJ496.A5 G65 NLM Class No.: WL340 G618d 1972 Dewey Class No.: 616.8/553

Goldish, Meish. Everything you need to know about dyslexia / Meish Goldish. Portion of

Dyslexia Edition Information: 1st ed. New York: Rosen Pub. Group, 1998. Description: 64 p.: ill. (some col.); 25 cm. ISBN: 0823925587 Summary: Explains the causes and symptoms of dyslexia and discusses how to overcome this disability and become a good reader and writer. LC Classification: LB1050.5.G645 1998 Dewey Class No.: 371.91/44 21

Goldsworthy, Candace L. Developmental reading disabilities: a language based treatment approach / Candace L. Goldsworthy. San Diego: Singular Pub. Group, c1996. Description: xiii, 301 p.: ill.; 23 cm. ISBN: 1565930851 LC Classification: LB1050.5.G65 1996 NLM Class No.: WL 340.6 G624d 1995 Dewey Class No.: 372.4/3 20

Goodman, Janna. The mystery at Haunted Ridge: a novel / Janna Goodman. American Fork, Utah: Covenant Communications, [1995] Description: 112 p.; 23 cm. ISBN: 1555036945 1555038255 Summary: Because twelve-year-old Carrie has dyslexia, she feels that she must solve the mystery behind the strange happenings at camp to prove that she's not stupid. LC Classification: PZ7.G61373 My 1995 Dewey Class No.: [Fic] 20

Goodman, Janna. The mystery of the third oak: a novel / Janna Goodman. American Fork, Utah: Covenant Communications, c1994. Description: 98 p.; 23 cm. ISBN: 1555036945 (pbk.): LC Classification: PZ7.G61373 Mys 1994 Dewey Class No.: [Fic] 20

Gordon, Melanie Apel. Let's talk about dyslexia / Melanie Apel Gordon. Edition Information: 1st ed. New York: PowerKids Press, 1999. Description: 24 p.: col. ill.; 19 cm. ISBN: 0823951995 Summary: Discusses a learning disability of approximately one in every ten people, including Albert Einstein, Thomas Edison, and how to cope with it. LC Classification: LB1050.5.G67 1999 Dewey Class No.: 371.91/44 21

Grammatism. Abstract: Findings from the literature on language development, dyslexia, and adult sentence processing provide a vehicle for comparing two models of the symptom complex associated with agrammatism. One model contends that agrammatism represents a deficit in linguistic structures. The other model maintains that the linguistic behavior associated with agrammatism is the result of a limitation in language processing. To adjudicate between the models, the present paper examines one linguistic construction, the restrictive relative clause. Crain S Ni W Shankweiler D Brain Lang 2001 Jun;77(3):294-304.

Grégoire, Jacques. Evaluer les troubles de la lecture: les nouveaux modèles théoriques et leurs implications diagnostiques / Jacques Grégoire, Bernadette Piérart; avec la contribution de Alégria... [et al.]. Bruxelles: De Boeck université, c1994. Piérart, Bernadette. Description: 272 p.: ill..; 24 cm. ISBN: 2804119165 LC Classification: LB1050.5.G695 1994 Dewey Class No.: 371.91/44 21

Griffin, John R, 1934- Therapy in dyslexia and reading problems: including vision, perception, motor skills / John R. Griffin, Howard N. Walton; with contributions by Y. Libbie Amsell. Los Angeles, Calif.: Instructional Materials & Equipment Distributors, c1985. Walton, Howard N. Amsell, Y. Libbie. Description: 105 p.: ill.; 28 cm. LC Classification: LB1050.5.G717 1985 Dewey Class No.: 428.4/2 19

Griffith, Joe, 1941- How dyslexic Benny became a star: a story of hope for dyslexic children and their parents / by Joe Griffith; [illustrated by Jenny Schulz]. Dallas, Tex.: Yorktown Press, c1998. Schulz, Jenny, ill. Description: xii, 113 p.: ill.; 22 cm. ISBN: 0965937909 Summary: A fifth-grader who is frustrated and humiliated because he can't read as well as his classmates becomes a star on the football field, and when he is diagnosed with dyslexia, he finds that he has a whole team of people ready to help. LC Classification:

PZ7.G881356 Ho 1998 Dewey Class No.: [Fic] 21 Other System No.: (OCoLC)37728378 NNRB (FS0360(00)) RC

Griffiths, Anita N. Teaching the dyslexic child / Anita N. Griffiths. Novato, Calif.: Academic Therapy Publications, c1978. Description: 128 p.: ill.; 22 cm. ISBN: 0878792058 LC Classification: LB1050.5.G72 Dewey Class No.: 371.9/14

Grissemann, Hans, Dr. Zur Anti-Legasthenie-Bewegung: sprach-, sozial- und neuropsychologische Hinweise zu neuen Ansätzen der Prävention, der Diagnostik und der Therapie der Lese- und Rechtschreibschwäche: gemeinsames Referat (leicht überarb.) an der Legasthenietagung vom 6./7. Oktober 1977 in Brugg-Windisch / Hans Grissemann, Emil E. Kobi. Bern: H. Huber, c1978. Kobi, Emil Erich, joint author. Description: 92 p.; 22 cm. ISBN: 3456806035 LC Classification: RJ496.A5 G75 Dewey Class No.: 618.92/68553 19 National Bib. No.: Sw***

Growing up dyslexic: a parent's view. Donawa W J Learn Disabil 1995 Jun-Jul;28(6):324-8.

Grüttner, Tilo, 1939- Legasthenie ist ein Notsignal: verstehen u. wirksam helfen / Tilo Grüttner; [Zeichn. von Rudi Scholz]. Edition Information: Orig.-Ausg. Reinbek bei Hamburg: Rowohlt, 1980. Description: 92 p.: ill.; 19 cm. ISBN: 3499173247: LC Classification: LB1050.5.G77 Dewey Class No.: 371.91/4 19 National Bib. No.: GFR80-A

Gutmann de Díaz, Hilde. [from old catalog] Sobre las dislexias adquiridas. [Caracas] Instituto de Psicología, Universidad Central de Venezuela [1968?] Description: 68 p. 28 cm. LC Classification: RC394.W6 G87

Hallgren, Bertil. Specific dyslexia ("congenital word-blindness") A clinical and genetic study. [Translated from the Swedish by Erica Odelberg] Stockholm, 1950.

Description: viii, 287 p. port, diagrs. 25 cm. LC Classification: RC383.A6 H33 Dewey Class No.: 616.855 Other System No.: (OCoLC)4900436

Hamilton-Fairley, Daphne. Dyslexia, speech therapy and the dyslexic / by Daphne Hamilton-Fairley. London: Helen Arkell Dyslexia Centre, 1976. Description: [2], 26 p.: ill.; 21 cm. ISBN: 0950362689 LC Classification: RJ496.S7 H35 Dewey Class No.: 371.9/14 National Bib. No.: GB77-02176

Hampshire, Susan, 1942- Susan's story: an autobiographical account of my struggle with words / Susan Hampshire. London: Sidgwick & Jackson, 1981. Description: 167 p.: ill.; 23 cm. ISBN: 0283987359: LC Classification: PN2598.H22 A37 1981 Dewey Class No.: 792/.028/0924 B 19

Handedness and cognitive abilities: findings in a representative sample of adolescents and young adults Abstract: Handedness and cognitive abilities in a representative sample of adolescents and young adults. The relationship between laterality and cognitive ability was examined in a representative sample of adolescents and young adults between 16 and 30 years of age. The study was designed as a possible replication of Annett's data supporting her right-shift theory (rst), but included other measures of laterality as well. Strehlow U Haffner J Parzer P Pfuller U Resch F Zerahn-Hartung C Z Kinder Jugendpsychiatr Psychother 1996 Dec;24(4):253-64.

Handedness and creativity in a sample of homosexual men. Abstract: A form concerning handedness, dyslexia, stuttering (self-report), and twinning was included in a study of sexual habits of homosexual men. Questions about interests in music, art, and creative writing were included. A questionnaire was sent out to male homosexuals. Out of 391 returned forms, 363 were suitable for data processing. Analysis showed 13.9% reported writing with the left hand, 6.5% with stuttering, and 8.6% with dyslexia.

The twin incidence was 1.2%. Gotestam KO Percept Mot Skills 2001 Jun;92(3 Pt 2):1069-74.

Hanja alexia with agraphia after left posterior inferior temporal lobe infarction: a case study. Abstract: Korean written language is composed of ideogram (Hanja) and phonogram (Hangul), as Japanese consists of Kanji (ideogram) and Kana (phonogram). Dissociation between ideogram and phonogram impairment after brain injury has been reported in Japanese, but few in Korean. We report a 64-yr-old right-handed man who showed alexia with agraphia in Hanja but preserved Hangul reading and writing after a left posterior inferior temporal lobe infarction. Interestingly, the patient was an expert in Hanja; he had been a Hanja calligrapher over 40 yr. Kwon JC Lee HJ Chin J Lee YM Kim H Na DL J Korean Med Sci 2002 Feb;17(1):91-5.

Hansen, Joyce. Yellow Bird and me / Joyce Hansen. New York: Clarion Books, c1986. Description: 155 p.; 22 cm. ISBN: 0899193358 Summary: Doris becomes friends with Yellow Bird as she helps him with his studies and his part in the school play and discovers that he has a problem known as dyslexia. LC Classification: PZ7.H19825 Ye 1986 Dewey Class No.: [Fic] 19

Hardwick, Paula. Books for the dyslexic / compiled and reviewed by Paula Hardwick. London: Helen Arkell Dyslexia Centre, [1976?] Description: [22] p.; 30 cm. LC Classification: Z1039.D94 H37 Dewey Class No.: 028.5/5 19 National Bib. No.: GB***

Harnois, Veronica D'Urso. The Harnois Program: decoding skills for dyslexic readers / Veronica D'Urso Harnois with E. Jeanne Harnois Furdyna. Edition Information: Teacher's ed. Pittsburgh, Pa.: Dorrance Pub. Co, c1994. Furdyna, E. Jeanne Harnois. Description: 87 p.: ill.; 28 cm. ISBN: 0805935401 LC Classification: LB1050.5.H27 1994 Dewey Class No.: 372.4/3 20

Hartmann, Gerlinde. Der Legastheniker auf der Unterstufe der Grundschule: unter welchen Gegebenheiten sollte er in eine ASO eingewiesen werden oder unter Hilfeleistung in d. VS verbleiben können / Gerlinde Hartmann. Wien: Ketterl, [1975] Description: 92 p.: ill.; 21 cm. LC Classification: LB1050.5.H33 National Bib. No.: Au75-22

Hasty, Ruth. How to teach dyslexics and other nonreaders: the Hasty way to reading / by Ruth Hasty. La Junta, Colo.: Springboard Press, c1987. Description: 57 p.; 23 cm. ISBN: 0945243006 (pbk.): LC Classification: LB1050.5.H34 1987 Dewey Class No.: 371.91/44 20

Hearing-impaired students' reading characteristics compared to dyslexic students (tested in Hebrew). Engel-Eldar R Rosenhouse J Int J Rehabil Res 2000 Dec;23(4):313-8.

Heaton, Pat. Dealing with dyslexia / Pat Heaton and Patrick Winterson; consultant in dyslexia, Margaret Snowling. Edition Information: 2nd ed. San Diego, CA: Singular Pub. Group, 1996. Winterson, Patrick. Snowling, Margaret J. Description: xv, 248 p.: ill.; 24 cm. ISBN: 1897635575 LC Classification: LC4708.H43 1996 Dewey Class No.: 371.91/44 21 Other System No.: (OCoLC)35300258

Heaton, Pat. Dyslexia: parents in need / Pat Heaton. London: Whurr Publishers, 1996. Description: xiii, 94 p.: ill.; 24 cm. ISBN: 1897635737 LC Classification: LC4708.H47 1996 Other System No.: (Uk)1897635737 (CStRLIN)UKBPGB9619760-B Cancelled Sys. No.: (Uk)D2270347

Helping children adjust--a Tri-Ministry Study: I. Evaluation methodology. Abstract: This report describes the evaluation methodology of the Tri-Ministry Study--a school-based trial evaluating the effectiveness of three universal programs: (a) a classwide social skills program (SS), (b) a partner reading program (RE); and,

(c) a combination of both (SS & RE), to reduce and prevent behavioural maladjustment among children in the primary division (up to grade 3) of Ontario schools. The trial was done between 1991 and 1995. Sixty schools in 11 boards of education took part and were assigned randomly to program(s) during the study. Contributing to the evaluation database are detailed follow-up assessments (observations, ratings, and standard tests) on 2439 children. Boyle MH Cunningham CE Heale J Hundert J McDonald J Offord DR Racine Y J Child Psychol Psychiatry 1999 Oct;40(7):1051-60.

Helping children adjust--a Tri-Ministry Study: II. Program effects. Abstract: This report describes program effects of the Tri-Ministry Study a school-based, longitudinal trial carried out over a 5-year period to assess the effectiveness of classwide social skills training (SS), partner reading (RE), and a combination of both (SS & RE) to reduce maladjustment among children in the primary division (up to grade 3) of Ontario schools. It places these effects in the context of other school-based prevention studies and discusses them in view of important methodological and programmatic issues Hundert J Boyle MH Cunningham CE Duku E Heale J McDonald J Offord DR Racine Y J Child Psychol Psychiatry 1999 Oct;40(7):1061-73.

Helping the child with dyslexia. Luiz N Indian Pediatr 1998 Mar;35(3):290.

Hemisphere-specific treatment of dyslexia subtypes: better reading with anxiety-laden words? Abstract: Twenty children (12 boys, 8 girls; mean age = 10.4 years) with P-type dyslexia (accurate but slow and fragmented reading) and 20 children (12 boys, 8 girls; mean age = 10.3 years) with L-type dyslexia (hurried, inaccurate reading) were treated with visual hemisphere-specific stimulation employing the HEMSTIM computer program. Stimulation was produced by presenting words to the left (L-dyslexia) or to the right (P-dyslexia) visual field. Children in the control condition received treatment with neutral words, whereas children in the experimental condition received treatment with anxiety-laden words. After treatment, the children with L-dyslexia in the experimental group made fewer substantive errors and more fragmentations on a text-reading task than did the children with L-dyslexia in the control group. Van Strien JW Stolk BD Zuiker S J Learn Disabil 1995 Jan;28(1):30-4.

Hemispheric processing characteristics for lexical decisions in adults with reading disorders. Abstract: The present study measured unilateral tachistoscopic vocal reaction times and error responses of reading-disordered and normally reading adults to single words and nonwords in a series of lexical decision tasks at two linguistic levels (concrete and abstract words). Analysis of variance on reaction times indicated that main effects of stimulus type, visual field, and the interaction of these variables were not significant for the reading-disordered group, but visual field and an interaction of visual field and stimulus type were for the normally reading adults. Walker MM Spires H Rastatter MP Percept Mot Skills 2001 Feb;92(1):273-87.

Hepworth, T. S. Dyslexia; the problem of reading retardation [by] T. S. Hepworth. [Sydney] Angus and Robertson [1971] Description: 100 p. illus. 22 cm. ISBN: 0207121826 LC Classification: RC394.W6 H46 Dewey Class No.: 616.85/53 National Bib. No.: Aus***

Historical trends in biological and medical investigations of reading disabilities: 1850-1915. Abstract: The theoretical roots of neuropsychological research lie in the case studies of reading disability completed during the late nineteenth and early twentieth centuries. This article reviews the methods, technologies, and operating tenets of these studies. The results suggest that the assumptions of anatomical and functional modularity for cortical processes became guiding principles for diagnosing and correcting reading difficulties. Pickle JM J Learn Disabil 1998 Nov-Dec;31(6):625-35.

Historical view of the influences of measurement and reading theories on the assessment of reading. Abstract: The purpose of this study is to briefly explore the interactions among measurement theories, reading theories, and measurement practices from an historical perspective. The assessment of reading provides a useful framework for examining how theories influence, and in some cases fail to influence, the practice of reading assessment as operationalized in reading tests. The first section describes a conceptual framework for examining the assessment of reading. Next I describe the major research traditions in measurement theory that have dominated measurement practice during the 20th century. Engelhard G Jr J Appl Meas 2001;2(1):1-26.

Høien, Torleiv, 1939- Dyslexia: from theory to intervention / by Torleiv Høien and Ingvar Lundberg. Dordrecht; Boston: Kluwer, 2000. Projected Pub. Date: 0007 Lundberg, Ingvar. Description: p.; cm. ISBN: 0792363094 (HB: alk. paper) LC Classification: RC394.W6 H65 2000 NLM Class No.: W1 NE342DG v.18 2000 WL 340.6 H719d 2000 Dewey Class No.: 616.85/53 21 Other System No.: (DNLM)100941729 Series:

Hornsby, Bevé. Overcoming dyslexia: a straightforward guide for families and teachers / Bevé Hornsby; foreword by Susan Hampshire and Angharad Rees. New York: Arco Pub, 1984. Description: 140 p.: ill. (some col.); 24 cm. ISBN: 0668056894: LC Classification: RJ496.A5 H67 1984 Dewey Class No.: 618.92/8553 19

How does vision affect learning? Part II. Abstract: 1. Dyslexia is a language-based learning disability in which phontiec analysis is genetically deficient. 2. Nonverbal learning differences are frequently overlooked in evaluating learning disabled children. 3. Children often have more than one category of learning difference, all of which must be diagnosed correctly to be effectively remediated. Koller HP J Ophthalmic Nurs Technol 1999 Jan-Feb;18(1):12-8.

How local is the impact of a specific learning difficulty on premature children's evaluation of their own competence? Abstract: The aim of this study was to determine whether children's perceptions of their own competence levels reflected their actual strengths and weaknesses (Specificity Hypothesis) or transcended these (Generality Hypothesis). Harter and Pike's measure of self-perception was administered to 163 prematurely born 6-year-olds with or without motor co-ordination and/or reading problems. Associations between children's self-perceptions and their scores on standardised tests of motor co-ordination and reading were assessed in three distinct ways. Jongmans M Demetre JD Dubowitz L Henderson SE J Child Psychol Psychiatry 1996 Jul;37(5):563-8.

How psychological science informs the teaching of reading. Abstract: This monograph discusses research, theory, and practice relevant to how children learn to read English. After an initial overview of writing systems, the discussion summarizes research from developmental psychology on children's language competency when they enter school and on the nature of early reading development. Subsequent sections review theories of learning to read, the characteristics of children who do not learn to read (i.e, who have developmental dyslexia), research from cognitive psychology and cognitive neuroscience on skilled reading, and connectionist models of learning to read. Rayner K Foorman BR Perfetti CA Pesetsky D Seidenberg MS Psychol Sci 2001 Nov;2(2 Suppl):31-74.

Human GABA(B) receptor 1 gene: eight novel sequence variants. Abstract: GABA (gamma-aminobutyric acid) is the principal inhibitory neurotransmitter in the brain. The human GABA(B) receptor (GABBR1) maps to the human leukocyte antigen (H Hum Mutat 2001 Apr;17(4):349-50.

Human gamma-aminobutyric acid B receptor gene: complementary DNA cloning, expression, chromosomal location, and genomic organization. Abstract: The 6p21.3 region of human chromosome 6 is a genetic locus for schizophrenia, juvenile myoclonic epilepsy, and dyslexia. Goei VL Choi J Ahn J Bowlus CL Raha-Chowdhury R Gruen JR Biol Psychiatry 1998 Oct 15;44(8):659-66.

Human verbal working memory impairments associated with thalamic damage. Abstract: Although animal studies, human neuroimaging studies, and numerous theoretical models suggest possible contributions of the thalamus to working memory, there are very few reported deficits in human working memory following thalamic lesions. The present study examined working memory performance in six individuals with isolated thalamic stroke and found evidence of impairment on a number of working memory span tasks, but not on a forward digit-span measure. Examination of additional aspects of working memory performance (e.g, spatial and object working memory), analysis of subjects with other sites of thalamic stroke, and functional neuroimaging suggest a role of the thalamus in working memory. Dagenbach D Kubat-Silman AK Absher JR Int J Neurosci 2001;111(1-2):67-87.

Hurford, Daphne. To read or not to read: answers to all your questions about dyslexia / Daphne M. Hurford. New York: Scribner, c1998. Description: 239 p.; 25 cm. ISBN: 0684839504 LC Classification: RC394.W6 H866 1998 Dewey Class No.: 616.85/53 21

Huston, Anne Marshall. Common sense about dyslexia / by Anne Marshall Huston. Lanham, MD: Madison Books, c1987. Description: xvi, 284 p.: ill.; 23 cm. ISBN: 0819156663 (pbk.: alk. paper):

0819163236 LC Classification: RC394.W6 H87 1987 NLM Class No.: WL 340.6 H842c Dewey Class No.: 616.85/53 19

Huston, Anne Marshall. Understanding dyslexia: a practical approach for parents and teachers / Anne Marshall Huston. Lanham: Madison Books: Distributed by National Book Network, c1992. Huston, Anne Marshall. Common sense about dyslexia. Description: xxii, 345 p.: ill.; 24 cm. ISBN: 0819178047 (cloth: alk. paper): 0819182494 (paper: alk. paper) LC Classification: RC394.W6 H87 1992 Dewey Class No.: 616.85/53 20

Hynd, George W. Dyslexia: neuropsychological theory, research, and clinical differentiation / George W. Hynd, Morris Cohen. New York: Grune & Stratton, c1983. Cohen, Morris. Description: xx, 270 p, [1] leaf of plates: ill.; 24 cm. ISBN: 0808915843 LC Classification: RC394.W6 H95 1983 NLM Class No.: WM 475 H997d Dewey Class No.: 616.85/53 19

Hyperactivity and reading disability: a longitudinal study of the nature of the association. Abstract: In order to investigate the possible causal relationships between hyperactivity and educational underachievement that might account for their frequent co-occurrence, four groups of boys, defined by the presence or absence of hyperactivity and specific reading retardation, were identified in an epidemiological study of 7 8-year-old children. They were examined in detail by means of parental interviews and psychological tests and reassessed 9 years later at the age of 16-18 years on a similar range of measures. Chadwick O Taylor E Taylor A Heptinstall E Danckaerts M J Child Psychol Psychiatry 1999 Oct;40(7):1039-50.

Hyperkinetic syndrome (attention deficit-/hyperactivity disorder) in adulthood Abstract: The clinical picture of adult hyperkinetic syndrome (HKS) or attention deficit/hyperactivity disorder is nearly unknown in Germany. It can be estimated, that approximately one third of affected children show symptoms as adults. In the combined type of the syndrome symptoms of inattention as well as of hyperactivity and impulsivity are present, a predominantly inattentive or hyperactive-impulsive type is possible. Retrospective diagnosis of HKS in childhood can be difficult. Disorganization, emotional disturbances and stress intolerance are common in adults with HKS as well as residual symptoms of learning disorders like dyslexia, dyscalculia and dysgraphia Krause KH Krause J Trott GE Nervenarzt 1998 Jul;69(7):543-56.

Hyperlexia in an adult patient with lesions in the left medial frontal lobe Abstract: A 69-year-old right-handed woman developed a transcortical motor aphasia with hyperlexia following resection of a glioma in the left medial frontal lobe. Neurological examination revealed grasp reflex in the right hand and underutilization of the right upper extremity. An MRI demonstrated lesions in the left medial frontal lobe including the supplementary motor area and the anterior part of the cingulate gyrus, which extended to the anterior part of the body of corpus callosum. Neuropsychologically she was alert and cooperative Suzuki K Yamadori A Kumabe T Endo K Fujii T Yoshimoto T Rinsho Shinkeigaku 2000 Apr;40(4):393-7.

Identification of side of seizure onset in temporal lobe epilepsy using memory tests in the context of reading deficits. Abstract: Sixty patients with temporal lobe epilepsy were classified into reading deficient (RD; n = 21) and non-reading deficient (non-RD; n = 39) groups. Selective deficits in verbal or nonverbal memory, consistent with side of seizure onset, were evident in the non-RD patients. Both verbal and nonverbal memory performance were reduced equivalently in individuals with RD, regardless of side of seizure onset. As a result, memory tests that were accurate in identifying side of seizure onset in the non-RD group were not as accurate in the RD group. Breier JI Brookshire BL Fletcher JM Thomas AB Plenger PM Wheless JW Willmore LJ Papanicolaou A J Clin Exp Neuropsychol 1997 Apr;19(2):161-71.

Identifying, assessing and helping dyspraxic children. Flory S Dyslexia 2000 Jul-Sep;6(3):205-8.

Immune disorders and handedness in dyslexic boys and their relatives. Abstract: Thirty dyslexic and 30 control boys aged 7-11 years were compared for frequency of immune disorders and handedness as well as for family history of immune disorders and learning disabilities (dyslexia and stuttering). They were compared for neurological status and for history of speech and language difficulties. There were no significant differences between the two groups in the frequency of immune disorders and in handedness. The results showed significantly more dyslexic boys with soft neurological signs and signs of speech and language disorders. Jariabkova K Hugdahl K Glos J Scand J Psychol 1995 Dec;36(4):355-62.

Immunogenetic studies in autism and related disorders. Abstract: The major histocompatibility complex comprises a number of genes that control the function and regulation of the immune system. One of these genes, the C4B gene, encodes a product that is involved in eliminating pathogens such as viruses and bacteria from the body. We previously reported that a deficient form of the C4B gene, termed the C4B null allele (no C4B protein produced) had an increased frequently in autism. Warren RP Singh VK Averett RE Odell JD Maciulis A Burger RA Daniels WW Warren WL Mol Chem Neuropathol 1996 May-Aug;28(1-3):77-81.

Impaired auditory frequency discrimination in dyslexia detected with mismatch evoked potentials. Abstract: Deficits in phonological skills appear to be at the heart of reading disability; however, the nature of this impairment is not yet known.

The hypothesis that dyslexic subjects are impaired in auditory frequency discrimination was tested by using an attention-independent auditory brain potential, termed mismatch negativity (MMN) while subjects performed a visual distractor task. In separate blocks, MMN responses to graded changes in tone frequency or tone duration were recorded in 10 dyslexic and matched control subjects. MMN potentials to changes in tone frequency but not to changes in tone duration were abnormal in dyslexic subjects. Baldeweg T Richardson A Watkins S Foale C Gruzelier J Ann Neurol 1999 Apr;45(4):495-503.

Impaired detection of variable duration embedded tones in ectopic NZB/BINJ mice. Abstract: Utilizing rodent models, prior research has demonstrated a significant association between focal neocortical malformations (i.e. induced microgyria, molecular layer ectopias), which are histologically similar to those observed in human dyslexic brains, and rate-specific auditory processing deficits as seen in language impaired populations. In the current study, we found that ectopic NZB/BINJ mice exhibit significant impairments in detecting a variable duration 5.6 kHz tone embedded in a 10.5 kHz continuous background, using both acoustic reflex modification and auditory event-related potentials (AERP). Peiffer AM Dunleavy CK Frenkel M Gabel Neuroreport 2001 Sep 17;12(13):2875-9.

Impaired processing of complex auditory stimuli in rats with induced cerebrocortical microgyria: An animal model of developmental language disabilities. Abstract: Individuals with developmental language disabilities, including developmental dyslexia and specific language impairment (SLI), exhibit impairments in processing rapidly presented auditory stimuli. It has been hypothesized that these deficits are associated with concurrent deficits in speech perception and, in turn, impaired language development. Additionally, postmortem analyses of human dyslexic brains have revealed the presence of focal neocortical malformations such as cerebrocortical microgyria. Clark MG Rosen GD Tallal P Fitch RH J Cogn Neurosci 2000 Sep;12(5):828-39.

Impaired recognition of traffic signs in adults with dyslexia. Abstract: Ten adults with dyslexia (4 women and 6 men, mean age: 26.8 years, range: 19-43 years) and 11 controls (5 women and 6 men, mean age: 20.5 years, range: 18-29 years) were tested on their ability to differentiate between real and false traffic signs. The stimuli, computer-presented color pictures, were chosen to minimize the applicability of verbal or written linguistic skills to the task. The adults with dyslexia recognized the traffic signs significantly less well than did the controls. Brachacki GW Nicolson RI Fawcett AJ J Learn Disabil 1995 May;28(5):297-301, 308.

Impaired short temporal interval discrimination in a dyslexic adult. Abstract: The ability to discriminate short temporal intervals was examined in a dyslexic adult (E.C.) and six matched controls. Listeners had to decide whether the second interval was shorter or longer than a standard (target) interval. Each interval was defined as the silent duration between two successive brief tones. Eight target intervals were used, ranging from 100 to 1,200 ms in duration. At each target interval, the differential threshold (DL) for duration was assessed, with the use of an adaptive psychophysical procedure. Rousseau L Hebert S Cuddy LL Brain Cogn 2001 Jun-Jul;46(1-2):249-54.

Impaired stimulus-driven orienting of attention and preserved goal-directed orienting of attention in unilateral visual neglect. Abstract: Neglect patients do not respond to stimuli presented on the side of space contralateral to the side of their brain lesions, indicating deficits to attentional or representational mechanisms. We describe a patient who shows a left neglect in normal reading and line bisection but an intact ability to locate the left end of the stimulus. Further tests showed that his seemingly intact ability to search into the "neglected" side was due to his ability to use local elements of the stimulus as cues in his serial search for the left end Luo CR Anderson JM Caramazza A Am J Psychol 1998 Winter;111(4):487-507.

Impaired temporal contrast sensitivity in dyslexics is specific to retain-and-compare paradigms. Abstract: Developmental dyslexia is a specific reading disability that affects 5-10% of the population. Recent studies have suggested that dyslexics may experience a deficit in the visual magnocellular pathway. The most extensively studied prediction deriving from this hypothesis is impaired contrast sensitivity to transient, low-luminance stimuli at low spatial frequencies. However, the findings are inconsistent across studies and even seemingly contradictory. University, Jerusalem, Israel. Ben-Yehudah G Sackett E Malchi-Ginzberg L Ahissar M Brain 2001 Jul;124(Pt 7):1381-95.

Impaired visual search in dyslexia relates to the role of the magnocellular pathway in attention. Abstract: We tested the hypothesis that in a cluttered visual scene, the magnocellular (M) pathway is crucial for focusing attention serially on the objects in the field. Since developmental dyslexia is commonly associated with an M pathway deficit, we compared reading impaired children and age-matched normal readers in a search task that required the detection of a target defined by the conjunction of two features, namely form and colour, that are processed by the parvocellular dominated ventral neocortical stream. Vidyasagar TR Pammer K Neuroreport 1999 Apr 26;10(6):1283-7.

Impaired visual word processing in dyslexia revealed with magnetoencephalography. Abstract: Dyslexia is most often attributed to phonological impairments, manifested in abnormal activation of the left temporal and temporoparietal cortex in response to auditorily presented language and possibly associated with anomalies in the cytoarchitecture and hemispheric symmetry of the plana temporale. The immediate cortical correlate of the severely impaired reading process has, however, remained obscure. Salmelin R Service E Kiesila P Uutela K Salonen O Ann Neurol 1996 Aug;40(2):157-62.

Improving perception of letters and visual structure of language. Abstract: Information about letters and the physical structure of language printed in Roman characters was given to children beginning to read. Experimental investigations coupled three alternative graphic modes of printing upper- and lower-case letters with an instructional intervention termed "Alpha-Beta" which provides practice in letter sorting, matching of letters, associative matching, and memory matching. In respect to graphics, Mode A letters were in standard alphabet form. Mode B provided standard letters with each backed by a unique half-tone (Visually Stippled Alphabet); Mode C provided standard letters with each backed by a unique visual texture (Visually Patterned Alphabet). Pre-posttest change in reading readiness was measured using the Metropolitan Readiness Test. Nelson TM Nilsson TH Piercey DJ Johnson T Frascara J Silva Delano S Susuki Sone E Villalon Bravo M Percept Mot Skills 1999 Apr;88(2):515-30.

Incidence of reading disability in a population-based birth cohort, 1976-1982, Rochester, Minn. Abstract: To report the incidence of reading disability among school-aged children. In this population-based birth cohort, reading disability was common among school-aged children and significantly more frequent among boys than girls, regardless of definition. Katusic SK Colligan RC Barbaresi WJ Schaid DJ Jacobsen SJ Mayo Clin Proc 2001 Nov;76(11):1081-92.

Increased levels of cytosolic phospholipase A2 in dyslexics. Abstract: Research findings are increasingly reporting evidence of physiological abnormalities in dyslexia and sites for dyslexia have been identified on three chromosomes. It has been suggested that genetic inheritance may cause phospholipid abnormalities in dyslexia somewhat similar to those found in schizophrenia. A key enzyme in phospholipid metabolism, Type IV, or cytosolic, phospholipase A2 (cP Prostaglandins Leukot Essent Fatty Acids 2000 Jul-Aug;63(1-2):37-9.

Independent genome-wide scans identify a chromosome 18 quantitative-trait locus influencing dyslexia. Abstract: Developmental dyslexia is defined as a specific and significant impairment in reading ability that cannot be explained by deficits in intelligence, learning opportunity, motivation or sensory acuity. It is one of the most frequently diagnosed disorders in childhood, representing a major educational and social problem. It is well established that dyslexia is a significantly heritable trait with a neurobiological basis. The etiological mechanisms remain elusive, however, despite being the focus of intensive multidisciplinary research. Fisher SE Francks C Marlow AJ MacPhie IL Newbury DF Cardon LR Ishikawa-Brush Y Richardson AJ Talcott JB Gayan J Olson RK Pennington BF Smith SD DeFries JC Stein JF Monaco AP Nat Genet 2002 Jan;30(1):86-91.

Indications for orthophony therapy in written language disorders in children. Work Group assembled by the National Agency for Health Accreditation and Evaluation (ANAES) Pouymayou C David L Ann Otolaryngol Chir Cervicofac 1998 Oct;115 Suppl 1:S75-88.

Individual differences in contextual facilitation: evidence from dyslexia and poor reading comprehension. Abstract: Ninety-two 7- to 10-year-old children read words presented in isolation or following a spoken sentence context. In absolute terms, poor readers showed more contextual facilitation than good readers. However, when the relative benefit of context was assessed, this was greater for children with better reading skills, and comprehension was a better predictor of contextual facilitation than decoding. Study 2 compared the performance of dyslexics with that of reading-age matched poor comprehenders and normal readers. Nation K Snowling MJ Child Dev 1998 Aug;69(4):996-1011.

Individual differences in story comprehension and recall of poor readers. Abstract: This study sought to identify poor readers and characterise weaknesses in their knowledge and use of story structure in comprehension and recall. Eighty year 3 children, 20 good readers and 60 poor readers, were selected from an initial pool of children based on factor analysis of scores from three measures of reading ability. The poor readers were then divided into relatively homogeneous subgroups, using eight additional measures of language-reading comprehension, by a numerical classification procedure. Wilkinson IA Elkins J Bain JD Br J Educ Psychol 1995 Dec;65 (Pt 4):393-407.

Information-processing patterns in specific reading disability. Abstract: This research investigated specific processing strengths and weaknesses among three groups of readers who ranged in age from 6 through 10 years. The first-grade unsuccessful and the older unsuccessful readers had similar information-processing patterns, whereas collectively they differed significantly from the first-grade successful readers on short-term auditory/working memory and decoding/encoding. When separately compared to the controls, the age-matched high-risk group showed additional weakness in rapid automatized naming, and the reading-level-matched older disabled group showed additional weakness in phonological coding as well as visual sequential memory. Watson C Willows DM J Learn Disabil 1995 Apr;28(4):216-31.

Inhibitory control of saccade generation mediated by various oculomotor regions in response to reading difficulty. Yang SN McConkie GW Ann N Y Acad Sci 2002 Apr;956:479-81.

Inhibitory deficits in reading disability depend on subtype: guessers but not spellers. Abstract: In this study, children with the guessing subtype of dyslexia (who read fast and inaccurately) were compared with children with the spelling subtype (who read slowly and accurately) on three aspects of executive functioning (EF): response inhibition, susceptibility to interference from irrelevant information, and planning. It was found that guessers were impaired in their ability to inhibit inappropriate responding on all tasks used to assess EF (the stop signal task, the Stroop task, and the Tower of London task). Sloot van der M Licht R Horsley TM Sergeant JA Neuropsychol Dev Cogn Sect C Child Neuropsychol 2000 Dec;6(4):297-312.

Inner-city adults with severe reading difficulties: a closer look. Abstract: Relatively little is known about the characteristics of inner-city adults who seek assistance from literacy programs. Increased knowledge about this population will enhance the development of more effective programs, as well as policy options. This study describes the characteristics of 280 adults, ages 16 to 63, who came to an adult literacy program that focused on severe reading difficulties. The program, located within a hospital complex in a large, urban area, attracted these individuals through an extensive multimedia outreach effort. Gottesman RL Bennett RE Nathan RG Kelly MS J Learn Disabil 1996 Nov;29(6):589-97.

Insights into brain function and neural plasticity using magnetic source imaging. Abstract: This review outlines the rationale for the use of magnetoencephalography (MEG) or magnetic source imaging (MSI), a noninvasive functional imaging technique, and the features that any imaging method should display to make a substantial contribution to cognitive neuroscience. After a brief discussion of the basic experimental approach used in the authors' studies, the use of early sensory components of brain magnetic responses is reviewed to address issues of the functional organization of the primary sensory cortices, followed by a comment on the clinical use of these components. Simos PG Papanicolaou AC Breier JI Fletcher JM Wheless JW Maggio WW Gormley W Constantinou JE Kramer L J Clin Neurophysiol 2000 Mar;17(2):143-62.

Instrument for locating students with suspected learning disabilities: a quantitative approach. Abstract: The instrument to locate students with learning disabilities was developed to create equality and uniformity, Journalthat such difficulties could be spotted independently of socialization factors, teachers and parents to whom the student had been exposed. The instrument was developed on the basis of research that defines the reading rate of students with reading disabilities in words per minute, the minimum number of errors for locating writing disabilities, and the number of answers and lines a student uses to reconstruct the content of a passage adapted to his or her age level. Engel R Int J Rehabil Res 1997 Jun;20(2):169-81.

Intact verbal description of letters with diminished awareness of their forms. Abstract: Visual processing and its conscious awareness can be dissociated. To examine the extent of dissociation between ability to read characters or words and to be consciously aware of their forms, reading ability and conscious awareness for characters were examined using a tachistoscope in an alexic patient. A right handed woman with 14 years of education presented with incomplete right hemianopia, alexia with kanji (ideogram) agraphia, anomia, and amnesia. Brain MRI disclosed cerebral infarction limited to the left lower bank of the calcarine fissure, lingual and parahippocampal gyri, and an old infarction in the right medial frontal lobe. Suzuki K Yamadori A J Neurol Neurosurg Psychiatry 2000 Jun;68(6):782-6.

Intelligence and dyslexia: implications for diagnosis and intervention. Abstract: In this paper we critically examine theoretical issues and practical consequences of including IQ in the definition of dyslexia. According to the discrepancy criterion individuals are classified as dyslexic if their reading skills are below what would be expected from their IQ scores. However, we argue that intelligence is a fuzzy concept and that there is no clear causal relationship between intelligence level and word decoding skills. Also, high and low IQ poor readers show the same reading performance patterns, indicating that both groups might benefit from the same remedial activities. Gustafson S Samuelsson S Scand J Psychol 1999 Jun;40(2):127-34.

Intensive training of phonological skills in progressive aphasia: a model of brain plasticity in neurodegenerative disease. Abstract: Three patients with a typical syndrome of nonfluent primary progressive aphasia (Mesulam's syndrome) were trained daily with a remediation protocol including auditory exercises specifically designed to involve several aspects of phonological processing, a domain known to be specifically affected in the condition. The speech content of the exercises was based on the temporal theory of phonological processes according to which increasing the duration of formant transition should facilitate phoneme discrimination and phoneomic awareness. Louis M Espesser R Rey V Daffaure V Di Cristo A Habib M Brain Cogn 2001 Jun-Jul;46(1-2):197-201.

Interhemispheric sensorimotor integration in pointing movements: a study on dyslexic adults. Abstract: In addition to reading disorders, numerous deficits have been found to be associated with dyslexia, suggesting that various neurological factors might be involved in its etiology. In the present study, we focused on three of the deficits that have been thought to accompany and to a certain extent, to explain dyslexia: an abnormal pattern of hemispheric asymmetry, abnormal hemispheric communication, and abnormal motor control. Velay JL Daffaure V Giraud K Habib M Neuropsychologia 2002;40(7):827-34.

International Association of Logopedics and Phoniatrics. Committee for School Questions. [from old catalog] Komplexe Sprachstörungen: Legasthenie = Handicaps multiples: Dyslexia: Bern: H. Huber, 1974. Kaiser, Eberhard, writer on speech problems, [from old catalog] ed. Kramer, Josefine, [from old catalog] ed. Related Titles: Handicaps multiples. Description: 219 p.: ill.; 22 cm. LC Classification: RJ496.S7 I5 1974

International Rodin Remediation Conference (7th: 1988: Wenner-Gren Center and Uppsala University) Brain and reading: structural and functional anomalies in developmental dyslexia with special reference to hemispheric interactions, memory functions, linguistic processes, and visual analysis in reading: proceedings of the 7th International Rodin Remediation Conference at the Wenner-Gren Center, Stockholm and Uppsala University, June 19-22, 1988 / edited by Curt von Euler, Ingvar Lundberg, and Gunnar Lennerstrand. Basingstoke, Hampshire: Macmillan; New York, NY: Stockton Press, 1989. Euler, Curt von, 1918- Lundberg, Ingvar. Lennerstrand, Gunnar. Description: xix, 390 p.: ill.; 24 cm. ISBN: 0935859691: LC Classification: RJ496.A5 I58 1988 NLM Class No.: W3 WE429 v. 54 WL 340.6 I61b 1988 Dewey Class No.: 616.85/53 20

International Study Group on Special Educational Needs. Seminar (3rd: 1983: Mayo Clinic) Understanding learning disabilities: international and multidisciplinary views / edited by Drake D. Duane and Che Kan Leong. New York: Plenum Press, c1985. Duane, Drake D, 1936- Leong, Che Kan. Description: xiii, 272 p.; 26 cm. ISBN: 0306419009 LC Classification: LC4704.I58 1985 NLM Class No.: W3 IN9075 3rd 1983u LC 4707 I61 1983u Dewey Class No.: 371.9 19

Interpreting the WISC-R subtest scores of reading impaired children--a structural approach. Abstract: The problem of characterising more specifically the cognitive requirements involved in subtests from standardised measures of intelligence represents a main problem in the research on exceptional populations. A new way of classifying tests of mental abilities is presented. Rather than focusing on the content of a given test, the present classification system focuses on their structures. The classification system is applied to the WISC-R (Wechsler Intelligence Scale for Children--Revised, Wechsler, 1974). Ottem E Scand J Psychol 1998 Mar;39(1):1-7.

Interview between Lindsay Peer and Bob Turney. Turney B Dyslexia 2001 Apr-Jun;7(2):85-96.

Intracranial arachnoidal cysts--localization, gender and sidedness Abstract: The aim of the present study was to investigate whether data on location and distribution of intracranial cysts in a large patient population may explain why and how such cysts are formed. We investigated 123 patients with 129 intracranial cysts, consecutively admitted to the Department of Neurosurgery in Bergen 1988-97. Data were analyzed with regard to intracranial location and gender distribution. Cysts were much more commonly located in the temporal fossae than one would expect if the distribution were random; 68.1% of patients had temporal cysts Wester K Svendsen F Hugdahl K Tidsskr Nor Laegeforen 1999 Nov 20;119(28):4162-4.

Intrafamilial association of pericentric inversion of chromosome 9, inv (9)(p11-q21), and rapid cycling bipolar disorder. Abstract: Association of a chromosome aberration and psychiatric disorder can be useful in highlighting a genomic region that can be profitably explored further using positional cloning. We report the case of a father and daughter both of whom have bipolar disorder II and a pericentric inversion of chromosome 9. McCandless F Jones I Harper K Craddock N Psychiatr Genet 1998 Winter;8(4):259-62.

Investigating semantic memory impairments: the contribution of semantic priming. Abstract: The semantic priming task is a valuable tool in the investigation of semantic memory impairments in patients with acquired disorders of language. This is because priming performance reflects automatic or implicit access to semantic information, unlike most other tests of semantic knowledge, which rely on explicit, voluntary access. Priming results are important for two main reasons: First, normal priming results may be observed in patients who perform poorly on other semantic memory tests, enabling us to distinguish between loss of, or damage to, information in semantic memory, and voluntary access to that information. Moss HE Tyler LK Memory 1995 Sep-Dec;3(3-4):359-95.

Investigation of quantitative measures related to reading disability in a large sample of sib-pairs from the UK. Abstract: We describe a family-based sample of individuals with reading disability collected as part of a quantitative trait loci (QTL) mapping study. Eighty-nine nuclear families (135 independent sib-pairs) were identified through a single proband using a traditional discrepancy score of predicted/actual reading ability and a known family history. Eight correlated psychometric measures were administered to each sibling, including single word reading, spelling, similarities, matrices, spoonerisms, nonword and irregular word reading, and a pseudohomophone test Marlow AJ Fisher SE Richardson AJ Francks C Talcott JB Monaco AP Stein JF Cardon LR Behav Genet 2001 Mar;31(2):219-30.

IQ tests. Pollock J Dyslexia 2001 Jul-Sep;7(3):172-3.

Irlen, Helen, 1945- Reading by the colors: overcoming dyslexia and other reading disabilities through the Irlen method / Helen Irlen. Garden City Park, N.Y.: Avery Pub. Group, c1991. Description: xiii, 195 p.: ill.; 23 cm. ISBN: 0895294761 (hardback): 0895294826 (pbk.): LC

Classification: RC394.W6 I75 1991 NLM Class No.: WL 340 I69r Dewey Class No.: 616.85/53 20

Is developmental dyslexia a disconnection syndrome? Evidence from PET scanning. Abstract: A rhyming and short-term memory task with visually presented letters were used to study brain activity in five compensated adult developmental dyslexics. Their only cognitive difficulty was in phonological processing, manifest in a wide range of tasks including spoonerisms, phonemic fluency and digit naming speed. PET scans showed that for the dyslexics, a subset only of the brain regions normally involved in phonological processing was activated: Broca's area during the rhyming task, temporo-parietal cortex during the short- term memory task. Paulesu E Frith U Snowling M Gallagher A Morton J Frackowiak RS Frith CD Brain 1996 Feb;119 (Pt 1):143-57.

Is dyslexia caused by a visual deficit? Skottun BC Vision Res 2001 Oct;41(23):3069-71.

Is English a dyslexic language? Abstract: McGuinness has suggested that there 'is no diagnosis and no evidence for any special type of reading disorder like dyslexia', and that poor teaching accounts for low levels of English literacy performance, rather than inherent personal deficits. Implicit in this is the assumption that some languages have simple grapheme-phoneme codes in which there is a one-to-one mapping, making them easy to teach and learn, while others have more complicated structures and are more difficult for teachers and students. Spencer K Dyslexia 2000 Apr-Jun;6(2):152-62.

Is memory loss without anatomical damage tantamount to a psychogenic deficit? The case of pure retrograde amnesia. Abstract: Following a car accident, a patient remained unconscious for approximately 20 min and confused for a few hours. When he could be questioned, he was found to have lost all past memories. The retrograde amnesia covered his whole life and concerned autobiographic events as well as famous facts and encyclopaedic knowledge. It partially involved the verbal and visual lexicon. Reading, writing and counting were no longer possible. Di Renzi E Lucchelli F Muggia S Spinnler H Neuropsychologia 1997 Jun;35(6):781-94.

Is preschool language impairment a risk factor for dyslexia in adolescence? Abstract: The literacy skills of 56 school leavers from the Bishop and Edmundson (1987) cohort of preschoolers with specific language impairment (SLI) were assessed at 15 years. The SLI group performed worse on tests of reading, spelling, and reading comprehension than age-matched controls and the literacy outcomes were particularly poor for those with Performance IQ less than 100. The rate of specific reading retardation in the SLI group had increased between the ages of 8 1/2 and 15 years and there had been a substantial drop in reading accuracy, relative to age. Snowling M Bishop DV Stothard SE J Child Psychol Psychiatry 2000 Jul;41(5):587-600.

Is the mind a cauliflower or an onion? British insights into cognitive organization from the study of abnormal function. Abstract: Clinical and normal psychology have had a long tradition of close interaction in British psychology. The roots of this interplay may predate the development of the British Psychological Society, but the Society has encouraged and supported this line of research since its inception. One fundamental British insight has been to consider the evidence from pathology as a potential constraint on theories of normal function. In turn, theories of normal function have been used to understand and illuminate cognitive pathology. McCarthy RA Br J Psychol 2001 Feb;92(Pt 1):171-92.

Is there a deficit of early vision in dyslexia? Abstract: A majority of dyslexic children have been found in many studies to show a deficiency of early vision, called transient deficit. A series of four experiments was conducted to test whether or not the performance in different tasks is affected by a transient deficit. However, no clear evidence of a transient deficit was found, although the reliability of the measurements was high and the power of the statistical tests was adequate. All previous findings regarding the transient deficit can be explained by a reduced amplitude of the transient response. Walther-Muller PU Perception 1995;24(8):919-36.

Is there a relationship between speech and nonspeech auditory processing in children with dyslexia? Abstract: A group of 8 young teenagers with dyslexia were compared to age-matched control participants on a number of speech and nonspeech auditory tasks. There were no differences between the control participants and the teenagers with dyslexia in forward and simultaneous masking, nor were there any differences in frequency selectivity as indexed by performance with a bandstop noise. Thresholds for backward masking in a broadband noise were elevated for the teenagers with dyslexia as a group. Rosen S Manganari E J Speech Lang Hear Res 2001 Aug;44(4):720-36.

Is there a visual deficit in dyslexia resulting from a lesion of the right posterior parietal lobe? Abstract: Dyslexia has conventionally been attributed to a left hemisphere deficit affecting language skills. However, it has recently been suggested that two-thirds of dyslexic people have a lesion of the right posterior parietal lobe (RPPL) resulting in poor oculo-motor control. It has been reported that neurological patients with RPPL lesions commonly manifest a neglect of the left side of space and this has been described in clinical observations of 'visual dyslexics'. We investigated this hypothesis with a sample of 53 dyslexic children and 53 controls using a line-bisection task Polikoff BR Evans BJ Legg CR Ophthalmic Physiol Opt 1995 Sep;15(5):513-7.

Is there an association between season of birth and reading disability? Abstract: Reported

associations between season of birth and reading failure suggest medical causation and prevention. The relationship between season of birth and two measures of reading outcome in two cohorts of children (n1 = 2411 and n2 = 1972) was studied using chi2 tests. None was significant. Logistic regression was used to investigate the joint associations of gender, age at school entrance, and season of birth with reading outcome. A significant interaction between reading failure and age category (overage at school entrance vs correct age) by season of birth was observed. Flynn JM Rahbar MH Bernstein AJ J Dev Behav Pediatr 1996 Feb;17(1):22-6.

Is ultrasound unsound? A review of epidemiological studies of human exposure to ultrasound. Abstract: We have reviewed the epidemiological studies of human exposure to diagnostic ultrasound during pregnancy. Studies have concentrated on possible associations between ultrasound exposure in utero and childhood malignancies, neurological maldevelopment, dyslexia, left-handedness, delayed speech development and low birth weight. It is concluded that no associations between ultrasound exposure in utero and childhood maldevelopment have been proven. Salvesen KA Eik-Nes SH Ultrasound Obstet Gynecol 1995 Oct;6(4):293-8.

Isolating the M(y)-cell response in dyslexia using the spatial frequency doubling illusion. Abstract: The contribution of M(y)-cell activity within a framework of a magnocellular-deficit theory of dyslexia is currently unknown. Twenty-one dyslexic readers and 19 control readers were compared on their threshold detection for the frequency doubling illusion - an index of M(y)-cell activity, coherent motion, and a visual acuity task. The dyslexic group performed more poorly on detection of the frequency doubling illusion and coherent motion compared to the control group, but both groups performed comparably on the visual acuity task. Pammer K Wheatley C Vision Res 2001 Jul;41(16):2139-47.

Issues in the assessment of reading disabilities in L2 children--beliefs and research evidence. Abstract: In bilingual and multilingual settings one is constantly challenged by the difficulty of teasing apart phenomena associated with normal second language (L2) reading acquisition from authentic warning signs of reading failure. The bulk of this paper focuses on a critical discussion of a cluster of beliefs that pertain to the issues concerning the diagnosis of reading disability in multilingual and bilingual settings among school children. Geva E Dyslexia 2000 Jan-Mar;6(1):13-28.

Janover, Caroline. How many days until tomorrow? / written by Caroline Janover; illustrated by Charlotte Fremaux. Bethesda, MD: Woodbine House, 2000. Fremaux, Charlotte, ill. Description: 173 p.: ill.; 21 cm. ISBN: 1890627224 (pbk.) Summary: Josh, who has dyslexia, spends the summer on an island off the coast of Maine and finds that he has much to prove to his gruff grandfather and his older brother. LC Classification: PZ7.J2445 Ho 2000 Dewey Class No.: [Fic] 21

Janover, Caroline. Josh: a boy with dyslexia / Caroline Janover; illustrated by Edward Epstein. Burlington, Vt.: Waterfront Books, c1988. Epstein, Edward, 1936- ill. Description: 100 p.: ill.; 22 cm. ISBN: 0914525107: Summary: Josh struggles to live down the stigma of his learning disability, dyslexia, and receive both respect and friendship from his peers. Includes information on the characteristics of dyslexia and a list of organizations that deal with learning disabilities. LC Classification: PZ7.J2445 Jo 1988 Dewey Class No.: [Fic] 19

Janover, Caroline. The worst speller in jr. high / by Caroline Janover; edited by Rosemary Wallner. Minneapolis, MN: Free Spirit, c1995. Wallner, Rosemary, 1964- Description: 202 p.; 19 cm. ISBN: 0915793768: Summary: Starting out in the seventh grade, Katie Kelso finds herself trying to cope with her dyslexia and form a friendship with a very bright boy at school,

while she and her family deal with her mother's cancer diagnosis. LC Classification: PZ7.J2445 Wo 1995 Dewey Class No.: [Fic] 20

Jiménez, Jaime M. Método antidisléxico para el aprendizaje de la lecto-escritura-cinematográfico / [por] Jaime M. Jiménez. [Madrid]: Ciencias de la Educación Preescolar y Especial, D.L. 1979. Description: 174 p.: ill.; 24 cm. ISBN: 8485252357: LC Classification: LB1050.5.J55 National Bib. No.: Sp

Joanette, Yves. Right hemisphere and verbal communication / Yves Joanette, Pierre Goulet, Didier Hannequin; with the collaboration of John Boeglin. Uniform [Contribution de l'hemisphere droit a la communication verbale. English New York: Springer-Verlag, c1990. Goulet, Pierre. Hannequin, Didier. Description: xiv, 228 p.; 25 cm. ISBN: 0387971017 (U.S.: alk. paper) LC Classification: QP399.J6213 1990 NLM Class No.: WL 340 J62c Dewey Class No.: 612.8/252 20

Johns Hopkins Conference on Research Needs and Prospects in Dyslexia and Related Aphasic Disorders, Johns Hopkins Medical Institutions, 1961. Reading disability; progress and research needs in dyslexia. Edited by John Money. Baltimore, Johns Hopkins Press, 1962. Money, John, 1921- Johns Hopkins University. Dept. of Pediatrics. Description: x, 222 p. illus. 24 cm. LC Classification: RC394.W6 J6 1961 Dewey Class No.: 616.8552

Jones, John. Dyslexia - there is a cure: the revolutionary home-teaching program / John Jones, Marianne Evan-Jones. Philadelphia, PA: Xlibris, 2000. Projected Pub. Date: 0003 Evan-Jones, Marianne. Description: p.; cm. ISBN: 0738812080 (cloth hardback: alk. paper) 0738812099 (trade paperback: alk. paper)

Jordan, Dale R. Dyslexia in the classroom / Dale R. Jordan. Edition Information: 2d ed. Columbus, Ohio: C. E. Merrill Pub. Co, c1977. Description: vii, 200 p.: ill.; 23

cm. ISBN: 0675084660 LC Classification: LB1050.5.J6 1977 Dewey Class No.: 371.9/14

Jordan, Dale R. Dyslexia in the classroom [by] Dale R. Jordan. Columbus, Ohio, C. E. Merrill Pub. Co. [1972] Description: ix, 194 p. 22 cm. ISBN: 0675091004 LC Classification: LB1050.5.J6 Dewey Class No.: 371.91/4

Jordan, Dale R. Overcoming dyslexia in children, adolescent, and adults / Dale R. Jordan. Edition Information: 3rd ed. Austin, Tx: Pro-Ed, 2002. Projected Pub. Date: 0201 Description: p. cm. ISBN: 0890798796 LC Classification: RC394.W6 J67 2002 Dewey Class No.: 616.85/53 21

Jordan, Dale R. Overcoming dyslexia in children, adolescents, and adults / Dale R. Jordan. Edition Information: 2nd ed. Austin, Tex.: Pro-ed, c1996. Description: xii, 367 p.: ill.; 23 cm. ISBN: 0890796424 (soft: alk. paper) LC Classification: RC394.W6 J67 1996 Dewey Class No.: 616.85/53 20

Jordan, Dale R. Overcoming dyslexia in children, adolescents, and adults / Dale R. Jordan. Austin, Tex.: Pro-Ed, c1989. Related Titles: Overcoming dyslexia. Description: ix, 245 p.: ill.; 23 cm. ISBN: 0890792046 LC Classification: RC394.W6 J67 1989 NLM Class No.: WM 475 J82o Dewey Class No.: 616.85/53 20

Jordan, Ian, 1957- Visual dyslexia: the missing links / Ian Jordan. London; Philadelphia: J. Kingsley Publishers, 2001. Projected Pub. Date: 0102 Description: p. cm. ISBN: 1853029629 (alk. paper) LC Classification: RJ496.A5 J67 2001 NLM Class No.: WL 340.6 J82v 2001 Dewey Class No.: 618.92/8553 21

Jornadas Chilenas de Dislexia, 1st, Santiago de Chile, 1969. Dislexia escolar. Montevideo: O.E.A, Instituto Interamericano del Niño, 1972. Interamerican Children's Institute.

Description: 105 p.; 24 cm. LC Classification: LB1050.5.J63 1969

Journal of reading, writing, and learning disabilities, international. Portion of Reading, writing, and learning disabilities Journal of reading, writing, and learning disabilities international J. read. writ. learn. disabil. int. New York, NY: American Library Pub. Co, c1984-c1991. Description: 7 v.; 26 cm. Vol. 1, no. 4- issued without seasonal designation. Vol. 1, no. 1 (fall 1984)-v. 7, no. 4 (Oct/Dec 1991). Current Frequency: Quarterly Continues: Chicorel abstracts to reading and learning disabilities 0149-533X (DLC) 81645006 (OCoLC)3488225 Continued by: Reading & writing quarterly 1057-3569 (DLC) 92643403 (OCoLC)24020427 ISSN: 0748-7630 Incorrect ISSN: 0149-533X Cancel/Invalid LCCN: sn 84007253 LC Classification: LB1050.5.J65 NLM Class No.: Z 5814.V4 C53 Dewey Class No.: 371.9 20 Other System No.: (OCoLC)ocm11007212 Acquisition Source: American Library Pub. Co, Inc, 275 Central Park West, New York, NY 10024

Journée pluridisciplinaire sur la dyslexie du développement (1st: 1999) Dyslexie, dyslexies: dépistage, remédiation et intégration: Première journée pluridisciplinaire sur la dyslexie du développement, 11 septembre 1999 / éditeurs Michel Habib, Véronique Rey. Aix-en-Provence: Publications de l'université de Provence, 2000. Habib, M. (Michel) Rey, Véronique. Description: 117 p.: ill. (some col.); 21 cm. ISBN: 285399466X LC Classification: RJ496.A5.J685 1999 Dewey Class No.: 618.92/8553 21

Kanji-predominant alexia in advanced Alzheimer's disease. Abstract: Oral reading is preserved until the late stage of Alzheimer's disease (AD). However, it is unknown whether reading of kanji and kana is differentially impaired in Japanese AD patients. The purpose of this study was to examine alexic pattern in AD as related to two script systems. As a result of multiple cognitive deficits, kanji reading is more impaired than kana reading in AD, but the difference is apparent only in the very late stage. Our findings suggest that kanji can be read correctly without meaning. Nakamura K Meguro K Yamazaki H Ishizaki J Saito H Saito N Shimada M Yamaguchi S Shimada Y Yamadori A Acta Neurol Scand 1998 Apr;97(4):237-43.

Karapetsas, A. V. H⁻e dyslexia sto paidi: diagn⁻os⁻e & therapia / A.V. Karapetsas. Ath⁻ena: Hell⁻enika grammata, 1991. Description: 110 p.: ill.; 22 cm. ISBN: 9607019318 LC Classification: RJ496.A5 K37 1991

Karnes, Lucia Rooney, comp. Dyslexia in special education. Pomfret, Conn, Orton Society [1965] Council for Exceptional Children. Description: 96 p. 22 cm. LC Classification: RC394.W6 K3 Dewey Class No.: 371.9 Other System No.: (OCoLC)1664278

Keates, Anita. Dyslexia and information and communications technology: a guide for teachers and parents / Anita Keates. London: D. Fulton Publishers, 2000. Description: vii, 88 p.: ill.; 30 cm. ISBN: 1853466514 LC Classification: RJ496.A5 K43 2000 Dewey Class No.: 616.85/5306 21

Kemp, Gene. Just Ferret / Gene Kemp; illustrated by Jon Davis. London; Boston: Faber and Faber, 1990. Davis, Jon, ill. Description: 126 p.: ill.; 21 cm. ISBN: 0571142869: Summary: The adventures of twelve-year-old Ferret as a new boy at Cricklepit Combined School where he begins to come to terms with his dyslexia, makes new friends, and deals with a bully. LC Classification: PZ7.K3055 Jv 1990 Dewey Class No.: [Fic] 20

Kennemore, Tim. Wall of words / Tim Kennemore. London: Faber and Faber, 1982. Description: 173 p.; 21 cm. ISBN: 0571118569: Summary: The eldest of four sisters, thirteen-year-old Kim tries to cope with the continued absence of her beloved author father and her favorite younger sister's terror of school. LC Classification: PZ7.K392 Wal 1982 Dewey Class No.: [Fic] 19

Kenny, Christine. Living and learning with dyslexia: the medusa's gaze / Christine Kenny. Salisbury: APS, 2001. Description: 95 p.: ill.; 22 cm. ISBN: 0953723437 (pbk.) LC Classification: LC4031.K46 1994 Dewey Class No.: 371.91 20 Series:

Klasen, Edith. The syndrome of specific dyslexia; with special consideration of its physiological, psychological, testpsychological, and social correlates. Uniform [Syndrom der Legasthenie. English Baltimore, University Park Press [1972] Description: xii, 235 p. 24 cm. ISBN: 0839107048 LC Classification: RJ496.A5 K5813 Dewey Class No.: 618.9/28/553

Knobloch-Gala, Anna. Asymetria i integracja pólkulowa a mowa i niektóre jej zaburzenia: problemy diagnozy psychologicznej dzieci z dysleksja / Anna Knobloch-Gala. Portion of Problemy diagnozy psychologicznej dzieci z dysleksja Edition Information: Wyd. 1. Kraków: Nakladem Uniwersytetu Jagiello´nskiego, 1995. Description: 93 p.: ill.; 24 cm. ISBN: 832330856X LC Classification: RC394.W6 K56 1995

Knowledge, implicit knowledge and metaknowledge in visual agnosia and pure alexia. Abstract: Residual or implicit knowledge has been observed in patients with object agnosia, optic aphasia and pure alexia. Previous investigators have considered implicit knowledge in these patients to be dissociated from awareness on the basis of intact semantic capabilities that are consistent with right hemisphere processing. The absence of explicit verbal identification is presumably dependent upon damaged left hemisphere systems. We describe a 72-year-old woman with a left occipital infarction, object agnosia and pure alexia who was unable to explicitly identify visual stimuli (objects and words), but was able to make reliable judgements of her residual knowledge on forced-choice matching tasks. While the patient could not consistently demonstrate awareness of knowledge prior to stimulus matching ('Do you know what this is?'), she was able to reliably demonstrate awareness of knowledge for response accuracy ('Are you sure?') assessed after stimulus matching. Further, the extent of the patient's metaknowledge corresponded to her degree of preserved knowledge. We propose that this pattern of performance suggests limited or partial access to preserved semantic knowledge which, though degraded, is not 'non-conscious'. Department of Neurology, Albert Einstein College of Medicine and Beth Israel Medical Center, New York, NY 10003, USA. Feinberg TE Dyckes-Berke D Miner CR Roane DM Brain 1995 Jun;118 (Pt 3):789-800.

Kobi, Emil Erich. Das legasthenische Kind: seine Erziehung und Behandlung / Emil E. Kobi. Edition Information: 4, erw. Aufl. Solothurn: Antonius-Verlag, 1978. Description: 152 p.: 20 ill.; 23 cm. LC Classification: LB1050.5.K57 1978 National Bib. No.: Sw78-9860

Kohler, Claude. [from old catalog] De la notion de dyslexie-dysorthographie à celle de dystopie, conférence du Dr Claude Kohler... 10 décembre 1968. Saint-Étienne, Centre départemental de documentation pédagogique, 16, rue Marcellin-Allard [1969?]. Description: 15 p. 27 cm. LC Classification: RJ496.A4 K6

Kowarik, Othmar. Legasthenie und ihre methodische Behandlung. [Von] Othmar Kowarik [und] Johann Kraft. (Illustr. v. Winfried Opgenoorth.) Wien, München, Jugend & Volk (1973). Kraft, Johann. Description: 179 p. 21 cm. ISBN: 3714153330 LC Classification: LB1050.5.K63 1973 National Bib. No.: Au73-11-203 Other System No.: (OCoLC)14637310

Kowarik, Othmar. Legasthenikerbetreuung in Gruppen und Kursen / Othmar Kowarik. Wien; München: Jugend & Volk, 1977.

Description: 243, [1] p.: ill.; 21 cm. ISBN: 3714153993: LC Classification: LB1050.5.K64 National Bib. No.: Au77-20

Kraiker, Christoph. [from old catalog] Hysterie. Volker Frenzel: Leistungsstörungen. München, Akademische Buchh. (1972). Frenzel, Volker. Leistungsstörungen. 1972. [from old catalog] Frenzel, Volker. Legasthenie. 1972. [from old catalog] Description: 104 p. 21 cm. LC Classification: RC532.K68 NLM Class No.: W6 P3.

Kuipers, Christine G. Behandeling van woordblindheid / Christine G. Kuipers en Kees Weggelaar, in samenwerking met E. Hulshoff Pol-Kars. 's-Gravenhage: Staatsuitgeverij, 1983. Weggelaar, Cornelis. Hulshoff Pol-Kars, E. Description: 280 p.: ill.; 24 cm. ISBN: 9012042151: LC Classification: RJ496.A5 K83 1983

Kuipers, Christine G. Woordblind / Christine G. Kuipers, in samenwerking met Cornelis Weggelaar 's-Gravenhage: Staatsdrukkerij, 1979. Weggelaar, Cornelis, joint author. Description: 235 p.: with ill.; 24 cm. ISBN: 9012024722: LC Classification: RJ496.A5 K84

Küspert, Petra, 1962- Phonologische Bewusstheit und Schriftspracherwerb: zu den Effekten vorschulischer Förderung der phonologischen Bewusstheit auf den Erwerb des Lesens und Rechtschreibens / Petra Küspert. Frankfurt am Main; New York: P. Lang, c1998. Description: 233 p.; 21 cm. ISBN: 3631325290 LC Classification: P118.K86 1998 Dewey Class No.: 371.91/44 21

Landau, Elaine. Dyslexia / by Elaine Landau. New York: F. Watts, 1991. Description: 62 p.: col. ill.; 23 cm. ISBN: 0531200302 (lib. bdg.) LC Classification: RC394.W6 L36 1991 Dewey Class No.: 616.85/53 20

Landerl, Karin, 1967- Legasthenie in Deutsch und Englisch / Karin Landerl. Frankfurt am Main; New York: P. Lang, c1996. Description: 182 p.: ill.; 21 cm. ISBN:

3631303033 LC Classification: RC394.W6 L365 1996 Dewey Class No.: 616.85/53 21

Lane, Kenneth A. Reversal errors: theories & therapy procedures / by Kenneth A. Lane. Edition Information: 1st ed. Santa Ana, CA: VisionExtension, 1988. Description: 154 p.: ill.; 28 cm. ISBN: 0929780000: LC Classification: RE48.2.C5 L36 1988 NLM Class No.: WW 105 L265r Dewey Class No.: 618.92/8553 19

Language abilities in children with attention deficit hyperactivity disorder, reading disabilities, and normal controls. Abstract: Research has demonstrated a high prevalence of language impairments (LI) and reading disabilities (RD) in children with attention deficit hyperactivity disorder (ADHD). Since RD is associated with LI, it is unclear whether the language impairments are specific to ADHD or associated with comorbid RD. The language abilities of ADHD children with and without RD were investigated in a task requiring recall of a lengthy narrative, and in tests assessing knowledge of the semantic aspects of language. Purvis KL Tannock R J Abnorm Child Psychol 1997 Apr;25(2):133-44.

Language acquisition problems and reading disorders: aspects of diagnosis and intervention / edited by Hannelore Grimm and Helmut Skowronek. Berlin; New York: W. de Gruyter, 1993. Grimm, Hannelore. Skowronek, Helmut. Description: xii, 360 p.: ill.; 25 cm. ISBN: 3110141205 (acid-free paper) LC Classification: RJ496.L35 L348 1993 Dewey Class No.: 618.92/855 20

Language and aphasias Abstract: Approximately 400,000 years ago men started to use language. Initially it was probably poor with few phonemes. With social evolution it became more complex, with the appearance of new phonemes and a more complete grammatical structure. The current concept of the processing of language dates, with little change, from the nineteenth century. The aphasias, as the expression of an alteration of language are an important support in the topographical localization of lesions, even before these can be shown on computerized tomography. Porta-Etessam J Nunez-Lopez R Balsalobre J Lopez E Hernandez A Luna A Rev Neurol 1997 Aug;25(144):1269-77.

Language and calculation within the parietal lobe: a combined cognitive, anatomical and fMRI study. Abstract: We report the case of a patient (ATH) who suffered from aphasia, deep dyslexia, and acalculia, following a lesion in her left perisylvian area. She showed a severe impairment in all tasks involving numbers in a verbal format, such as reading aloud, writing to dictation, or responding verbally to questions of numerical knowledge. In contrast, her ability to manipulate non-verbal representations of numbers, i.e, Arabic numerals and quantities, was comparatively well preserved, as evidenced for instance in number comparison or number bisection tasks Cohen L Dehaene S Chochon F Lehericy S Naccache L Neuropsychologia 2000;38(10):1426-40.

Language deficits in dyslexic children: speech perception, phonology, and morphology. Abstract: We investigated the relationship between dyslexia and three aspects of language: speech perception, phonology, and morphology. Reading and language tasks were administered to dyslexics aged 8-9 years and to two normal reader groups (age-matched and reading-level matched). Three dyslexic groups were identified: phonological dyslexics (PD), developmentally language impaired (LI), and globally delayed (delay-type dyslexics). The LI and PD groups exhibited similar patterns of reading impairment, attributed to low phonological skills Joanisse MF Manis FR Keating P Seidenberg MS J Exp Child Psychol 2000 Sep;77(1):30-60.

Language development and symbolic play in children with and without familial risk for dyslexia. Abstract: The purposes of this study were to investigate (a) whether children in families with a positive history of dyslexia were more likely to show delays in language development than children without family risk and (b) whether a delayed onset of expressive language (late talking) predicted later language development. We analyzed the language development of 200 children longitudinally at 14, 24, 30, and 42 months and assessed their symbolic play at 14 months. Half of the children (N = 106) were from families with a history of dyslexia (the Dyslexia Risk [DR] group), and other children served as age-matched controls Lyytinen P Poikkeus AM LaakJournalML Eklund K Lyytinen H J Speech Lang Hear Res 2001 Aug;44(4):873-85.

Language learning impairments: integrating basic science, technology, and remediation. Abstract: One of the fundamental goals of the modern field of neuroscience is to understand how neuronal activity gives rise to higher cortical function. However, to bridge the gap between neurobiology and behavior, we must understand higher cortical functions at the behavioral level at least as well as we have come to understand neurobiological processes at the cellular and molecular levels. This is certainly the case in the study of speech processing, where critical studies of behavioral dysfunction have provided key insights into the basic neurobiological mechanisms relevant to speech perception and production. Tallal P Merzenich MM Miller S Jenkins W Exp Brain Res 1998 Nov;123(1-2):210-9.

Language problems in poor readers. Abstract: In recent definitions of dyslexia there is agreement on the following: dyslexia is a language (-based) disorder restricted to difficulties in phonological processing abilities. This causes primary problems in word decoding and spelling, and, as a consequence, in reading comprehension. This is in accordance with the widely accepted reading model, which regards decoding as a prerequisite for reading comprehension. Naucler K Magnusson E Logoped Phoniatr Vocol 2000;25(1):12-21.

Lapses of concentration and dyslexic performance on the Ternus task. Abstract: Recently, Cestnick and Coltheart (Cognition 71 (1999) 231) have reported evidence of abnormal performance on the Ternus apparent motion task in dyslexics. We demonstrate that some aspects of their data may be accounted for by more frequent lapses of concentration in the dyslexic group than in controls. We then report on a study in which a modification of the Ternus procedure was employed to simplify the task and to control for the effects of inattention. The results suggest that dyslexics do genuinely differ from normal readers in their perceptual processing. Davis C Castles A McAnally K Gray J Cognition 2001 Sep;81(2):B21-31.

Late cognitive brain potentials, phonological and semantic classification of spoken words, and reading ability in children. Abstract: Event-related potential (ERP), reaction time, and response accuracy measures were obtained during rhyming and semantic classification of spoken words in 10 average (mean age 11.64 years) and 9 impaired reading (mean age 12.10 years) children. The behavioral measures of classification did not distinguish the groups. In the ERPs, rhyme processing produced more pronounced group differences than did semantic processing at about 480 ms, with a relatively more negative distribution for the impaired readers at centroparietal sites. Lovrich D Cheng JC Velting DM J Clin Exp Neuropsychol 1996 Apr;18(2):161-77.

Laterality and types of dyslexia. Abstract: The right shift theory of handedness and cerebral specialization suggests that there is an underlying substrate of random lateral asymmetries in all higher animals and a specific factor in humans which increases the probability of left hemisphere advantage. The specific factor displaces the random distribution along a continuum of asymmetry in favour of the left hemisphere and the right hand. The distribution of handedness in families can be explained if the shift to dextrality depends on a single gene, rs +, when the frequency of the gene is estimated from the proportion of dysphasics with unilateral lesions of the left versus the right hemisphere. Annett M Neurosci Biobehav Rev 1996 Winter;20(4):631-6.

Laterality in animals: relevance to schizophrenia. Abstract: Anomalies in the laterality of numerous neurocognitive dimensions associated with schizophrenia have been documented, but their role in the etiology and early development of the disorder remain unclear. In the study of normative neurobehavioral organization, animal models have shed much light on the mechanisms underlying and the factors affecting adult patterns of both functional and structural asymmetry. Nonhuman species have more recently been used to investigate the environmental, genetic, and neuroendocrine factors associated with developmental language disorders in humans. Cowell PE Fitch RH Denenberg VH Schizophr Bull 1999;25(1):41-62.

Lateralized cognitive deficits in children following cerebellar lesions. Abstract: The aim of this preliminary study was to examine the developing cognitive profiles of children with cerebellar tumours in a consecutive series of clinical patients. MRI and longitudinal intellectual profiles were obtained on seven children (two females, five males; mean age 3 years at diagnosis; mean age 7 years at first assessment). Tumours in three of the children were astrocytomas; of the remaining tumours, two were medulloblastomas, one low-grade glioma, and one ependymoma. Scott RB Stoodley CJ Anslow P Paul C Stein JF Sugden EM Mitchell CD Dev Med Child Neurol 2001 Oct;43(10):685-91.

Lateralized word recognition: assessing the role of hemispheric specialization, modes of lexical access, and perceptual asymmetry. Abstract: The processing advantage for words in the right visual field (RVF) has often been assigned to parallel orthographic analysis by the left hemisphere and sequential by the right. The authors investigated this notion using the Reicher-Wheeler task to suppress influences of guesswork and an eye-tracker to ensure central fixation. RVF advantages obtained for all serial positions and identical U-shaped serial-position curves obtained for both visual fields (Experiments 1-4). Jordan TR Patching GR Milner AD J Exp Psychol Hum Percept Perform 2000 Jun;26(3):1192-208.

Learning disabilities and dyslexia. ASHA 1995 Jan;37(1):63-4.

Learning disabilities just don't add up. Accardo P Lindsay RL J Pediatr 1998 Sep;133(3):320-1.

Learning disabilities sourcebook: basic information about disorders such as dyslexia, visual and auditory processing deficits, attention deficit/hyperactivity disorder, and autism, along with statistical and demographic data, reports on current research initiatives, an explanation of the assessment process, and a special section for adults with learning disabilities / edited by Linda M. Shin. Detroit, MI: Omnigraphics, c1998. Shin, Linda M. Description: xi, 579 p.; 24 cm. ISBN: 0780802101 (lib. bdg.: alk. paper) LC Classification: LC4705.L434 1998 Dewey Class No.: 371.92/6 21

Learning disabilities, dyslexia, and vision: a subject review. Committee on Children with Disabilities, American Academy of Pediatrics (AAP) and American Academy of Ophthalmology (AAO), American Association for Pediatric Ophthalmology and Strabismus (AAPOS). Abstract: Learning disabilities are common conditions in pediatric patients. The etiology of these difficulties is multifactorial, reflecting genetic influences and abnormalities of brain structure and function. Early recognition and referral to qualified educational professionals is critical for the best possible outcome.

Visual problems are rarely responsible for learning difficulties. No scientific evidence exists for the efficacy of eye exercises ("vision therapy") or the use of special tinted lenses in the remediation of these complex pediatric developmental and neurologic conditions. Pediatrics 1998 Nov;102(5):1217-9.

Learning disabilities, employment discrimination, and the ADA. Abstract: The Americans with Disabilities Act (ADA) of 1990 was intended to prohibit discrimination against individuals with disabilities. Although the scope of this legislation is broad, there are aspects of Title I and Title II of the ADA that may be of particular interest to persons with learning disabilities who are preparing for employment. This article discusses those aspects and presents case studies to demonstrate how the ADA could potentially be applied to typical situations. Suggestions are given for individuals with learning disabilities, their parents, and teachers with regard to employment preparation in secondary and postsecondary settings. Anderson PL Kazmierski S Cronin ME J Learn Disabil 1995 Apr;28(4):196-204.

Learning disabilities: implications for psychiatric treatment / edited by Laurence L. Greenhill. Washington, DC: American Psychiatric Press, c2000. Greenhill, Laurence L. Description: xxi, 182 p.: ill. (some col.); 23 cm. ISBN: 0880483830 (alk. paper) LC Classification: RC394.L37 L43 2000 NLM Class No.: WS 110 L43752 2000 Dewey Class No.: 616.85/889 21 Other System No.: (DNLM)100929103

Learning disorders with a special emphasis on reading disorders: a review of the past 10 years. Abstract: To review the past 10 years of clinical and research reports on learning disorders. Much progress has been made in our understanding of learning disabilities, especially in reading disabilities. Resolution of definitional and conceptual issues will greatly assist research into assessment, treatment, and long-term outcome of learning disabilities with and without concurrent psychiatric disorders. Further research into the nature, extent, and correlates of comorbid learning disabilities and their treatment is much needed. Beitchman JH Young AR J Am Acad Child Adolesc Psychiatry 1997 Aug;36(8):1020-32.

Learning to read in Williams syndrome: looking beneath the surface of atypical reading development. Abstract: In this paper, we make a fundamental distinction between literacy attainment scores and the actual process of learning to read, and examine these two aspects of reading in atypical development. Reading skills in a group of children and adults with the genetic disorder Williams syndrome (WS) were compared to a group of typically developing children matched for reading age and receptive vocabulary scores. Study 1 focused on the product of reading and explored the relationship between reading, general cognition, and phonological skills. Laing E Hulme C Grant J Karmiloff-Smith A J Child Psychol Psychiatry 2001 Sep;42(6):729-39.

Lefavrais, Pierre. Les mécanismes de la lecture: étude analytique et expérimentale de la lecture rapide et de la dyslexie: principes fondamentaux de la rééducation des déficients en lecture / Pierre Lefavrais. Issy-les-Moulineaux, France: Editions EAP, [1983] Description: 309 p.: ill.; 22 cm. ISBN: 2864910268 LC Classification: LB1050.5.L375 1983 Dewey Class No.: 371.91/4 19

Left hemisphere of the brain is underactive in dyslexic people. Abdulla S BMJ 1998 Apr 18;316(7139):1189.

Left minineglect in dyslexic adults. Abstract: We searched for a core mechanism underlying the diverse behavioural and sensorimotor deficits in dyslexic subjects. In psychophysical temporal order judgement and line motion illusion tasks, adult dyslexics processed stimuli in the left visual hemifield significantly (approximately 15 ms) more slowly than normal readers, indicating a left-sided 'minineglect'. Furthermore, abrupt stimuli captured attention in both visual hemifields less effectively in dyslexics than in normal readers. Hari R Renvall H Tanskanen T Brain 2001 Jul;124(Pt 7):1373-80.

Left neglect dyslexia and the processing of neglected information. Abstract: A patient (ES) with a right fronto-temporo-parieto-occipital lesion, and left neglect dyslexia, is reported. ES performed reading and association tasks on written words, composed of two embedded words, one to the left and one to the right of the division point. The meaning of the whole stimulus differed from that of the embedded words, and could not be inferred from either of them. ES produced appropriate associations even to those stimuli on which she made neglect paralexic errors. Vallar G Guariglia C Nico D Tabossi P J Clin Exp Neuropsychol 1996 Oct;18(5):733-46.

Legasthenie, neue Wege der Heilung: Vorbeugungs- u. Behandlungsvorschläge / hrsg. von Dierk Trempler. Edition Information: Orig.-Ausg. Freiburg im Breisgau; Basel; Wien: Herder, 1976. Trempler, Dierk, 1944- Description: 155 p.: ill.; 18 cm. ISBN: 3451090414: LC Classification: LB1050.5.L383 National Bib. No.: GFR76-A

Less developed corpus callosum in dyslexic subjects--a structural MRI study. Abstract: Based on previous studies and due to the characteristics of dyslexia as an auditory phonological decoding disorder, we predicted that the shape of the posterior corpus callosum (CC) would differ between dyslexic and control subjects. A clear shape difference in the posterior midbody of the CC was found between dyslexic and control subjects. This fits with recent other studies that have reported a strong growth factor in this CC region during the late childhood years, coinciding with literacy acquisition. Our results show that the dyslexic group has not undergone the same growth pattern as the normal reading group. von Plessen K Lundervold A Duta N Heiervang E Klauschen F Smievoll AI Ersland L Hugdahl K Neuropsychologia 2002;40(7):1035-44.

Lessons from the follow-up of developmental dyslexics. Abstract: The follow-up of developmental dyslexics from childhood to maturity reveals interesting and important facts. One of the main conclusions which can be reached on considering these facts is that reading and writing can be acquired without phonology. Many developmental dyslexics manage to reach high levels of literacy while remaining seriously handicapped in their phonological skills. The suggestion presented in this paper advocates the adoption of the practical strategies employed by the dyslexics as the basis of the remedial methods to be used in schools. Daryn E Med Hypotheses 2000 Mar;54(3):434-7.

Lester, Tyler. Welcome to Dyslexic Park / by Tyler Lester; illustrations by Diane Russell; graphics by Toby Alice Delaney. Fresno, CA: Poppy Lane Pub, c1999. Russell, Diane, ill. Delaney, Toby Alice. Description: 1 v. (unpaged): col. ill.; 27 cm. ISBN: 0938911163 LC Classification: PZ7.L56345 We 1999 Dewey Class No.: [E] 21

Letter dyslexia in a letter-by-letter reader. Abstract: We describe a letter-by-letter patient who produced misreading errors in both letters in isolation and in words. All errors were visual in nature. We hypothesized an access deficit to the abstract visual representation of letters that prevents letter identification. This deficit could account for the patient's letter-by-letter behavior, since each letter constituted a potential identification problem. An access deficit, moreover, could explain the patient's letter visual errors. Perri R Bartolomeo P Silveri MC Brain Lang 1996 Jun;53(3):390-407.

Letter-by-letter alexia after left hemispheral lesion without hemianopsia nor callosal involvement. 2 cases Abstract: We describe two patients suffering from a letter-by-letter reading following an infarct in the left posterior cerebral artery's territory. Unlike most of the verbal alexics, this strategy was particularly fast and effective. Two other features distinguished these patients from verbal alexics: the absence of hemianopia and the sparing of the corpus callosum. A study of the reading of letters and words by each hemisphere was performed. In the first case, the left hemisphere was unable to identify any letter or word Verstichel P Cambier J Rev Neurol (Paris) 1997 Oct;153(10):561-8.

Levinson, Harold N. A scientific Watergate, dyslexia: how and why countless millions are deprived of breakthrough medical treatment / Harold N. Levinson. Lake Success, NY: Stonebridge Pub, c1994. Description: xxiii, 455 p.: ill.; 24 cm. ISBN: 0963930303 LC Classification: RC394.W6 L478 1994 Dewey Class No.: 616.85/53 20 Other System No.: (OCoLC)30493827

Levinson, Harold N. A solution to the riddle dyslexia / Harold N. Levinson. New York: Springer-Verlag, c1980. Description: xii, 398 p.: ill.; 25 cm. ISBN: 0387905154 LC Classification: RJ496.A5 L48 Dewey Class No.: 616.85/53 19 Series:

Levinson, Harold N. Smart but feeling dumb / Harold N. Levinson. Edition Information: Rev. ed. New York: Warner Books, c1994. Description: xx, 299 p.; 21 cm. ISBN: 0446395455 LC Classification: RC394.W6 L48 1994 Dewey Class No.: 616.85/53 20

Levinson, Harold N. Smart but feeling dumb / Harold N. Levinson. New York, NY: Warner Books, c1984. Description: xvii, 236 p.: ill.; 24 cm. ISBN: 0446513075 LC Classification: RC394.W6 L48 1984 Dewey Class No.: 616.85/53 19

Levinson, Harold N. The discovery of cerebellar-vestibular syndromes & therapies: a solution to the riddle - dyslexia / Harold N. Levinson. Edition

Information: 2nd ed. Lake Success, NY: Stonebridge Publishing, Ltd, 2000. Projected Pub. Date: 0003 Description: p.; cm. ISBN: 0963930311

Levinson, Harold N. The upside-down kids: helping dyslexic children understand themselves and their disorder / Harold N. Levinson and Addie Sanders. New York, N.Y.: M. Evans, c1991. Sanders, Addie. Description: xvii, 150 p.: ill.; 22 cm. ISBN: 0871316250: LC Classification: LC4708.L48 1991 Dewey Class No.: 371.91/44 20

Levinson, Harold N. Turning around the upside-down kids: helping dyslexic kids overcome their disorder / Harold Levinson and Addie Sanders. Variant Half Turning around New York: M. Evans & Co, c1992. Sanders, Addie. Description: xiv, 156 p.: ill.; 22 cm. ISBN: 0871317001: LC Classification: LC4708.L48 1992 Dewey Class No.: 371.91/44 20

Lexical access via letter naming in a profoundly alexic and anomic patient: a treatment study. Abstract: We report the results of a letter naming treatment designed to facilitate letter-by-letter reading in an aphasic patient with no reading ability. Patient M.R.'s anomia for written letters reflected two loci of impairment within visual naming: impaired letter activation from print (a deficit commonly seen in pure alexic patients who read letter by letter) and impaired access to phonology via semantics (documented in a severe multimodality anomia). Remarkably, M.R. retained an excellent ability to pronounce orally spelled words, demonstrating that abstract letter identities could be activated normally via spoken letter names, and that lexical phonological representations were intact when accessed via spoken letter names. Greenwald ML Gonzalez Rothi LJ J Int Neuropsychol Soc 1998 Nov;4(6):595-607.

Lexical and semantic processing in the absence of word reading: evidence from neglect dyslexia. Abstract: Nine patients with left-sided neglect and nine matched control patients performed three tasks on horizontal (either normal or mirror-reversed) letter strings. The tasks were: reading aloud, making a lexical decision (word vs non-word), and making a semantic decision (living vs non-living item). Relative to controls, neglect patients performed very poorly in the reading task, whereas they performed nearly normally in the lexical and semantic tasks. This was considered to be a dissociation between direct tasks, rather than a dissociation between explicit and implicit knowledge. Ladavas E Umilta C Mapelli D Neuropsychologia 1997 Aug;35(8):1075-85.

Lexical factors in the word-superiority effect. Abstract: In the Reicher-Wheeler paradigm, fluent readers can identify letters better when they appear in a word than when they appear in either a pronounceable pseudoword (a lexicality effect) or a single letter (a word-letter effect). It was predicted that if both of these effects involve a lexical factor, then adult acquired dyslexic subjects whose deficit prevents access to visual word form should show disruptions of the normal effects on the Reicher-Wheeler task. Hildebrandt N Caplan D Sokol S Torreano L Mem Cognit 1995 Jan;23(1):23-33.

Lexical representation and processing of morphologically complex words: evidence from the reading performance of an Italian agrammatic patient. Abstract: The study of patients with acquired language disorders has provided crucial evidence for contemporary theories on mental lexical representation. This is particularly true for the representation of morphologically complex words. In this paper we analyzed the performance of a patient (M.B.) affected by agrammatism and dyslexia. M.B. was required to read aloud simple and morphologically complex words. The patient's pattern of errors was interpreted as the result of a predominant use of the lexical routine (phonological dyslexia). Luzzatti C Mondini S Semenza C Brain Lang 2001 Dec;79(3):345-59.

Ligeti, Róbert. [from old catalog] Gyermekek olvasászavarai (dyslexia). Budapest, Adadémiai Kiadó, 1967. Description: 100 p. illus. 19 cm. LC Classification: LB1105.P7 Köt 8

Linguistic evaluation of Profet II: a pilot project. Abstract: Profet, a word prediction program, was designed to accelerate the writing process and to minimize the writing effort of persons with motor dysfunction. It has proved to be beneficial in text construction for persons with linguistic impairment such as dyslexia. With increasing linguistic demands on support for individuals with severe reading and writing difficulties/dyslexia, the need for an improved version of Profet arose. Thus, Profet II was designed. In this study, a procedure for evaluating Profet II has been developed. Results from a single-case evaluation study with a person with dyslexia are presented Magnuson T Hunnicutt S Logoped Phoniatr Vocol 2000;25(3):105-14.

Linkage analysis and genetic models in dyslexia--considerations pertaining to discrete trait analysis and quantitative trait analyses. Abstract: We used simulation studies to assess the relative powers of various autosomal-dominant models of inheritance for dyslexia. Muller-Myhsok B Grimm T Eur Child Adolesc Psychiatry 1999;8 Suppl 3:40-2.

Linkage analysis in heterogeneous and complex traits. Abstract: Linkage analysis is generally carried out under single-gene models, while complex traits are thought to be under the control of multiple interacting genes. Current issues related to linkage analysis for complex traits are discussed. It is argued that linkage analyses should be carried out for sub-phenotypes, in addition to classical "affected-unaffected" phenotypes. Correlations for phenotypes among family members are often computed on the basis of extreme phenotypes of a proband, which results in biased estimates. Ott J Bhat A Eur Child Adolesc Psychiatry 1999;8 Suppl 3:43-6.

Linkage studies suggest a possible locus for developmental dyslexia on chromosome 1p. Abstract: Eight extended dyslexic families with at least four affected individuals were genotyped with twelve genetic markers spanning the Rh (rhesus factor) locus. Eleven of these markers were located on the short arm and the other was on the long arm of chromosome 1. Five theoretically derived phenotypes were used in the linkage analyses: 1) phonemic awareness; 2) phonological decoding; 3) rapid automatized naming; 4) single word reading; and 5) vocabulary. In addition, a lifetime diagnosis of dyslexia was used as a phenotype. Both parametric and non-parametric genetic analyses were completed. Grigorenko EL Wood FB Meyer MS Pauls JE Hart Am J Med Genet 2001 Jan 8;105(1):120-9.

Linkage study of polymorphisms in the gene for myelin oligodendrocyte glycoprotein located on chromosome 6p and attention deficit hyperactivity disorder. Abstract: Family and twin studies have shown that there is a substantial genetic contribution to both reading disabilities (RD) and attention deficit hyperactivity disorder (ADHD), and recent twin studies have suggested that the overlap between these phenotypes is largely due to common genetic influences. Studies using a linkage approach to search for genes for susceptibility to RD and ADHD have identified regions linked to each of these phenotypes separately, with recent studies suggesting that some chromosomal regions may contribute to both. Linkage to the human leukocyte antigen (H Am J Med Genet 2001 Apr 8;105(3):250-4.

Linksz, Arthur. On writing, reading, and dyslexia. New York, Grune & Stratton [1973] Description: viii, 256 p. illus. 24 cm. ISBN: 0808907891 LC Classification: LB1576.L54 Dewey Class No.: 428/.4

Lire, écrire et compter aujourd'hui: heurs et malheurs des premiers apprentissages scolaires / sous la direction de Roger Salbreux; [ont collaboré à cet ouvrage Alegria, Jesus... et al.]. Paris: ESF, c1995.

Salbreux, Roger. Alegria, Jesus. Description: 122 p.: ill.; 24 cm. ISBN: 2710111322 LC Classification: LB1050.5.L57 1995

Litchman, Kristin Embry. The wrong side of the pattern / Kristin E. Litchman. Unionville, N.Y.: Royal Fireworks Press, c1997. Description: 154 p.; 22 cm. ISBN: 0880923814 (pbk.) 0880923822 (lib. bdg.) LC Classification: PZ7.L69735 Wr 1997 Dewey Class No.: [Fic] 21

Lobrot, Michel. Troubles de la langue écrite et remèdes. Paris, Éditions ESF [1972] Description: 215 p. illus. 24 cm. LC Classification: LB1050.5.L58 NLM Class No.: WL 340 L799t 1972 Other System No.: (OCoLC)5181872 Series: LC Classification: RC394.W6 RYA 0567

Looking with one's mind's eye. Abstract: On the basis of clinical cases reported in the literature, an attempt is made to show that conscious mental representations of written words have a left-right dimension similar to their counterparts in the physical world. They may, therefore, be affected by unilateral neglect in much the same way as words on a written or printed page. Usually, real words and their representations run in the same direction. However, in some cases, they appear to run in opposite directions and this may result in the production of mirror writing. Lebrun Y Eur J Disord Commun 1995;30(3):279-302.

Loss of silent reading in frontotemporal dementia: unmasking the inner speech. Vercueil L Klinger H J Neurol Neurosurg Psychiatry 2001 May;70(5):705.

Lulham, Margaret. Dyslexia: books for the dyslexic. Edition Information: Revised ed. / reviewed by Margaret Lulham. London: Helen Arkell Dyslexia Centre, 1978. Hardwick, Paula. Books for the dyslexic. Description: [2], 43 p.; 21 cm. ISBN: 0950362697: LC Classification: Z5346.L84 1978 HV1743.G7 Dewey Class No.: 028.52 National Bib. No.: GB78-19792

Lundgren, Torbjörn, 1949- På spaning efter ordblindheten: en stridsskrift / av Torbjörn Lundgren. Stockholm: Carlsson, c1991. Description: 132 p.: ill.; 21 cm. ISBN: 9177984269: LC Classification: LB1050.5.L86 1991

Lyman, Donald E. Making the words stand still / Donald E. Lyman; foreword by Robert S. Sloat. Boston: Houghton Mifflin, 1986. Description: xv, 272 p.: ill.; 22 cm. ISBN: 0395362199: LC Classification: LC4704.L96 1986 Dewey Class No.: 371.9 19

MacCracken, Mary. Turnabout children: overcoming dyslexia and other learning disabilities / Mary MacCracken. Edition Information: 1st ed. Boston: Little, Brown and Co, c1986. Description: ix, 258 p.: ill.; 22 cm. ISBN: 0316555401: LC Classification: LC4705.M33 1986 Dewey Class No.: 371.91/4 19

Madison, Sigrid, 1918- Hoppande bokstäver: en bok om dyslexi / Sigrid Madison. Stockholm: Tiden/Folksam, c1988. Description: 153 p.: ill.; 21 cm. ISBN: 9155034802 LC Classification: LB1050.5.M25 1988

Magnetic source imaging and the neural basis of dyslexia. Poeppel D Rowley HA Ann Neurol 1996 Aug;40(2):137-8.

Magnetoencephalographic mapping of the language-specific cortex. Abstract: In this paper the authors introduce a novel use of magnetoencephalography (MEG) for noninvasive mapping of language-specific cortex in individual patients and in healthy volunteers. Findings include: 1) receptive language-specific areas can be reliably activated by simple language tasks and this activation can be readily recorded in short MEG sessions; 2) MEG-derived maps of each individual are reliable because they remain stable over time and are independent of whether auditory or visual stimuli are used to activate the brain; and 3) these maps are valid because they concur with results of the Wada procedure in assessing hemispheric dominance for language and with the results of cortical stimulation in identifying the precise topography of receptive language regions within the dominant hemisphere. Although the MEG mapping technique should be further refined, it has been shown to be efficacious by correctly identifying the language-dominant hemisphere and specific language-related regions within this hemisphere. Further development of the technique may render it a valuable adjunct for routine presurgical planning in many patients who harbor tumors or have epilepsy. Papanicolaou AC Simos PG Breier JI Zouridakis G Willmore LJ Wheless JW Constantinou JE Maggio WW Gormley WB J Neurosurg 1999 Jan;90(1):85-93.

Magnocellular visual function and children's single word reading. Abstract: Recent research has shown that reading disabled children find it unusually difficult to detect flickering or moving visual stimuli, consistent with impaired processing in the magnocellular visual stream. Yet, it remains controversial to suggest that reduced visual sensitivity of this kind might affect children's reading. Here we suggest that when children read, impaired magnocellular function may degrade information about where letters are positioned with respect to each other, leading to reading errors that contain sounds not represented in the printed word. Cornelissen PL Hansen PC Hutton JL Evangelinou V Stein JF Vision Res 1998 Feb;38(3):471-82.

Male prevalence for reading disability is found in a large sample of black and white children free from ascertainment bias. Abstract: Male vulnerability to neurodevelopmental disorders remains controversial. For one disorder, reading disability, this sex bias has been interpreted as an artifact of referral bias. We investigated sex differences for the incidence of reading disability within a large prospective sample of White (N = 16,910) and Black (N = 15,313) children derived from the National Collaborative Perinatal Project (NCPP). Children were classified as having either moderate or severe reading disability when they had reading scores lower than 1.5 or 2.0 standard errors of prediction, respectively, given their age and intelligence. Flannery KA Liederman J Daly L Schultz J J Int Neuropsychol Soc 2000 May;6(4):433-42.

Management of childhood lead poisoning: clinical impact and cost-effectiveness. Abstract: No consensus exists regarding the preferred treatment of childhood lead poisoning. The authors used decision analysis to compare the clinical impacts and cost-effectiveness of four management strategies for childhood lead poisoning, and to investigate how effective chelation therapy must be in reducing neuropsychologic sequelae to warrant its use. Treatment strategies for childhood lead poisoning vary in clinical impact, cost, and cost-effectiveness. Chelation of the 1.4% of United States preschoolers whose blood lead levels are 2.21 mumol/L (25 micrograms/dL) or higher could prevent more than 45,000 cases of reading disability, and save more than $900 million per year in overall costs when the costs of remedial education are considered. Glotzer DE Freedberg KA Bauchner H Med Decis Making 1995 Jan-Mar;15(1):13-24.

Management of reading and spelling problems in children and adults. Funnell E Br J Clin Psychol 1996 Nov;35 (Pt 4):643-4.

Managing the clumsy and non-reading child. Waterston T Practitioner 1999 Sep;243(1602):675-7.

Manilla, George T. Dyslexia: a reading and writing correction method / George T. Manilla. Edition Information: 1st ed. Elko, Nev.: High Desert Pub, c1990. Description: v, 91 p.: 31 ill.; 22 cm. ISBN: 0962887919 (pbk.) 0962887900 (hard) LC Classification: LC4708.M36 1990 Dewey Class No.: 371.91/44 20

Marburg Spelling Training program--results of a brief intervention Abstract: The Marburg Spelling Training Program was administered to a sample of 10 spelling-disabled primary school pupils (2nd-4th graders) over three months in an individual setting The Marburg Spelling Training Program has now proven to be effective not only in long-term, but in short-term intervention. Schulte-Korne G Deimel W Hulsmann J Seidler T Remschmidt H Z Kinder Jugendpsychiatr Psychother 2001 Feb;29(1):7-15.

Marchiafava-Bignami disease: computed tomographic scan, 99mTc HMPAO-SPECT, and F Arch Neurol 1999 Jan;56(1):107-10.

Marek, Margot. Different, not dumb / by Margot Marek; photographs by Barbara Kirk. New York: F. Watts, 1985. Kirk, Barbara, ill. Description: 32 p.: ill.; 20 x 26 cm. ISBN: 0531047229 (lib. bdg.) Summary: Because he gets some letters mixed up or reversed, Mike is assigned to a special class in which he learns the basic reading skills he eventually uses to avert a serious accident. LC Classification: PZ7.M3352 Di 1985 Dewey Class No.: [E] 19

Martin, Ann M, 1955- Yours turly, Shirley / Ann M. Martin. Edition Information: 1st ed. New York: Holiday House, c1988. Description: 133 p.; 22 cm. ISBN: 0823407195 Summary: Shirley, a fourth-grader with dyslexia, struggles with her feelings of inferiority as she compares herself to her intellectually gifted older brother and newly adopted Vietnamese sister. LC Classification: PZ7.M3567585 Yo 1988 Dewey Class No.: [Fic] 19

Martin, William Lee. A psico-avaliação da eficiência viso-mnemônica motora em crianças com distúrbios de aprendizagem: um estudo do valor discriminatório do teste MFD de Graham-Kendall / William Lee Martin. João Pessoa, Paraíba: Editora Universitária, [1979] Description: 149 p.: ill.; 22 cm. LC Classification: MLCS 92/12679 (B)

Maryland. Governor's Commission on Dyslexia. Report to the Governor and

General Assembly of Maryland. [Cockeysville] 1972. Description: v, 62 p. 23 cm. LC Classification: LB1050.5.M36 Dewey Class No.: 371.9/14

Matejcek, Zdenek. [from old catalog] Vývojové poruchy ctení. Edition Information: 1. vyd. Praha, SPN, t. Tisk 4, Prerov, 1972. Description: 238, [1] p. with photos and tables. 21 cm. LC Classification: RJ496.A5 M37

Mathematics and dyslexia--an overlooked connection. Abstract: This paper describes various kinds of learning disability. It is suggested that the connection between mathematical difficulties and dyslexia has been largely overlooked by educators. Students' failure to understand how the number system works and the resultant failure to appreciate place values account for many of the mathematical difficulties experienced by dyslexic learners. Malmer G Dyslexia 2000 Oct-Dec;6(4):223-30.

Mathematics and the brain: uncharted territory? Abstract: The prevalence of disorders of arithmetic skills in children of circa 6 % calls for intensive consideration of the subject by health care providers and researchers. The necessity of interdisciplinary cooperation is evident. The current classifications by the ICD-10 (Specific disorder of arithmetic skills) and DSM-IV (Mathematics disorder) represent different viewpoints. A developmental dyscalculia is exclusively diagnosed according to clinical presentation. Arithmetic and its disorders are brain functions, determined and influenced by the (cerebral) human development Neumarker KJ Eur Child Adolesc Psychiatry 2000;9 Suppl 2:II2-10.

Matthys-Egle, Markus, 1962- Diagnose "Legasthenie": Konzepte systemischer Beratung in der Schulpsychologie als Alternative zur Praxis der Symptomkonstruktion / Markus Matthys-Egle. Bern; New York: P. Lang, c1996. Description: 264 p.: ill.; 21 cm. ISBN: 390675622X LC Classification: RJ496.A5

M37 1996 Dewey Class No.: 618.92/8553 21

McCurty, Darlene M. I'm special, too! / Darlene M. McCurty; [cover and text illustrations by Napoleon Wilkerson]. Edition Information: 1st ed. Chicago, Ill.: African American Images, c1992. Wilkerson, Napoleon, ill. Description: 55 p.: ill.; 22 cm. ISBN: 0913543276 (pbk.): Summary: Nehemiah, who feels like a failure because he is always being put down and told he is no good, gains the respect of his classmates when his essay is chosen to represent the school in a statewide creative writing contest. LC Classification: PZ7.M47841634 Im 1992 Dewey Class No.: [Fic] 20 Other System No.: (OCoLC)26197144

McLeod, John. Handbook for dyslexia schedule and school entrance check list. [St. Lucia, Queensland] University of Queensland Press [1969] Description: 28 p. 27 cm. LC Classification: LB1050.M32 Dewey Class No.: 372.4/13 National Bib. No.: Aus68-1756

Mellansjo school-home. Psychopathic children admitted 1928-1940, their social adaptation over 30 years: a longitudinal prospective follow-up. Abstract: The school-home for "psychopathic" children, Mellansjo, was founded in 1928. The initiator was Alice Hellstrom, a teacher and physician. She was a child psychiatric pioneer in Sweden. She had no formal education in child and adolescent psychiatry but with support from Professor of Paediatrics Isaac Jundell she received education in pediatrics and from Professor of Psychiatry Bror Gadelius she was trained in psychiatry. Hellstrom made a study trip to Europe where she visited child psychiatry clinics. She visited Summerhill in England and professors Aichhorn and Lazar in Austria. Fried I Acta Paediatr Suppl 1995 Apr;408:1-42.

Memory span, naming speed, and memory strategies in poor and normal readers. Abstract: Eleven-year-old severely impaired poor readers failed to show a word length effect with pictorial presentation, but showed an effect of equal magnitude to that of reading age and chronological age controls with auditory presentation. The lack of a pictorial word length effect was unlikely to be due to slow speed of naming skills, as in one study these were at least as fast as those of the reading age controls. It is possible that the poor readers failed to verbally encode the pictures. However, they reported using verbal rehearsal, and lip movements were often observed during presentation, suggesting that they did verbally encode the items. Johnston RS Anderson M Memory 1998 Mar;6(2):143-63.

Mental and somatic health and social adjustment in ordinary school children during childhood and adolescence related to central nervous functions as expressed by a complex reaction time. Abstract: A cohort of ordinary Swedish children were followed up from school entry through childhood and adolescence and checked retrospectively from birth to the age of 6 years regarding psychiatric and physical health and contact with the social welfare authorities. The children were allocated to different risk groups at age 7 on the basis of their psycho-physical development expressed as complex reaction time (CRT). Frisk M Eur Child Adolesc Psychiatry 1995 Jul;4(3):197-208.

Mental development in polysomy X Klinefelter syndrome (47,XXY; 48,XXXY): effects of incomplete X inactivation. Abstract: The child with XXY or a variant form is a fertile ground for scientific investigation because of the homogeneity of the disorder and the increased prevalence of learning disorders associated with it. However, the research studies of boys with XXY (Klinefelter syndrome) have been plagued by a variety of factors from small sample size, methodological flaws, and ascertainment bias. In spite of these shortcomings, there remains some consistency to the neurobehavioral profile of this disorder Samango-Sprouse C Semin Reprod Med 2001 Jun;19(2):193-202.

Mental disease a heritage. New genetic knowledge can reveal "public diseases" such as autism, dyslexia, alcoholism, anorexia, schizophrenia Abstract: Family and adoption studies indicate that genetic factors play a role in the development of many psychiatric disorders. A variable number of possible interacting genes predisposing to the diseases is likely. The genetic dissection has been hampered by genetic complexity as well as by difficulties in defining the phenotypes. Genetic mapping efforts using sib pairs, twins and individual large families has revealed preliminary or tentative evidence for susceptibility loci for a number of psychiatric disorders. Wetterberg L Lakartidningen 2000 Feb 9;97(6):558-62, 565-7.

Meredith, Patrick. Dyslexia and the individual. London, Elm Tree Books Ltd, 1972. Description: 190 p. illus. 23 cm. ISBN: 0241023106 LC Classification: RC429.M47 1972 Dewey Class No.: 371.9/14 National Bib. No.: B72-30515

Mesker, Pierre, 1905- De menselijke hand: een onderzoek naar de ontwikkeling van de handvaardigheid in relatie tot die van de cerebrale organisatie gedaan bij leesgestoorde kinderen / P. Mesker. Edition Information: 3e druk. Nijmegen: Dekker & Van de Vegt, 1977. Description: viii, 226 p.: ill.; 20 cm. ISBN: 9025596185: LC Classification: RJ496.A5 M47 1977 National Bib. No.: Ne77-17

Messerschmitt, Paul. Ils ne savent pas lire-- et s'ils étaient dyslexiques? / Paul Messerschmitt; [avec] Catherine Flohic, Marielle Génot-Delbecque, Danièle Legrain. Variant Subtitle on cover: Réponses aux parents Spine Et s'ils étaient dyslexiques? [Paris]: Flohic, c1993. Description: 130 p.; 21 cm. Cancelled ISBN: 9782907958928 LC Classification: LB1050.5.M43 1993 Dewey Class No.: 371.91/44 20

Metabolic abnormalities in developmental dyslexia detected by 1H magnetic resonance spectroscopy. Abstract:

Neurological and physiological deficits have been reported in the brain in developmental dyslexia. The temporoparietal cortex has been directly implicated in dyslexic dysfunction, and substantial indirect evidence suggests that the cerebellum is implicated. We wanted to find out whether the neurological and physiological deficits manifested as biochemical changes in the brain. We suggest that the observed differences reflect changes in cell density in the temporo-parietal lobe in developmental dyslexia and that the altered cerebral structural symmetry in dyslexia is associated with abnormal development of cells or intracellular connections or both. The cerebellum is biochemically asymmetric in dyslexic men, indicating altered development of this organ. These differences provide direct evidence of the involvement of the cerebellum in dyslexic dysfunction. Rae C Lee MA Dixon RM Blamire AM Thompson CH Styles P Talcott J Richardson AJ Stein JF Lancet 1998 Jun 20;351(9119):1849-52.

Methods of investigating a visual deficit in dyslexia. Abstract: The evidence for a visual deficit in dyslexia is inconclusive. We have developed several tests to investigate the parallel pathways of the visual system that can be applied to dyslexic subjects. Using the techniques of electroretinography, visual evoked potentials, adaptometry and contrast sensitivity, special protocols have been designed to elicit responses from these parallel pathways. These techniques are applicable in the investigation of many pathological conditions, and of interest for pure research. Greatrex JC Drasdo N Ophthalmic Physiol Opt 1998 Mar;18(2):160-6.

Microstructure of temporo-parietal white matter as a basis for reading ability: evidence from diffusion tensor magnetic resonance imaging. Abstract: Diffusion tensor magnetic resonance imaging (MRI) was used to study the microstructural integrity of white matter in adults with poor or normal reading ability. Subjects with reading difficulty exhibited decreased diffusion anisotropy bilaterally in temporoparietal white matter. Axons in these regions were predominantly anterior-posterior in direction. No differences in T1-weighted MRI signal were found between poor readers and control subjects, demonstrating specificity of the group difference to the microstructural characteristics measured by diffusion tensor imaging (DTI Klingberg T Hedehus M Temple E Salz T Gabrieli JD Moseley ME Poldrack RA Neuron 2000 Feb;25(2):493-500.

Miles, T. R. (Thomas Richard) Dyslexia at college / T.R. Miles and Dorothy E. Gilroy; with contributions from C.R. Wilsher... [et al.]. London; New York: Methuen, 1986. Gilroy, Dorothy E. Description: x, 144 p.: ill.; 20 cm. ISBN: 0416396704 LC Classification: LB1050.5.M514 1986 Dewey Class No.: 371.91/4 19

Miles, T. R. (Thomas Richard) Dyslexia, the pattern of difficulties / T.R. Miles. Springfield, Ill.: Thomas, c1983. Description: viii, 225 p.: ill.; 24 cm. ISBN: 0398047472 LC Classification: RJ496.A5 M537 1983 Dewey Class No.: 618.92/8553 19

Miles, T. R. (Thomas Richard) Dyslexia: a hundred years on / T.R. Miles and Elaine Miles. Edition Information: 2nd ed. Buckingham; Philadelphia: Open University Press, 1999. Miles, Elaine. Description: vii, 198 p.: port.; 23 cm. ISBN: 0335200346 (pbk.) LC Classification: RC394.W6 M55 1999 NLM Class No.: WM 475.6 M643d 1998 Dewey Class No.: 616.85/53 21

Miles, T. R. (Thomas Richard) Dyslexia: a hundred years on / T.R. Miles and Elaine Miles. Milton Keynes; Philadelphia: Open University Press, 1990. Miles, Elaine. Description: ix, 124 p.; 23 cm. ISBN: 0335095410: 0335095402 (pbk.): LC Classification: RC394.W6 M55 1990 NLM Class No.: WM 475 M643da Dewey Class No.: 616.85/53 20

Miles, T. R. (Thomas Richard) More help for dyslexic children / [by] T. R. Miles and Elaine Miles. London: Methuen, 1975. Miles, Elaine, joint author. Description: vi, 74 p.: ill.; 21 cm. ISBN: 0423497502: LC Classification: LB1050.5.M515 Dewey Class No.: 371.9/14 National Bib. No.: GB75-14087

Miles, T. R. (Thomas Richard) On helping the dyslexic child, by T. R. Miles. London, Methuen Educational, 1970. Description: ix, 70 p. illus, facsims. 21 cm. ISBN: 042343070X LC Classification: LB1050.5.M516 Dewey Class No.: 371.91/1 National Bib. No.: B70-23870

Miles, T. R. (Thomas Richard) Recognising the dyslexic child: notes for parents and teachers / [by T. R. Miles with the assistance of others]. [Staines]: Dyslexia Institute, [1974] Dyslexia Institute. Description: 8 p.; 21 cm. ISBN: 0950391506: LC Classification: LB1050.5.M517 NLM Class No.: WL340 N643r 1974 Dewey Class No.: 618.9/28/553075 National Bib. No.: GB 75-03516

Miles, T. R. (Thomas Richard) The dyslexic child / [by] T. R. Miles; foreword by Oliver Zangwill. London: Priory Press, 1974. Description: 140 p.: facsims.; 23 cm. ISBN: 0850780969: LC Classification: RJ496.A5 M54 Dewey Class No.: 371.9/14 National Bib. No.: GB 75-03393

Miles, T. R. (Thomas Richard) The dyslexic child / T. R. Miles; foreword by Oliver Zangwill. Westport, Conn.: Technomic Pub. Co, 1976, c1974. Description: 140 p.; 23 cm. ISBN: 0877621977 LC Classification: RJ496.A5 M54 1976 Dewey Class No.: 371.9/14

Miles, T. R. (Thomas Richard) Understanding dyslexia / [by] T. R. Miles; foreword by Oliver Zangwill. Edition Information: [New ed.]. Sevenoaks: Teach Yourself Books, 1978. Description: 125 p.: ill.; 18 cm. ISBN: 0340226323: LC Classification: RJ496.A5 M54 1978

Dewey Class No.: 371.9/14 National Bib. No.: GB78-30560

Millichap, J. Gordon. Dyslexia: as the neurologist and educator read it / by J. Gordon Millichap and Nancy M. Millichap. Springfield, Ill, U.S.A.: Thomas, c1986. Millichap, Nancy M. Description: xi, 144 p.: ill.; 24 cm. ISBN: 0398052395 LC Classification: RJ496.A5 M55 1986 NLM Class No.: WL 340.6 M654d Dewey Class No.: 618.92/8552 19

Minicolumnar pathology in dyslexia. Abstract: The minicolumn is an anatomical and functional unit of the brain whose genesis accrues from germinal cell divisions in the ventricular zone of the brain. Disturbances in the morphometry of minicolumns have been demonstrated recently for both autism and Down's syndrome. We report minicolumnar abnormalities in the brain of a dyslexic patient. The corresponding developmental disturbance (ie, large minicolumns) could account for the perceptual errors observed in dyslexia. Casanova MF Buxhoeveden DP Cohen M Switala AE Roy EL Ann Neurol 2002 Jul;52(1):108-10.

Misreading dyslexia. Researchers debate the causes and prevalence of the disorder. Tashman B Sci Am 1995 Aug;273(2):14, 16.

Molecular approaches to the genetic analysis of specific reading disability. Abstract: Specific reading disability is a complex phenotype that is under both genetic and environmental influences. There is evidence for at least one major gene, which may be detectable by parametric linkage analysis, but detection of other quantitative trait loci may require nonparametric methods. Phenotype definition may be critical in identifying genes that affect different components of the reading process. Current research from two separate laboratories supports the localization of one gene influencing reading disability to the histocompatibility region of chromosome 6p and suggests that another gene may be located on chromosome 15 Smith SD Kelley PM Brower AM Hum Biol 1998 Apr;70(2):239-56.

Money, John, 1921- ed. The disabled reader; education of the dyslexic child. John Money, editor. Gilbert Schiffman, advisory editor. Baltimore, Johns Hopkins Press [1966] Schiffman, Gilbert B, joint ed. Description: xiii, 421 p. illus. 23 cm. LC Classification: LB1050.5.M6 Dewey Class No.: 372.413

Monocular occlusion can improve binocular control and reading in dyslexics. Abstract: Developmental dyslexia is a neurodevelopmental condition which causes 5-10% of children to have unexpected difficulty learning to read. Many dyslexics have impaired development of the magnocellular component of the visual system, which is important for timing visual events and controlling eye movements. Poor control of eye movement may lead to unstable binocular fixation, and hence unsteady vision; this could explain why many dyslexics report that letters appear to move around, causing visual confusion. Previous research has suggested that such binocular confusion can be permanently alleviated by temporarily occluding one eye. Stein JFss Richardson AJ Fowler MS Brain 2000 Jan;123 (Pt 1):164-70.

Mono-ocular occlusion for treatment of dyslexia. Fawcett AJ Lancet 2000 Jul 8;356(9224):89-90.

Mono-ocular occlusion for treatment of dyslexia. Soothill JF Lancet 2000 Sep 2;356(9232):856.

Montenegro, Aura. Dislexia-disortografia: investigação psicopedagógica na escola primaria / Aura Montenegro. Coimbra [Portugal: s.n.], 1974. Description: xx, 361 p.; 24 cm. LC Classification: LB1050.5.M66 1974

Moragne, Wendy. Dyslexia / Wendy Moragne. Brookfield, Conn.: MillBrook Press, c1997. Description: 96 p.: ill.; 24 cm.

ISBN: 0761302069 (lib. bdg.) Summary: Explains the nature of dyslexia, the various forms of treatment, and the many challenges faced by those living with this condition. Includes case studies and interviews. LC Classification: RJ496.A5 M66 1997 Dewey Class No.: 616.85/53 20

Morphological alteration of temporal lobe gray matter in dyslexia: an MRI study. Abstract: Functional imaging studies of developmental dyslexia have reported reduced task-related neural activity in the temporal and inferior parietal cortices. To examine the possible contribution of subtle anatomic deviations to these reductions, volumes were measured for the major lobes of the brain, the subcortical nuclei, cerebellum, and lateral ventricles on magnetic resonance imaging (MRI) scans from 16 right-handed dyslexic men, ages 18 to 40, and 14 matched controls, most of whom had previously undergone PET imaging. A Eliez S Rumsey JM Giedd JN Schmitt JE Patwardhan AJ Reiss AL J Child Psychol Psychiatry 2000 Jul;41(5):637-44.

Morris, John C. The Education Act, how it provides for handicapped children: basic legal information which applies to the education of all handicapped pupils and to the dyslexic in particular / by John C. Morris. A dyslexic child in the family: a psychiatrist's sensitive and helpful consideration of the emotional tight-rope to be negotiated by parents / by A. F. Cheyne. London: London Dyslexia Association, [1977] Cheyne, A. F. Dyslexic child in the family. 1977. North London Dyslexia Association. Description: [12] p.; 30 cm. LC Classification: KD3664.M67 Dewey Class No.: 371.9/14 National Bib. No.: GB77-17400

Mosse, Hilde L. The complete handbook of children's reading disorders: a critical evaluation of their clinical, educational, and social dimensions / Hilde L. Mosse. New York: Human Sciences Press, c1982. Related Titles: Children's reading disorders. Description: 2 v. (714 p.): ill.;

24 cm. ISBN: 0898850770 (set) 0898850215 (v. 1) 0898850266 (v. 2) LC Classification: RJ496.A5 M67 NLM Class No.: WM 475 M913c Dewey Class No.: 618.92/8553 19

Mosse, Hilde L. The complete handbook of children's reading disorders: you can prevent or correct learning disorders / Hilde L. Mosse. Beaverton, Or.: Riggs Institute Press, [1987, c1982] Related Titles: You can prevent or correct learning disorders. Description: 714 p.: ill.; 23 cm. ISBN: 0942311000 (pbk.): LC Classification: RJ496.A5 M67 1987 Dewey Class No.: 618.92/8553 19

Motion sickness amelioration induced by prism spectacles. Abstract: A side effect of the prescription of prism glasses according to the principle of Utermohlen to improve mechanical reading skills of certain types of learning disabled children was the alleviation of car sickness. Besides a decrease in reported symptoms after prescription of these glasses, the effect is quantified by a decrease in estimated number of emeses per year per patient. A placebo effect is unlikely because alleviation of car sickness was not the original intention of the prescription, and the symptoms returned as soon as the spectacles were discontinued. Vente PE Bos JE de Wit G Brain Res Bull 1998 Nov 15;47(5):503-5.

Moynihan, Lauren E. Taking dyslexia to school / Lauren E. Moynihan. Edition Information: 1st ed. Plainview, NY: JayJo Books, 2002. Projected Pub. Date: 0201 Description: p. cm. ISBN: 1891383175 Series: Special kids in school; eleventh book in our special kids in school series Other System No.: (DLC) 01097487

Mozota Ortiz, José Ramón. Chequeo a la dislexia / José Ramón Mozota Ortiz. [Zaragoza]: Instituto de Ciencias de la Educación, Universidad de Zaragoza, [1979] Description: 290 p.: ill.; 21 cm. ISBN: 8460015165 LC Classification: LB1050.5.M69 Dewey Class No.: 371.91/7 19 National Bib. No.: Sp***

Mucchielli-Bourcier, Arlette. Traitement de la dyslexie; à l'usage des parents, des instituteurs et des rééducateurs. Paris, Éditions sociales françaises [1966] Description: 190 p, 30 l. illus. 24 cm. LC Classification: LB1050.5.M82 Dewey Class No.: 371.9/14

Multidisciplinary investigation is best for children with learning disabilities. Too critical attitude to diagnoses can keep the disorders hidden Abstract: This article presents evidence of the importance of multidisciplinary assessment of students with learning disabilities. Multidisciplinary collaboration between different professions provides a more complete picture of each person's unique requirements, thereby facilitating more appropriate teaching. A critical attitude toward diagnosing students with learning disabilities may result in exaggeration of psychosocial problems, thereby running the risk that genuine learning disabilities, neurological problems or other disorders are being overlooked. Fohrer U Westholm L Lakartidningen 2001 Mar 21;98(12):1374-6.

Multilingualism and dyslexia: challenges for research and practice. Abstract: Over the last two decades there has been an expansion of activity and substantial progress in research on dyslexia and research on bilingualism and multilingualism. But the study of dyslexia has generally focused on monolingual learners and the study of bilingualism has tended to focus on speakers who do not have special educational needs. This paper will review the strands of research to date that have a bearing on multilingualism and dyslexia and attempt to identify the major challenges that face researchers and teachers. Cline T Dyslexia 2000 Jan-Mar;6(1):3-12.

Multilingualism, literacy, and dyslexia: a challenge for educators / edited by Lindsay Peer and Gavin Reid; foreword by David Blunkett. London: D. Fulton Publishers, 2000. Peer, Lindsay. Reid, Gavin, 1950- British Dyslexia Association. Description:

xiv, 304 p.: ill.; 24 cm. ISBN: 1853466964 (pbk.) LC Classification: LC4708.5.M85 2000 Dewey Class No.: 371.91/44 21 Other System No.: (UkLWHE)b000066161

Multiple-domain dissociation between impaired visual perception and preserved mental imagery in a patient with bilateral extrastriate lesions. Abstract: A brain-damaged patient is described whose pattern of performance provides insight into both the functional mechanisms and the neural structures involved in visual mental imagery. The patient became severely agnosic, alexic, achromatopsic and prosopagnosic following bilateral brain lesions in the temporo-occipital cortex. However, her mental imagery for the same visual entities that she could not perceive was perfectly preserved. paolo@broca.inserm.fr Bartolomeo P Bachoud-Levi AC De Gelder B Denes G Dalla Barba G Brugieres P + Degos JD Neuropsychologia 1998 Mar;36(3):239-49.

Multivariate behavioral genetic analysis of achievement and cognitive measures in reading-disabled and control twin pairs. Abstract: In recent years behavioral genetic studies have provided conclusive evidence that reading disability and related learning disorders, such as mathematics disability, are due at least in part to heritable factors (DeFries et al. 1987; Alarcon et al. 1997). Although the observed relationship between performance in these areas may be due substantially to genetic influences (Light and DeFries 1995; Thompson et al. 1991), relatively few studies have examined the genetic and environmental etiology of this covariation in a multivariate framework Light JG Defries JC Olson RK Hum Biol 1998 Apr;70(2):215-37.

Multivariate genetic analysis of Wechsler Intelligence Scale for Children--Revised (WISC-R) factors. Abstract: Wechsler Intelligence Scale for Children--Revised (WISC-R) factor scores (Verbal Comprehension, Perceptual Organization,

and Freedom from Distractibility) were obtained from 574 twin pairs in the Colorado Reading Project and subjected to multivariate genetic analysis. Variances were partitioned into components common to the three WISC-R factors and to those specific to each factor. Substantial commonality, both genetic and environmental, was found among the three factors. Casto SD DeFries JC Fulker DW Behav Genet 1995 Jan;25(1):25-32.

Music alexia in a patient with mild pure alexia: disturbed visual perception of nonverbal meaningful figures. Abstract: A 26-year-old female pianist suffered from an intracerebral hematoma caused by an arteriovenous malformation of the left occipital parasplenial region, which was operated on seven months after the onset. Incomplete right hemianopsia, mild pure alexia, and partially disturbed naming of visual objects persisted several months after the removal of the malformation. Evaluation of musical ability one and three months after surgery showed that her auditory recognition of music was intact, Horikoshi T Asari Y Watanabe A Nagaseki Y Nukui H Sasaki H Komiya K Cortex 1997 Mar;33(1):187-94.

Naidoo, Sandhya. Specific dyslexia: the research report of the ICAA Word Blind Centre for Dyslexic Children; introduction by Alfred White Franklin. London, Pitman, 1972. Invalid Children's Aid Association, London. Word Blind Centre for Dyslexic Children. Description: xv, 165 p. illus, forms. 23 cm. ISBN: 0273360930 LC Classification: RJ496.A5 N34 NLM Class No.: WL340 N155s 1972 Dewey Class No.: 618.9/28/553 National Bib. No.: B72-11459

Naidoo, Sandhya. Specific dyslexia; the research report of the ICAA Word Blind Centre for Dyslexic Children [by] Sandhya Naidoo. Introd. by Alfred White Franklin. New York, J. Wiley [1973, c1972] Invalid Children's Aid Association, London. Word Blind Centre for Dyslexic Children. Description: xv, 165 p. 23 cm. ISBN: 0470629150 LC Classification: RJ496.A5

N34 1973 NLM Class No.: WL340 N155s 1973 Dewey Class No.: 618.9/28/553

Naming and verbal memory skills in adults with Attention Deficit Hyperactivity Disorder and Reading Disability. Abstract: Research suggests that children with Attention Deficit Hyperactivity Disorder (ADHD) and Reading Disability (RD) can be differentiated based on their performance on measures of naming and verbal memory. It is not known whether this same pattern characterizes adults with these disorders. In this study, adults with and without ADHD and RD were compared on naming and verbal memory abilities. Rashid FL Morris MK Morris R J Clin Psychol 2001 Jun;57(6):829-38.

Naming speed performance and stimulant effects indicate effortful, semantic processing deficits in attention-deficit/hyperactivity disorder. Abstract: This study investigated rapid automatized naming and effects of stimulant medication in school-age children with attention-deficit/hyperactivity disorder (ADHD) with and without concurrent reading disorder (RD). Two ADHD groups (67 ADHD only; 21 ADHD + RD) and a control group of 27 healthy age-matched peers were compared on four variables: color naming speed, letter naming speed, phonologic decoding, and arithmetic computation. Discriminant function analysis (DFA) was conducted to predict group membership. Tannock R Martinussen R Frijters J J Abnorm Child Psychol 2000 Jun;28(3):237-52.

National Conference on Dyslexia, Philadelphia, 1966. Dyslexia; diagnosis and treatment of reading disorders. Edited by Arthur H. Keeney [and] Virginia T. Keeney. Saint Louis, Mosby, 1968. Keeney, Arthur H. (Arthur Hail), 1920- Keeney, Virginia T, ed. American Committee on Optics and Visual Physiology. United States. Public Health Service. Neurological and Sensory Disease Service Program. Description: xii, 182 p. illus. 26 cm. LC Classification:

LB1050.5.N3 1966aa Dewey Class No.: 372.4/13

National Institute of Mental Health Conference on Dyslexia, Rockville, Md, 1977. Dyslexia: an appraisal of current knowledge / edited by Arthur L. Benton, David Pearl. New York: Oxford University Press, 1978. Benton, Arthur Lester, 1909- Pearl, David, 1921- National Institute of Mental Health (U.S.) Description: xvii, 544 p.: ill.; 24 cm. ISBN: 0195023846: LC Classification: RJ496.A5 N37 1977 NLM Class No.: WM47.3 N277d 1977 Dewey Class No.: 616.8/553

NATO Advanced Study Institute on Developmental and Acquired Disorders of Reading and Writing Systems in Different Languages: a Cognitive Neuropsychological Perspective (1987: Il Ciocco, Italy) Reading and writing disorders in different orthographic systems / edited by P.G. Aaron and R. Malatesha Joshi. Dordrecht; Boston: Kluwer Academic Publishers, c1989. Aaron, P. G. Joshi, R. Malatesha. NATO Advanced Study Institute. Description: x, 416 p.: ill.; 25 cm. ISBN: 0792304616 LC Classification: LB1050.5.N33 1987 Dewey Class No.: 371.91/44 20

NATO Advanced Study Institute on Dyslexia: a Global Issue (1982: Maratea, Italy) Dyslexia: a global issue / edited by R.N. Malatesha and H.A. Whitaker. The Hague; Boston: Published in cooperation with NATO Scientific Affairs Division [by] M. Nijhoff; Hingham, MA, USA: distributors for the U.S. and Canada, Kluwer Boston, 1984. Malatesha, R. N. Whitaker, Harry A. North Atlantic Treaty Organization. Scientific Affairs Division. Description: ix, 590 p.: ill.; 24 cm. ISBN: 9024729092 LC Classification: RJ496.A5 N38 1982 Dewey Class No.: 616.85/53 19 Series:

NATO Advanced Study Institute on Neuropsychology and Cognition (1980: Augusta, Ga.) Neuropsychology and cognition: proceedings of the NATO Advanced Study Institute on

Neuropsychology and Cognition, Augusta, Georgia, U.S.A, September 8-18, 1980 / edited by R.N. Malatesha and L.C. Hartlage. The Hague; Boston: M. Nijhoff Publishers; Hingham, MA: Distributors for the U.S. and Canada, Kluwer Boston, 1982. Malatesha, R. N. Hartlage, Lawrence C. Description: 2 v.: ill.; 25 cm. ISBN: 9024727278 (v. 1) 9024727286 (v. 2) LC Classification: QP360.N37 1980 NLM Class No.: W1 102 N279n 1980 Dewey Class No.: 612/.82 19

Need for serious debate on remedial and dyslexia-classes Gulfe A Lakartidningen 1995 Oct 18;92(42):3869.

Neocortical ectopias are associated with attenuated neurophysiological responses to rapidly changing auditory stimuli. Abstract: Developmental dyslexia has been separately associated with the presence of ectopic collections of neurons in layer I of neocortex (ectopias) and with alterations in processing rapidly changing stimuli. We have used BXSB/MpJ-Yaa mice, some of which have neocortical ectopias, to directly test the hypothesis that ectopias may alter auditory processing. Auditory event related potentials (AERPs) were elicited by pairs of 10.5 kHz tones separated by silence, 0.99 kHz, or 5.6 kHz tones of variable duration Frenkel M Sherman GF Bashan KA Galaburda AM LoTurco JJ Neuroreport 2000 Feb 28;11(3):575-9.

Neural systems affected in developmental dyslexia revealed by functional neuroimaging. Eden GF Zeffiro TA Neuron 1998 Aug;21(2):279-82.

Neuroanatomical, neuroradiological and functional magnetic resonance imaging correlates of developmental dyslexia Abstract: Neuropathological data in dyslexia has demonstrated alterations in the symmetry normally present in the planum temporale, as well as microdysgenesis in superficial cortical layers and disruption of the cytoarchitecture in subcortical structures. Neuroradiological and functional neuroimaging studies in dyslexia are consistent with localization of dysfunction to the temporoparietal junction. Present neuropathological and neuroimaging data support the concept that the fundamental problem in developmental dyslexia is a phonologic deficit. Tuchman RF Rev Neurol 1999 Aug 16-31;29(4):322-6.

Neurobehavioral phenotype of Klinefelter syndrome. Abstract: A defined genetic syndrome with neurobehavioral components offers an unusual paradigm for the correlation of genetic defects with neurodevelopmental abnormalities. The power of the combination of detailed behavioral, neuroanatomical, and genetic studies has been demonstrated in studies of other conditions involving the sex chromosomes, such as Fragile X syndrome (Mazzocco [2000] Ment Retard Develop Disabil Res Rev. 6:96-106) and Turner syndrome (Ross [2000] Ment Retard Develop Disabil Res Rev. 6:135-141 Ment Retard Dev Disabil Res Rev 2000;6(2):107-16.

Neurobiologic correlates of developmental dyslexia: how do dyslexics' brains differ from those of normal readers? Filipek PA J Child Neurol 1995 Jan;10 Suppl 1:S62-9.

Neurobiological studies of reading and reading disability. Abstract: Evidence from neuroimaging studies, including our own, suggest that skilled word identification in reading is related to the functional integrity of two consolidated left hemisphere (LH) posterior systems: a dorsal (temporo-parietal) circuit and a ventral (occipito-temporal) circuit. This posterior system appears to be functionally disrupted in developmental dyslexia. Relative to nonimpaired readers, reading-disabled individuals demonstrate heightened reliance on both inferior frontal and right hemisphere posterior regions, presumably in compensation for the LH posterior difficulties. Pugh KR Mencl WE Jenner AR Katz L Frost SJ Lee JR Shaywitz SE Shaywitz BA J Commun Disord 2001 Nov-Dec;34(6):479-92.

Neurobiology of learning disabilities. Abstract: Learning disabilities are the product of neurological damage which occurs during fetal development. The malformations produced are unique to each individual and do not resemble acquired neurological damage. Consequently, models of developmental disorders must be developed independently and cannot be based on acquired adult aphasia or dyslexia literature. Neurological conditions of adults with developmental disorders are difficult to interpret since aberrations that occur early during fetal development can have a cascading effect, disrupting neural organization in other brain regions. Chase CH Semin Speech Lang 1996 Aug;17(3):173-81.

Neurocognitive and pharmacological approach to specific learning disorders Abstract: Specific learning disorders are distinguished from general development disorders since, in general, only a certain number of processing mechanisms are involved whilst the remainder are unaffected. Etchepareborda MC Rev Neurol 1999 Feb;28 Suppl 2:S81-93.

Neurocognitive stability in Asperger syndrome, ADHD, and reading and writing disorder: a pilot study. Abstract: Boys with Asperger syndrome (n=20), attention-deficit-hyperactivity disorder (n=20), and reading and writing disorder (n=20) were followed up and retested on several neuropsychological measures 1 to 2 years after initial assessments. Wechsler Intelligence Scale for Children (WISC-III) Full Scale, Verbal, and Performance IQ scores remained stable for all diagnostic groups. Kaufman factors and 'fluid' and 'crystallized' abilities were stable measures. Subtest stability over time, was slightly more variable. Nyden A Billstedt E Hjelmquist E Gillberg C Dev Med Child Neurol 2001 Mar;43(3):165-71.

Neuroimaging findings in a patient recovering from global alexia to spelling dyslexia. Abstract: The authors report findings in a 67-year-old right-handed man who had an ischemic infarct in the territory of the left posterior cerebral artery. The clinical manifestation consisted mainly of total alexia without agraphia. The patient gradually recovered, subsequently showing the syndrome of spelling dyslexia. Cerebral MR-images revealed a circumscript infarction of medial and basal parts of left temporal lobe. Lanzinger S Weder B Oettli R Fretz C J Neuroimaging 1999 Jan;9(1):48-51.

Neuroimaging in child and adolescent neuropsychiatric disorders. Abstract: To review the major findings and pathophysiological implications of imaging studies of neuropsychiatric disorders that onset in childhood or adolescence. Neuroimaging data regarding pathological central nervous system development in childhood are still sparse, and many of the findings in developmental disorders of childhood onset concern the study of adult subjects with those disorders. Nevertheless, imaging modalities previously used only in adults are with increasing frequency being applied to the study of children, which will likely continue to contribute to the understanding of pathological brain structure and function throughout childhood and to the improved treatment of these disorders. Peterson BS J Am Acad Child Adolesc Psychiatry 1995 Dec;34(12):1560-76.

Neuroimaging in the developmental disorders: the state of the science. Abstract: The developmental disorders of childhood autistic, developmental language, reading (dyslexia), and attention deficit-hyperactivity disorders-manifest with deficits in the traditional behavioral domains of cognition, language, visual-spatial function, attention, and socialization. However, none of these disorders has been associated with characteristic discrete focal lesions or recognized encephaloclastic processes. Developmental cognitive neuroscientists must therefore begin with the spectrum of sometimes divergent behaviors occurring within these disorders and work backward in an attempt to identify the responsible anomalous neural systems. Since the advent of "brain imaging" two decades ago, much effort has focused on identifying brain-behavior correlates in these disorders. Filipek PA J Child Psychol Psychiatry 1999 Jan;40(1):113-28.

Neurological assessment for learning disability Abstract: Learning disabilities present a diagnostic and therapeutic management challenge that requires an interdisciplinary approach initiated and coordinated by the child neurologist. An optimal evaluation for these conditions must include an extensive knowledge of the types and range of these disorders, a complete neurological and laboratory examination, a neuropsychological assessment tailored to the individual needs of the patient, a speech pathological evaluation when pertinent, and special attention to the frequent co-occurrence of more than one condition susceptible of interfering with learning. Kuljis RO Rev Neurol 1999 Aug 16-31;29(4):326-31.

Neurological assessment of learning disorders Abstract: The neurological concept of learning is approached from a cybernetic point of view, taking into account that a child should recognize a fact, learn it semantically and decided whether it is worth storing; the dynamic aspect of memory is the true motor of the ability to learn and all this is modulated by the attention factor. The contribution of neurological assessment is considered as part of the functions of a multi-disciplinary team which should deal with the diagnosis and treatment of children with learning disorders. Campos-Castello J Rev Neurol 1998 Aug;27(156):280-5.

Neuronal asymmetries in primary visual cortex of dyslexic and nondyslexic brains. Abstract: Dyslexic brains exhibit histologic changes in the magnocellular (magno) cells of the lateral geniculate nucleus, and consistent with these changes, dyslexics demonstrate abnormal visually evoked potentials and brain activation to magno-specific stimuli. The current study was aimed at determining whether these findings were associated with changes in the primary visual cortex with the prediction that magno components of this cortex would be affected. We measured cross-sectional neuronal areas in primary visual cortex (area 17) in dyslexic and nondyslexic autopsy specimens. Jenner AR Rosen GD Galaburda AM Ann Neurol 1999 Aug;46(2):189-96.

Neurophysiological measures of reading difficulty in very-low-birthweight children. Abstract: Twenty-four 8-10-year-old children (13 very low birthweight, 11 control) performed a lexical decision and a semantic classification task while event-related potentials (ERPs) were recorded. Both groups were within normal range on standardized reading tests, but the very-low-birthweight group had lower scores. There were no differences between groups in reaction times or accuracy for ERP tasks. On analyses of P2a (246 ms anteriorly), P2p (336 ms posteriorly), N2a (356 ms anteriorly), and N2p (396 ms posteriorly) peaks and a late positive component, control children showed greater right than left asymmetry at P2p and greater left than right asymmetry at N2a. Very-low-birthweight children showed less asymmetry. Khan SC Frisk V Taylor MJ Psychophysiology 1999 Jan;36(1):76-85.

Neurophysiology of fluent and impaired reading: a magnetoencephalographic approach. Abstract: This article reviews a series of magnetoencephalographic (MEG) experiments aimed at identifying cortical areas and time windows relevant or even critical for fluent reading. The approach was to compare single-word processing in fluent and dyslexic readers. The activations which differed between the two groups were then studied in more detail to determine their functional roles. In fluent reading, overall visual feature processing occurs about 100 milliseconds (ms) after seeing a word, in the posteromedial extrastriate cortex bilaterally. Salmelin R Helenius P Service E J Clin Neurophysiol 2000 Mar;17(2):163-74.

Neuropsychiatric problems among children are signigicantly underdiagnosed. Intervention programs result in better and less expensive care Abstract: Neuropsychiatric problems (Asperger syndrome, ADHD, reading and writing disorders) affect 6-10 per cent of all children in Sweden. Many of these disorders are never diagnosed. As a consequence, secondary behaviour problems and impaired family relations often follow. A study of 60 families with at least one child affected by one of the above mentioned disorders shows that quality of life can be increased and problems reduced if parents and children are informed of the child's disabilities and the child receives a special education programme. Nyden A Paananen M Gillberg C Lakartidningen 2000 Nov 29;97(48):5634-9, 5641.

Neuropsychological and cognitive processes in reading / edited by Francis J. Pirozzolo, Merlin C. Wittrock. New York: Academic Press, 1981. Pirozzolo, Francis J. Wittrock, M. C. (Merlin C.), 1931- Description: xvii, 344 p.: ill.; 24 cm. Cancelled ISBN: 012577360X: LC Classification: BF456.R2 N43 NLM Class No.: WM 475 N494 Dewey Class No.: 153.6 19

Neuropsychological approach to the learning disability: the correlation between neuropsychological findings and rCBF Abstract: We investigated the relationship between a disorder of higher brain function and the area of reduced regional cerebral blood flow (rCBF) in learning disabled (LD) children. Subjects consisted of two LD children with a specific Kanji writing disorder, one with dyslexia and dysgraphia and two with a specific verbal semantic disorder. Neuropsychological assessment batteries were used to detect higher brain disorders, and single photon emission tomography to measure rCBF. We found that the area of reduced rCBF in LD children correspond to that in adults with an acquired brain damage showing similar symptoms. Uno A No To Hattatsu 1999 May;31(3):237-43.

Neuropsychological correlates of childhood attention-deficit/hyperactivity disorder: explainable by comorbid disruptive behavior or reading problems? Abstract: Questions remain as to whether neuropsychological processing deficits associated with child attention-deficit/hyperactivity disorder (ADHD) are accounted for by co-occurring disorders, especially in clinical samples. The authors examined ADHD and comorbid oppositional defiant, conduct, and reading disorders. Boys with ADHD displayed hypothesized deficits on effortful neuropsychological tasks regardless of categorical or dimensional control of comorbid antisocial behavior problems. Nigg JT Hinshaw SP Carte ET Treuting JJ J Abnorm Psychol 1998 Aug;107(3):468-80.

Neuropsychological evidence for case-specific reading: multi-letter units in visual word recognition. Abstract: We describe a patient (GK) who shows symptoms associated with Balint's syndrome and attentional dyslexia. GK was able to read words, but not nonwords. He made many misidentification and mislocation errors when reporting letters in words, suggesting that his word-naming ability did not depend upon preserved position-coded, letter identification. We show that GK was able to read lower-case words better than upper-case words, but upper-case abbreviations better than lower-case abbreviations. Hall DA Humphreys GW Cooper AC Q J Exp Psychol A 2001 May;54(2):439-67.

Neuropsychological long-term outcome of rolandic EEG traits. Abstract: Long-term outcome of rolandic epilepsy (RE) is associated with a diversity of neuropsychological deficits in childhood, although RE is historically considered as a benign epileptic disorder. Dyslexia and other developmental disorders are associated with rolandic EEG traits. In general, both dyslectic groups did not show significant neuropsychological deficits as compared to standard controls. However, there were more reading errors and a tendency to attention impairments in the group with rolandic EEG trait as compared to the dyslectic group with normal EEG. Possible pathogenic factors are discussed. Carlsson G Igelbrink-Schulze N Neubauer BA Stephani U Epileptic Disord 2000;2 Suppl 1:S63-6.

Neuropsychological profiles of adults with Klinefelter syndrome. Abstract: Children and adolescents with Klinefelter syndrome (XXY) have been reported to show deficits in language processing including VIQ < PIQ and a learning disability in reading and spelling. However, whether this is characteristic of adults with Klinefelter syndrome has not been established. Thirty-five men with Klinefelter syndrome, aged 16 to 61, and 22 controls were evaluated with a comprehensive neuropsychological battery. J Int Neuropsychol Soc 2001 May;7(4):446-56.

Neuropsychology of normal pressure hydrocephalus Abstract: Although dementia is described as one of the constituent characteristics of normal pressure hydrocephalus (NPH), alongside gait disturbances and urinary incontinence, there is a rather limited number of controlled studies concerning neuropsychological deficits in the disease. A wide range of psychopathologically relevant symptoms have been described, but the common features of most cases include mental and motor slowing, apathy, emotional indifference, anosognosia, memory and attentional impairment. Merten T Nervenarzt 1999 Jun;70(6):496-503.

Neuroscience. Dyslexia: same brains, different languages. Helmuth L Science 2001 Mar 16;291(5511):2064-5.

Nevada. Legislature. Legislative Commission. Study of dyslexia and other specific learning disabilities / Legislative Commission of the Legislative Counsel Bureau, State of Nevada. [Carson City, Nev.]: The Commission, [1984] Description: x, 64 p.; 28 cm. LC Classification: RC394.W6 N48 1984

New gene targets related to schizophrenia and other psychiatric disorders: enzymes, binding proteins and transport proteins involved in phospholipid and fatty acid metabolism. Abstract: Phospholipids make up about 60% of the brain's dry weight. In spite of this, phospholipid metabolism has received relatively little attention from those seeking genetic factors involved in psychiatric and neurological disorders. However, there is now increasing evidence from many quarters that abnormal phospholipid and related fatty acid metabolism may contribute to illnesses such as schizophrenia, bipolar disorder, depression and attention deficit hyperactivity disorder. To date the possible specific proteins and genes involved have been relatively ill-defined. Horrobin DF Bennett CN Prostaglandins Leukot Essent Fatty Acids 1999 Mar;60(3):141-67.

Newton, Margaret, M.Sc. Dyslexia: a guide for teachers and parents / Margaret Newton, Michael Thomson. London: University of London Press, 1975. Thomson, Michael E., joint author. Description: viii, 56 p.; 20 cm. ISBN: 0340200499: LC Classification: LB1050.5.N48 Dewey Class No.: 371.9/14 National Bib. No.: GB 75-09534

Niemeyer, Wilhelm. Legastenie und Milieu: ein Beitr. z. Ätiologie u. Therapie d. Lese-Rechtschreibschwäche (LRS) / Wilhelm Niemeyer. Hannover; Dortmund; Darmstadt; Berlin: Schroedel, 1974. Description: 226 p.; 23 cm. ISBN: 3507391023: LC Classification: LB1050.5.N53 National Bib. No.: GFR74-A

Niemeyer, Wilhelm. Lese- und Rechtschreibschwäche: Theorie, Diagnose, Therapie u. Prophylaxe / Wilhelm Niemeyer. Edition Information: 1. Aufl. Stuttgart; Berlin; Koln; Mainz: Kohlhammer, 1978. Description: 176 p.; 21 cm. ISBN: 3170043609: LC Classification: LB1050.5.N54 National Bib. No.: GFR78-A

Nithsdale schizophrenia surveys 21: a longitudinal study of National Adult Reading Test stability. Abstract: The stability of the National Adult Reading Test (NART) as a measure of pre-morbid intelligence in schizophrenia has not yet been satisfactorily established despite the widespread use of the NART in schizophrenia research. Our results provide the necessary evidence that the NART can be used as a stable measure of pre-morbid intelligence in schizophrenia. Morrison G Sharkey V Allardyce J Kelly RC McCreadie RG Psychol Med 2000 May;30(3):717-20.

Nitsopoulos, M‾enas. Vo‾etheiste to paidi sas / M‾ena Nitsopoulou. Thessalonik‾e: Ekdotik‾e Homada, 1987. Description: 93 p.: ill.; 21 cm. LC Classification: RC394.W6 N5 1987

No confirmation of Geschwind's hypothesis of associations between reading disability, immune disorders, and motor preference in ADHD. Abstract: Geschwind and colleagues have proposed an association among reading disability, immune disorder, and motor preference. Although reading disability commonly overlaps with attention deficit hyperactivity disorder (ADHD), ADHD has not been previously examined in studies evaluating Geschwind's hypothesis. In this paper we evaluate whether ADHD is associated with either asthma or left motor preference and whether asthma and left motor preference are associated with each other. Subjects were 6- to 17-year-old boys with DSM-III-R ADHD (n = 140) and normal controls (n = 120). Biederman J Milberger S Faraone SV Lapey KA Reed ED Seidman LJ J Abnorm Child Psychol 1995 Oct;23(5):545-52.

No deficits at the point of hemispheric indecision. Abstract: This study attempted to replicate a recent finding by Crow et al. [Neuropsychologia 36 (1998) 1275] showing that about equal skill of right and left hand (i.e. hemispheric indecision) is associated with deficits in cognitive and scholastic achievement. The present study assessed hemispheric indecision by using Annett's [Left, Right, Hand and Brain: The Right Shift Theory, Lawrence Erlbaum, London, 1985] peg moving test and by assessing the consistency of hand preference at school entrance. Non-verbal intelligence, reading and spelling accuracy were assessed about three years later. Mayringer H Wimmer H Neuropsychologia 2002;40(7):701-4.

Non-impaired auditory phase locking in dyslexic adults. Abstract: Dyslexic adults have profound difficulties in discriminating rapidly presented sound sequences. To test whether these deficits might be caused by impaired neuronal phase locking to the envelopes of the sound stimuli, 20 normal-reading and 13 dyslexic adults discriminated pitches of pure tones at approximately 1 kHz (producing spectral pitch due to place coding in the cochlea) and of approximately 80 Hz amplitude modulations of white noise (producing periodicity pitch based on temporal information only. Hari R Saaskilahti A Helenius P Uutela K Neuroreport 1999 Aug 2;10(11):2347-8.

Nonlinguistic perceptual deficits associated with reading and language disorders. Abstract: Recent behavioral evidence supports the idea that some individuals with reading and language disorders are impaired in their perception of nonlinguistic auditory and visual information. More sophisticated measurement paradigms and analysis techniques are leading to a clearer understanding of these deficits and to possibilities for their remediation. Wright BA Bowen RW Zecker SG Curr Opin Neurobiol 2000 Aug;10(4):482-6.

Noradrenergic mechanisms in ADHD children with and without reading disabilities: a replication and extension. Abstract: To examine noradrenergic (NA) function in children with attention-deficit hyperactivity disorder (ADHD) by replicating and expanding upon a previous finding that ADHD children with and without reading disabilities (RD) differ in plasma levels of the NA metabolite 3-methoxy-4-hydroxyphenylglycol (MHPG). These data indicate that children with ADHD are not homogeneous with regard to NA function and that neurochemical variation is closely associated with differences in clinical characteristics of the children. Halperin JM Newcorn JH Koda VH Pick L McKay KE Knott P J Am Acad Child Adolesc Psychiatry 1997 Dec;36(12):1688-97.

Normal planum temporale asymmetry in dyslexics with a magnocellular pathway deficit. Abstract: Developmental dyslexia has been associated with both abnormal hemispheric symmetry of the planum temporale (PT) and a deficit in the magnocellular visual pathway. We examined the relationship between these two abnormalities. Using sagittal magnetic resonance images and three methods, we measured the PT in dyslexic subjects with a documented magnocellular deficit and controls. Dyslexic subjects did not deviate from normal leftward PT asymmetry, but both groups became less left-lateralized with methods that excluded sulcul tissue. Best M Demb JB Neuroreport 1999 Feb 25;10(3):607-12.

Nosek, Kathleen. Dyslexia in adults: taking charge of your life / Kathleen Nosek. Dallas, Tex.: Taylor Pub. Co, c1997. Description: xiv, 192 p.; 23 cm. ISBN: 0878339485 (pb) LC Classification: RC394.W6 N67 1997 Dewey Class No.: 616.85/53 21

Not all dyslexics are created equal. Abstract: Dyslexia is a common disorder that has traditionally been treated as a homogeneous condition. However, recent evidence indicates that it is a heterogenous condition with several subtypes. For example, studies of the visual system indicate that not all dyslexics have a normal visual pathway. Approximately 75% have a processing deficit in the magnocellular pathway. Our previous study indicated that dysphoneidetic but not dyseidetic dyslexics exhibit a

magnocellular pathway defect These results suggest that treatment strategies for dyslexics may need to be modified to take into account their specific subtype. Ridder WH 3rd Borsting E Cooper M McNeel B Huang E Optom Vis Sci 1997 Feb;74(2):99-104.

Number processing and calculation in a case of visual agnosia. Abstract: We describe the performance of a brain-damaged subject who suffered from visual agnosia leading to major difficulties in generating and exploiting visual representations from long-term memory. His performance in a physical judgement task in which he was required to answer questions about the visual shapes of Arabic numerals reflected his agnosic problems. However, he showed no impairment in usual number processing and calculation tasks. Pesenti M Thioux M Samson D Bruyer R Seron X Cortex 2000 Jun;36(3):377-400.

Nursing students with disabilities: a survey of baccalaureate nursing programs. Abstract: In an effort to raise awareness of critical issues regarding the obligations of institutions of higher learning to accept and accommodate qualified disabled students, this study surveyed 247 baccalaureate nursing programs to determine their responses and reactions to applicants and students with disabilities. Almost half of the programs responding to the survey reported admitting students with disabilities, the most prevalent of which were dyslexia and other learning disabilities. Watson PG J Prof Nurs 1995 May-Jun;11(3):147-53.

Objective improvement from base-in prisms for reading discomfort associated with mini-convergence insufficiency type exophoria in school children. Abstract: To determine whether base-in prism glasses could diminish asthenopia, and improve reading abilities (speed, accuracy and comprehension). Base-in prism glasses improve subjective reading comfort and abilities (speed, accuracy and comprehension) in these patients. Stavis M Murray M Jenkins P Wood R Brenham B

Jass J Binocul Vis Strabismus Q 2002 Summer;17(2):135-42.

Objects and properties: a study of the breakdown of semantic memory. Abstract: This paper reports a study of the breakdown of semantic memory in the case of a subject with semantic dementia. The first experiment shows that the subject failed to comprehend words of low familiarity and word frequency, even though the spoken word forms were recognised as familiar. Experiments 2 and 3 showed (a) that the recall of word meanings in definition tasks did not vary with the generality of the word meaning (e.g. category, basic level, or subordinate property) but varied instead with the concept familiarity and frequency of the name; (b) that the ability to verify properties of basic-level objects was not affected by the ability to comprehend the property name, but depended instead on the degree of knowledge demonstrated for the object name in definition tasks; (c) that properties were frequently verified correctly when the object had been defined only to the superordinate level. Funnell E Memory 1995 Sep-Dec;3(3-4):497-518.

Ocular manifestations of pediatric disease. Abstract: A review of the ocular manifestations of pediatric disease is in some ways a review of pediatrics itself. A paper this size cannot hope to be comprehensive in scope or encyclopedic in detail. Instead, we have chosen to touch on recent developments in pediatrics that we feel may be of particular interest to the ophthalmologist, as well as certain areas of pediatric ophthalmology that make it clear that a child's ocular disease takes place in the larger context of the growing child. Kelly CJ Calhoun JH Curr Opin Ophthalmol 1998 Dec;9(6):111-5.

Oehrle, Brigitte D. Visuelle Wahrnehmung und Legasthenie: Literaturbericht u. empir. Untersuchung z. Theorie d. visuellen Formauffassungsstörungen bei Legasthenikern / Brigitte D. Oehrle. Weinheim; Basel: Beltz, 1975. Description: 201 p.: ill.; 21 cm. ISBN:

3407545185: LC Classification: LB1050.5.O33 National Bib. No.: GFR75-A

Oliver, Diana. Tough luck, Ronnie / by Diana Oliver. New York: Random House, c1994. Description: 124 p.; 20 cm. ISBN: 0679854754 (pbk.): LC Classification: PZ7.O4686 To 1994 Dewey Class No.: [Fic] 20 Other System No.: (OCoLC)29898823

On a failure to replicate: methodologically close, but not close enough. A response to hogben et al. Abstract: Williams, Brannan and Lartigue (1987) (Clinical Vision Science, 1, 367-371) reported that poor readers took significantly longer to search letter arrays for a target than did good readers. In addition, they reported that blurring the letter arrays leads to faster search times for poor readers and a loss of the significant differences between the groups seen with unblurred displays. In a recent attempt to replicate these findings, Hogben et al. (1996) (Vision Research, 36, 1503-1507) found no differences in search rates between good and poor readers using unblurred arrays, and no differences in search rate between the groups when blurred arrays were used. Vision Res 1996 May;36(10):1509-11.

On being dyslexic. An inside view. Simon CS ASHA 1999 Mar-Apr;41(2):18-23.

On subtypes of developmental dyslexia: evidence from processing time and accuracy scores. Abstract: Phonological dyslexics (Ph-DYS) are characterized by a phonological deficit, while surface dyslexics (S-DYS) are characterized by an orthographic deficit. Four issues were addressed in this study. First, we determined the proportion of Ph-DYS and S-DYS in a population of French dyslexics by applying Castles and Coltheart's (1993) regression method to two previously unused diagnostic measures: pseudo-word and irregular-word processing time. Thirty-one dyslexics were matched to 19 average readers of the same age (10 years, CA controls) and to 19 younger children of the same reading level (8 years, RL controls). Sprenger-Charolles L Cole P Lacert P Serniclaes W Can J Exp Psychol 2000 Jun;54(2):87-104.

On the "specifics" of specific reading disability and specific language impairment. Abstract: The reading and oral language scores of 110 children with a specific reading disability (SRD) and 102 children with a specific language impairment (SLI) indicated that approximately 53% of children with an SRD and children with an SLI could be equally classified as having an SRD or an SLI, 55% of children with an SRD have impaired oral language, and 51% of children with an SLI have a reading disability. Finding that a large percentage of children can be equally classified as SRD or SLI has repercussions for the criteria used to define an SRD, for conceptualising subgroups of learning disability, and for estimates of the incidence of SRD. McArthur GM Hogben JH Edwards VT Heath SM Mengler ED J Child Psychol Psychiatry 2000 Oct;41(7):869-74.

On the bases of two subtypes of developmental [corrected] dyslexia. Abstract: This study examined whether there are different subtypes of developmental dyslexia. The subjects were 51 dyslexic children (reading below the 30th percentile in isolated word recognition), 51 age-matched normal readers, and 27 younger normal readers who scored in the same range as the dyslexics on word recognition. Using methods developed by Castles and Coltheart (1993), we identified two subgroups who fit the profiles commonly termed "surface" and "phonological" dyslexia. Surface subjects were relatively poorer in reading exception words compared to nonwords; phonological dyslexics showed the opposite pattern. Manis FR Seidenberg MS Doi LM McBride-Chang C Petersen A Cognition 1996 Feb;58(2):157-95.

On the benefits of direct teaching of spelling in children's language arts instruction. Abstract: Three studies involved 5 children, ages 6 to 8 years, who were experiencing difficulty in learning skills in reading. Each participated in several spelling tasks which led to improved reading skills, perhaps because stimulus were formed. Stromer R Percept Mot Skills 1996 Oct;83(2):701-2.

On the production and correction of involuntary prosaccades in a gap antisaccade task. Abstract: In an antisaccade task, where saccades in the direction opposite of a suddenly presented stimulus are required, certain numbers of prosaccades can occur. The hypothesis is put forward that poor fixation and poor voluntary saccade control constitute two independent sources for the errors. This possibility is investigated by including the corrections of the errors in the analysis. First, the eye movements of 346 normal subjects (group N) performing a gap antisaccade and an overlap prosaccade task were measured. For each subject the proportion of express saccades in the overlap prosaccade task and the proportion of prosaccades in the gap antisaccade task were determined. Fischer B Gezeck S Hartnegg K Vision Res 2000;40(16):2211-7.

On the use of metacontrast to assess magnocellular function in dyslexic readers. Abstract: It has been proposed that dyslexia is the result of a deficit in the magnocellular system. Reduced metacontrast masking in dyslexic readers has been taken as support for this view. In metacontrast, a masking stimulus reduces the visibility of a spatially adjacent target stimulus when the target stimulus precedes the masking stimulus by about 30-100 msec. Recent evidence indicates that the latency difference between the magnocellular and parvocellular subcortical pathways is at most 20 msec and may be as small as only 5 msec, or even less. Skottun BC Percept Psychophys 2001 Oct;63(7):1271-4.

On the use of the Ternus test to assess magnocellular function. Abstract: Ternus stimuli give rise to two mutually exclusive visual experiences: with long interstimulus intervals (ISIs) the elements in the stimulus are perceived as moving together as a group ('group movement'), while at shorter ISIs only a single element appears to be moving ('element movement' or 'end-to-end movement'). It has been hypothesized that group and element movements, respectively, reflect magnocellular and parvocellular activity. On this basis, Ternus tests have been used to assess magnocellular function in dyslexic individuals. Skottun BC Perception 2001;30(12):1449-57.

Optic aphasia with pure alexia: a mild form of visual associative agnosia? A case study. Abstract: A single-case study is reported of a naming disorder selective to the visual modality. The patient showed intact access to structural knowledge of objects and letters, but impaired access to complete semantic knowledge of objects and alphabetical knowledge of letters from visual input. The impairment was most striking when the patient had to discriminate between semantically similar objects or within a given symbolic repertoire, i.e. letters. The co-occurrence of a partial deficit of visual recognition for objects and for letters indicated features of optic aphasia and pure alexia. Chanoine V Ferreira CT Demonet JF Nespoulous JL Poncet M Cortex 1998 Jun;34(3):437-48.

Optic aphasia: evidence of the contribution of different neural systems to object and action naming. Abstract: Visual stimulus naming was studied in a 66-year-old male patient with optic aphasia subsequent to left occipito-temporal infarction. While having difficulty in naming objects perceived visually, he was able to name objects by viewing gestures illustrating their use, and to name actions shown in pictures. These results suggest that naming performance depends on the kind of stimulus that is visually presented (object vs. action. Ferreira CT Giusiano B Ceccaldi M Poncet M Cortex 1997 Sep;33(3):499-513.

Optometric correlates of Meares-Irlen syndrome: a matched group study. Abstract: People who report visual perceptual distortions, typically when reading, that are alleviated by using coloured filters are described as suffering from 'Meares-Irlen Syndrome'. A recent double-masked placebo-controlled trial showed that this condition cannot be solely explained as a placebo effect and that the beneficial filter is idiosyncratic and sometimes needs to be highly specific. Several mechanisms have been suggested for Meares-Irlen Syndrome including ocular motor (binocular and accommodative) anomalies, a sensitivity to patterned stimuli (pattern glare), and a deficit of the transient visual sub-system. Evans BJ Busby A Jeanes R Wilkins AJ Ophthalmic Physiol Opt 1995 Sep;15(5):481-7.

Optometric management of reading dysfunction / John R. Griffin... [et al.]. Boston: Butterworth-Heinemann, 1996. Griffin, John R, 1934- Description: viii, 254 p.: ill.; 27 cm. ISBN: 0750695161 LC Classification: RJ61.O68 1996 NLM Class No.: WL 340.6 O62 1996 Dewey Class No.: 616.85/5306 20

Optometric vision therapy and training for learning disabilities and dyslexia: DVD surgery; curing complications of strabismus surgery. Romano PE Binocul Vis Strabismus Q 2002 Spring;17(1):12-4.

Optometric vision therapy. Gallaway M Binocul Vis Strabismus Q 2002 Summer;17(2):82.

Oral hygiene dyslexia. A fresh approach to a frustrating problem. Waese S Ont Dent 1996 Apr;73(3):29-30.

Oral reading in Chinese: evidence from dementia of the Alzheimer's type. Abstract: The traditional view of oral reading ability in patients with dementia holds that it is a preserved skill even if there is a general impairment to lexico-semantic processing ability. Recently, this view has been challenged by studies showing that the oral reading ability of patients with dementia can deteriorate over the course of the disease. These studies have found that the oral reading of irregular English words is more prone to error than the oral reading of regular words by patients with dementia suggesting that the oral reading of irregular words depends upon support from semantic memory Weekes B Int J Lang Commun Disord 2000 Oct-Dec;35(4):543-59.

Orienting of visual attention in dyslexia: evidence for asymmetric hemispheric control of attention. Abstract: The control of attentional orienting was studied in children with specific reading disorder (SRD) or dyslexia, and it was compared with that of normal readers. We used the covert orienting paradigm to measure subjects' reaction times for target detection both in valid and invalid cue conditions, either in the left or in the right visual fields. In experiment 1, we investigated exogenous orienting. The cue consisted of a peripheral abrupt onset and the cue-target delay was 350 ms. As compared with normal readers, in dyslexics the cue effect was absent in the right visual field, whereas in the left visual field a greater cue effect was observed. Facoetti A Turatto M LorusJournalML Mascetti GG Exp Brain Res 2001 May 1;138(1):46-53.

Orthographic analogies and developmental dyslexia. Abstract: Goswami (1986, 1988) has demonstrated that children can use orthographic analogies (particularly at the onset-rime level) between the spelling patterns in words to help to decode new words (e.g. using 'beak' to read 'peak'). This strategy has been shown in children as young as six years old. Since it is known that children with developmental dyslexia find it particularly difficult to read words that they have not been specifically taught (Lovett, Warren-Chaplin, Ransby & Borden, 1990), the present study investigated whether dyslexic children might be unable to use analogies. Hanley JR Reynolds CJ Thornton A Br J Psychol 1997 Aug;88 (Pt 3):423-40.

Orthographies and reading: perspectives from cognitive psychology, neuropsychology, and linguistics / edited by Leslie Henderson. London; Hillsdale, N.J.: L. Erlbaum Associates, c1984. Henderson, Leslie. Description: 143 p.: ill.; 24 cm. ISBN: 0863770096 LC Classification: LB1050.O75 1984 Dewey Class No.: 428.4 19

Orthography, reading, and dyslexia / edited by James F. Kavanagh and Richard L. Venezky. Baltimore: University Park Press, c1980. Kavanagh, James F. Venezky, Richard L. National Institute of Child Health and Human Development (U.S.) Description: xvii, 325 p.: ill.; 24 cm. ISBN: 0839115598 LC Classification: P240.2.O77 Dewey Class No.: 411 19

Orton, Samuel Torrey, 1879-1948. Word-blindness in school children and other papers on strephosymbolia (specific language disability-dyslexia) 1925-1946. Compiled by June Lyday Orton. Pomfret, Conn, Orton Society, 1966. Description: viii, 280 p. illus, port. 23 cm. LC Classification: RC394.W6 O7 Dewey Class No.: 616.85/5 Other System No.: (OCoLC)965783

Osmond, John. The reality of dyslexia / John Osmond. Edition Information: U.S. ed. Cambridge, Mass.: Brookline Books, 1995. Description: x, 150 p.: ill.; 23 cm. ISBN: 1571290176 (pbk.) LC Classification: RC394.W6 O86 1995 Dewey Class No.: 616.85/53 20

Osmond, John. The reality of dyslexia / John Osmond; with a foreword by T.R. Miles. London: Cassell in association with Channel Four Television, 1993. Channel Four (Great Britain) Description: xii, 132 p.: ill.; 22 cm. ISBN: 0304327638 (pbk) 030432762X (cased) LC Classification: RC394.W6 O86 1993 Dewey Class No.: 616.85/53 20 Other System No.: (OCoLC)29182039

Outpatient treatment of dyslexia through stimulation of the cerebral hemispheres. Abstract: Although a number of experimental investigations into the effects of hemisphere stimulation on the reading performance of individuals with dyslexia are currently available, only a few studies have addressed the effects of treatment in the setting of an outpatient clinic. The present study reports on the reading results after a treatment that was based on the balance model and incorporated notions from cognitive psychological origin in 80 children with severe dyslexia who were referred to the outpatient clinic of the Paedological Institute in Amsterdam. Kappers EJ J Learn Disabil 1997 Jan-Feb;30(1):100-25.

Outstanding questions about phonological processing in dyslexia. Abstract: It is widely accepted that developmental dyslexia results from some sort of phonological deficit. Yet, it can be argued that phonological representations and their processing have been insufficiently tested in dyslexia research. Firstly, claims about how tasks tap into certain kinds of representations or processes are best appreciated in the light of an explicit information-processing model. Here, a cognitive model of lexical access is described, incorporating speech perception, reading and object recognition. Ramus F Dyslexia 2001 Oct-Dec;7(4):197-216.

Overcoming dyslexia. Morris B Fortune 2002 May 13;145(10):54-8, 62, 64 passim.

Paine, Richmond S. Dyslexia and reading disabilities; papers, by Richmond Paine, Helmer Myklebust, Deso Weiss, et al. New York, MSS Information Corp. [1972] Myklebust, Helmer R, joint author. Weiss, Deso A. (Deso Arthur), joint author. Description: 224 p. illus. 24 cm. ISBN: 0842270051 LC Classification: RJ496.A5 P35 Dewey Class No.: 618.9/28/533

Paradis, Michel. Neurolinguistic aspects of the Japanese writing system / Michel Paradis, Hiroko Hagiwara, Nancy Hildebrandt;

foreword by John C. Marshall. Orlando, Fla.: Academic Press, 1985. Hagiwara, Hiroko. Hildebrandt, Nancy. Description: xvi, 222 p.; 24 cm. ISBN: 0125449658 (pbk.: alk. paper) LC Classification: RC394.W6 P37 1985 Dewey Class No.: 616.85/53/0089956 19

PASS neurocognitive dysfunction in attention deficit Abstract: Attention deficit disorder shows both cognitive and behavioral patterns. According to PASS pattern, planning deficiency is a relevant factor. Neurological planning is not exactly the same than neurological executive function. The behavioral pattern is mainly linked to planning deficiency, but to other PASS processing deficits and even to no processing deficit. Perez-Alvarez F Timoneda-Gallart C Rev Neurol 2001 Jan 1-15;32(1):30-7.

Payne, Esamel. See-think-say: reading method for dyslexics / by Esamel Payne. Fredericksburg, Va.: Payne Pub. Co, c1977. Related Titles: Reading method for dyslexics. Description: 3 v.; 28 cm. LC Classification: LB1050.5.P3 Dewey Class No.: 371.9/14

Payne, Trevor, 1948- Dyslexia: a parents' and teachers' guide / Trevor Payne and Elizabeth Turner. Clevedon, England; Philadelphia: Multilingual Matters, 1998. Projected Pub. Date: 9812 Turner, Elizabeth, 1947- Description: p. cm. ISBN: 1853594113 (hardcover: alk. paper) 1853594105 (pbk.: alk. paper) LC Classification: LC4710.G7 P39 1998 Dewey Class No.: 371.91/44 21

Peaks of linkage are localized by a BAC/PAC contig of the 6p reading disability locus. Abstract: A gene for reading disability has been localized by nonparametric linkage to 6p21.3-p22 in several published reports. However, the lack of an uninterrupted genomic clone contig has made it difficult to determine accurate intermarker distances, precise marker order, and genetic boundaries and hinders direct comparisons of linkage. The search and discovery of the hemochromatosis gene

(HFE) led to the creation of a bacterial artificial chromosome (BAC) and P-1 derived artificial chromosome (PAC) contig that extended physical maps 4 Mb from the MHC toward pter and localized new markers in that region [10-12]. Ahn J Won TW Zia A Reutter H Kaplan DE Sparks R Gruen JR Genomics 2001 Nov;78(1-2):19-29.

People with dyslexia are quite capable of nursing. Shepherd K Nurs Stand 2002 May 22-28;16(36):30.

Perceiving left and imagining right: dissociation in neglect. Abstract: Signor Piazza, a patient with a left parieto-occipital haemorrhage and a right thalamic stroke, showed severe right personal neglect (e.g. touching own body parts) and right perceptual neglect in tasks with (e.g. cancelling tasks) or without (e.g. description of a complex picture) motor response. He had right-sided neglect dyslexia (including single words), without language impairments. However, the patient presented with a clear left-sided deficit in the representational domain (e.g. imagery tasks). Beschin N BasJournalA Della Sala S Cortex 2000 Jun;36(3):401-14.

Perception of voice and tone onset time continua in children with dyslexia with and without attention deficit/hyperactivity disorder. Abstract: Tasks assessing perception of a phonemic contrast based on voice onset time (VOT) and a nonspeech analog of a VOT contrast using tone onset time (TOT) were administered to children (ages 7.5 to 15.9 years) identified as having reading disability (RD; n = 21), attention deficit/hyperactivity disorder (ADHD; n = 22), comorbid RD and ADHD (n = 26), or no impairment (NI; n = 26). Children with RD, whether they had been identified as having ADHD or not, exhibited reduced perceptual skills on both tasks as indicated by shallower slopes on category labeling functions and reduced accuracy even at the endpoints of the series where cues are most salient Breier JI Gray L Fletcher JM Diehl RL Klaas P Foorman BR Molis MR J Exp Child Psychol 2001 Nov;80(3):245-70.

Perceptual auditory gap detection deficits in male BXSB mice with cerebrocortical ectopias. Abstract: Underlying impairments in rapid auditory processing may contribute to disrupted phonological processing, which in turn characterizes developmental language impairment (LI). Identification of a neurobiological feature of LI that is associated with auditory deficits would further support this model. Accordingly, we found that adult male rats with induced cortical malformations were impaired in rapid auditory processing. Since 40-60% of BXSB mice exhibit spontaneous focal cerebrocortical ectopias (as seen in dyslexics brains), we assessed auditory gap detection in adult male BXSB mice. Clark MG Sherman GF Bimonte HA Fitch RH Neuroreport 2000 Mar 20;11(4):693-6.

Perceptual discrimination of speech sounds in developmental dyslexia. Abstract: Experiments previously reported in the literature suggest that people with dyslexia have a deficit in categorical perception. However, it is still unclear whether the deficit is specific to the perception of speech sounds or whether it more generally affects auditory function. In order to investigate the relationship between categorical perception and dyslexia, as well as the nature of this categorization deficit, speech specific or not, the discrimination responses of children who have dyslexia and those of average readers to sinewave analogues of speech sounds were compared. Serniclaes W Sprenger-Charolles L Carre R Demonet JF J Speech Lang Hear Res 2001 Apr;44(2):384-99.

Perez, Tony. Albert N.: a case study / by Tony Perez. [s.l.: s.n.], c1976 ([Manila], Philippines: Journal Press) Description: 182 p.; 18 cm. LC Classification: RC464.A38 P47 Dewey Class No.: 618.92/8588 B 19

Perinatal gonadectomy affects corticocortical connections in motor but not visual cortex in adult male rats. Abstract: Sexual dimorphisms and/or hormone modifiability have been documented for numerous structural endpoints in the cerebral cortex, including cortical thickness and dendrite morphology. The present study asked whether gonadal steroids might sculpt cortical circuit organization. Accordingly, neonatal gonadectomy, with and without testosterone propionate replacement, was followed by fine-grained microcircuit tract tracing analyses of the organization of corticocortical circuits of identified layers of primary motor and primary visual cortices in the same animals in adulthood. Venkatesan C Kritzer MF J Comp Neurol 1999 Dec 13;415(2):240-65.

Perinatal gonadectomy exerts regionally selective, lateralized effects on the density of axons immunoreactive for tyrosine hydroxylase in the cerebral cortex of adult male rats. Abstract: The catecholamine innervation of the cerebral cortex is essential for its normal operations and is implicated in cortical dysfunction in mental illness. Previous studies in rats have shown that the maturational tempo of these afferents is highly responsive to changes in gonadal hormones. The present findings show that perinatal hormone manipulation has striking, region- and hemisphere-specific consequences for cortical catecholamines in adulthood. Kritzer MF J Neurosci 1998 Dec 15;18(24):10735-48.

Persistence of dyslexia: the Connecticut Longitudinal Study at adolescence. Abstract: The outcome in adolescence of children diagnosed as dyslexic during the early years of school was examined in children prospectively identified in childhood and continuously followed to young adulthood. This sample offers a unique opportunity to investigate a prospectively identified sample of adolescents for whom there is no question of the childhood diagnosis and in whom highly analytic measures of reading and language can be administered in adolescence. Deficits in phonological coding continue to characterize dyslexic readers even in adolescence; performance on phonological processing measures contributes most to discriminating dyslexic and average readers, and average and superior readers as well. These data support and extend the findings of previous investigators indicating the continuing contribution of phonological processing to decoding words, reading rate, and accuracy and spelling. Children with dyslexia neither spontaneously remit nor do they demonstrate a lag mechanism for catching up in the development of reading skills. In adolescents, the rate of reading as well as facility with spelling may be most useful clinically in differentiating average from poor readers. Department of Pediatrics, Yale University School of Medicine, New Haven, CT 06510-8064, USA. sally.shaywitz@yale.edu Shaywitz SE Fletcher JM Holahan JM Shneider AE Marchione KE Stuebing KK Francis DJ Pugh KR Shaywitz BA Pediatrics 1999 Dec;104(6):1351-9.

Perspectives on dyslexia / edited by George Th. Pavlidis. Chichester; New York: Wiley, c1990. Pavlidis, George Th. Description: 2 v.: ill.; 24 cm. ISBN: 0471922048 (v. 1): 0471924849 (v. 2): LC Classification: RC394.W6 P47 1990 NLM Class No.: WM 475 P467 Dewey Class No.: 616.85/53 20

Pesetsky, Bette, 1932- Stories up to a point / Bette Pesetsky. Edition Information: 1st ed. New York: Knopf, 1981. Description: 113 p.; 22 cm. ISBN: 0394520793 LC Classification: PS3566.E738 S75 1981 Dewey Class No.: 813/.54 19

Petersen, Jørgen, 1944- Visuel perception og læsning: opstilling og afprøvning af et testbatteri til undersøgelse af visuel perception / af Jørgen Petersen. København: Institut for dansk sprog og litteratur, Danmarks lærerhøjskole, 1987- Description: <v. 1; in 3: ill.; 30 cm. ISBN:

8788295427 (v. 1, set) LC Classification: LB1067.5.P48 1987

Phonemes, rhymes, and intelligence as predictors of children's responsiveness to remedial reading instruction: evidence from a longitudinal intervention study. Abstract: We present an analysis of data from a longitudinal intervention study with 7-year-old poor readers (Hatcher, Hulme, & Ellis, 1994). A battery of cognitive and phonological tasks administered before the intervention began revealed five separate factors: Phoneme Manipulation, Rhyme, Verbal Ability, Nonverbal Ability and Phonological Memory. We assessed the extent to which these factors were predictive of children's responsiveness to the teaching interventions they received Hatcher PJ Hulme C J Exp Child Psychol 1999 Feb;72(2):130-53.

Phonological and semantic information in word and nonword reading in a deep dyslexic patient. Abstract: Deep dyslexia is diagnosed when brain-injured, previously literate adults make reading errors that include hallmark semantic paralexias (e.g, reading HEART as BLOOD) and are impaired at reading nonwords (e.g, FRIP). The diversity of these symptoms have led most researchers to conclude that there are multiple sources of impairment in this syndrome and that one of the most critical is a failure to process phonological information at a sublexical level. Buchanan L Kiss I Burgess C Brain Cogn 2000 Jun-Aug;43(1-3):65-8.

Phonological and visuo-spatial working memory alterations in dyslexic children. Abstract: Working memory allows the retention of a limited amount of information for a brief period of time and the manipulation of that information. This study was undertaken to compare possible differences in working memory between dyslexic and control children. Present results suggest the importance of visuo-spatial and phonological loop alterations in dyslexic children that may result in difficulties with similar words and spatial information. Poblano A Valadez-Tepec T

de Lourdes Arias M Garcia-Pedroza F Arch Med Res 2000 Sep-Oct;31(5):493-6.

Phonological awareness deficits in developmental dyslexia and the phonological representations hypothesis. Abstract: The claim that the well-documented difficulties shown by dyslexic children in phonological awareness tasks may arise from deficits in the accuracy and the segmental organization of the phonological representations of words in their mental lexicons is receiving increasing interest from researchers. In this experiment, two versions of the phonological representations hypothesis were investigated by using a picture naming task and a battery of phonological measures at three linguistic levels (syllable, onset-rime, phoneme). Swan D Goswami U J Exp Child Psychol 1997 Jul;66(1):18-41.

Phonological awareness in French-speaking children at risk for reading disabilities. Abstract: We report the phonological awareness abilities of preliterate French-speaking children. The performance of a group of children identified At Risk (n = 26) for reading disabilities was compared to that of normally developing age-matched controls (n = 22) on a range of standardised and experimental tests. Results showed the At Risk children to have a selective impairment in expressive relative to receptive language, whereas Controls performed at equivalent levels on both measures. Courcy A Beland R Pitchford NJ Brain Cogn 2000 Jun-Aug;43(1-3):124-30.

Phonological dyslexia and phonological dysgraphia following left and right hemispherectomy. Abstract: Four adults who had hemispherectomies because of severe epilepsy following infantile of childhood damage to one hemisphere of the brain, are assessed on their reading and spelling abilities in an attempt to see if the two hemispheres are equipotential for these abilities in infancy. The psycholinguistic assessments of language processing in aphasia (PALPA) are used, and the results are interpreted from the viewpoint of hypotheses of "normal" right and left hemisphere reading abilities Ogden JA Neuropsychologia 1996 Sep;34(9):905-18.

Phonological impairment in dyslexic children with and without early speech-language disorder. Abstract: This study examines phonological awareness in a group of 10 dyslexic children, compared with two groups of children (a reading-equivalent control group and a group of beginning readers). Five of the dyslexic children exhibited an early speech-language impairement, and five others were not language-impaired. The experimental design consisted of a set of 10 tasks involving sensitivity to phonological strings, phonetic identification, and phoneme segmentation and manipulation. Plaza M Eur J Disord Commun 1997;32(2):277-90.

Phonological processes and brain mechanisms / Harry A. Whitaker, editor. New York: Springer-Verlag, c1988. Whitaker, Harry A. Description: xii, 184 p.; 24 cm. ISBN: 0387966048: LC Classification: QP399.P48 1988 NLM Class No.: WL 340.5 P5745 Dewey Class No.: 616.85/52 19

Phonological processing in dyslexic children: a study combining functional imaging and event related potentials. Abstract: Difficulties in phonological processing are currently considered one of the major causes for dyslexia. Nine dyslexic children and eight control children were investigated using functional magnetic resonance imaging (fMRI) during non-oral reading of German words. All subjects silently read words and pronounceable non-words in an event related potentials (ERP) investigation, as well. The fMRI showed a significant difference in the activation in the left inferior frontal gyrus between the dyslexic and control groups, resulting from a hyperactivation in the dyslexics. Georgiewa P Rzanny R Gaser C Gerhard UJ Vieweg U Freesmeyer D Mentzel HJ Kaiser WA Blanz B Neurosci Lett 2002 Jan 18;318(1):5-8.

Phonological processing, not inhibitory control, differentiates ADHD and reading disability. Abstract: To test for the distinctiveness of attention-deficit hyperactivity disorder (ADHD) and reading disability (RD) and the independence of the cognitive domains, inhibition and phonological processing, which are proposed as central to ADHD and RD, respectively, using a classic double dissociation design These findings question the role of inhibitory control as a unique cognitive marker for ADHD and suggest true comorbidity for children with both ADHD and RD. Hospital for Sick Children, Toronto, Ontario, Canada. Purvis KL Tannock R J Am Acad Child Adolesc Psychiatry 2000 Apr;39(4):485-94.

Phonological representations, reading development and dyslexia: towards a cross-linguistic theoretical framework. Abstract: This paper attempts to integrate recent research findings in phonological development, reading development and dyslexia into a coherent theoretical framework that can provide a developmental account of reading and reading difficulties across languages. It is proposed that the factors governing phonological development across languages are similar, but that important differences in the speed and level of phonological development are found following the acquisition of alphabetic literacy. Goswami U Dyslexia 2000 Apr-Jun;6(2):133-51.

Phonological spelling errors among dyslexic children learning a transparent orthography: the case of Czech. Abstract: Substantial evidence from studies of English-speaking dyslexic children's spelling suggests that these individuals have a persistent impairment in representing the phonological structure and content of words in writing. In contrast, several studies of German dyslexic children (Landerl & Wimmer,

2000) suggest that, among learners of transparent orthographies, the above impairment is transient and resolves by the end of grade 2; instead dyslexic spelling is characterised by a persistent impairment in learning inconsistent spelling patterns. Caravolas M Volin J Dyslexia 2001 Oct-Dec;7(4):229-45.

Phonology, reading acquisition, and dyslexia: insights from connectionist models. Abstract: The development of reading skill and bases of developmental dyslexia were explored using connectionist models. Four issues were examined: the acquisition of phonological knowledge prior to reading, how this knowledge facilitates learning to read, phonological and nonphonological bases of dyslexia, and effects of literacy on phonological representation. Compared with simple feedforward networks, representing phonological knowledge in an attractor network yielded improved learning and generalization. Harm MW Seidenberg MS Psychol Rev 1999 Jul;106(3):491-528.

Pictogram naming in dyslexic and normal children assessed by SLO. Abstract: We measured pictogram naming (PN) and text reading in dyslexic and normally reading young teenagers. Eye movements were monitored by scanning laser ophthalmoscope, revealing positions of fovea, stimuli on the retina, and speech simultaneously. While text reading speed showed the expected difference between groups, PN speeds overlapped widely. PN was mainly controlled by retrieval time in both groups and correlated with age in dyslexics. During PN, only backward saccades occurred more frequently in dyslexics. Trauzettel-Klosinski S MacKeben M Reinhard J Feucht A Durrwachter U Klosinski G Vision Res 2002 Mar;42(6):789-99.

Picture naming deficits in developmental dyslexia: the phonological representations hypothesis. Abstract: The picture and word naming performance of developmental dyslexics was compared to the picture and word naming performance of non-dyslexic ("garden variety") poor readers, reading age, and chronological age-matched controls. The stimulus list used for both tasks was systematically manipulated for word length and word frequency. In order to examine picture naming errors in more depth, an object name recognition test assessed each subject's vocabulary knowledge of those names which they were unable to spontaneously label in the picture naming task. Swan D Goswami U Brain Lang 1997 Feb 15;56(3):334-53.

Planar asymmetry tips the phonological playground and environment raises the bar. Abstract: Reading readiness varies as a function of family and environmental variables. This study of 11-year-old children (N = 39) was designed to determine if there was an additional or interactive contribution of brain structure. Evidence is presented that both environmental and biological variables predict phonological development. Temporal lobe (planar) asymmetry, hand preference, family history of reading disability, and SES explained over half of the variance in phonological and verbal performance. Eckert MA Lombardino LJ Leonard CM Child Dev 2001 Jul-Aug;72(4):988-1002.

Plantier, Gisèle. Les malheurs d'un enfant dyslexique / Gisèle Plantier; présenté par Pierre Debray-Ritzen. Paris: A. Michel, c1981. Description: 229 p.; 21 cm. ISBN: 2226010874 LC Classification: LB1050.5.P55 Dewey Class No.: 371.91/4 19 National Bib. No.: F***

Planum temporale asymmetry and ear advantage in dichotic listening in Developmental Dyslexia and Attention-Deficit/Hyperactivity Disorder (ADHD). Abstract: The planum temporale is clearly involved in language processing, for it serves as the auditory association cortex. Research has consistently demonstrated that 60 to 70% of the population has leftward asymmetry of the planum temporale. Research has suggested that dyslexic individuals tend to have either rightward asymmetry or symmetrical plana. Moreover, many studies have found a relationship between the presence of dyslexia and/or language impairment and deficits in the normal right ear advantage found in dichotic listening paradigms. Foster LM Hynd GW Morgan AE Hugdahl K J Int Neuropsychol Soc 2002 Jan;8(1):22-36.

Planum temporale, planum parietale and dichotic listening in dyslexia. Abstract: A reduction or reversal of the normal leftward asymmetry of the planum temporale (PT) has been claimed to be typical of dyslexia, although some recent studies have challenged this view. In a population-based study of 20 right-handed dyslexic boys and 20 matched controls, we have measured the PT and the adjacent planum parietale (PP) region in sagittal magnetic resonance images. For the PT, mean left and right areas and asymmetry coefficients were compared. Since a PP area often could not be identified in one or both hemispheres, a qualitative comparison was used for this region. Heiervang E Hugdahl K Steinmetz H Inge Smievoll A Stevenson J Lund A Ersland L Lundervold A Neuropsychologia 2000;38(13):1704-13.

Plastic neural changes and reading improvement caused by audiovisual training in reading-impaired children. Abstract: This study aimed at determining whether audiovisual training without linguistic material has a remediating effect on reading skills and central auditory processing in dyslexic children. It was found that this training resulted in plastic changes in the auditory cortex, indexed by enhanced electrophysiological mismatch negativity and faster reaction times to sound changes. Importantly, these changes were accompanied by improvement in reading skills. The results indicate that reading difficulties can be ameliorated by special training programs and, further, that the training effects can be observed in brain activity. Kujala T Karma K Ceponiene R Belitz S Turkkila P Tervaniemi M Naatanen R Proc Natl Acad Sci U S A 2001 Aug 28;98(18):10509-14.

Politics and reading. Hall SL Pediatrics 2002 Jul;110(1 Pt 1):193-5; discussion 193-5.

Pollock, Joy. Day-to-day dyslexia in the classroom / Joy Pollock and Elisabeth Waller. London; New York: Routledge, 1994. Waller, Elisabeth. Description: xiv, 171 p.: ill.; 24 cm. ISBN: 0415111323 LC Classification: LC4708.P65 1994 Dewey Class No.: 371.91/44 20

Pollock, Joy. Dyslexia: the problem of spelling / by Joy Pollock. Edition Information: Revised ed. London: The Helen Arkell Dyslexia Centre, 1975. Description: [2], 25 p.: ill, facsims.; 21 cm. ISBN: 0950362662: LC Classification: LB1574.P64 Dewey Class No.: 371.9/14 National Bib. No.: GB76-01000

Poor saccadic control correlates with dyslexia. Abstract: A large group of subjects, either average readers or reading/spelling disabled subjects (n = 185; age between 8-25 years; M = 13 +/- 4 years), were tested in various standardized cognitive tasks including reading/spelling assessment and in non-cognitive saccadic eye movement tasks. Dyslexics were separated into a subgroup (D1) with deficits in the serial auditory short-term memory and a subgroup (D2) with an isolated low achievement in reading/writing. Control subjects had no relevant cognitive deficit of any type. Saccadic eye movements were measured in a single target and in a sequential-target task. Biscaldi M Gezeck S Stuhr V Neuropsychologia 1998 Nov;36(11):1189-202.

Possible relevance of phospholipid abnormalities and genetic interactions in psychiatric disorders: the relationship between dyslexia and schizophrenia. Abstract: The fatty acids of cell membrane phospholipids are essential for normal membrane structures, for the functioning of membrane-bound and membrane-associated proteins and for normal cell-signalling responses. In dyslexia, there is evidence for reduced incorporation of docosahexaenoic acid and arachidonic acid into cell membranes, while in schizophrenia, there is evidence for an increased rate of docosahexaenoic acid and arachidonic acid loss from membranes because of enhanced phospholipase A2 activity. Horrobin DF Glen AI Hudson CJ Med Hypotheses 1995 Dec;45(6):605-13.

Posterior alexia after right occipitotemporal infarction. Gomez-Tortosa E Del Barrio A J Neurol Neurosurg Psychiatry 2001 May;70(5):702-3.

Postgeniculate afferent visual system and visual higher cortical function, 1995-1996. Wall M J Neuroophthalmol 1997 Sep;17(3):209-17.

Potential diagnostic aids for abnormal fatty acid metabolism in a range of neurodevelopmental disorders. Abstract: Disorders of neurodevelopment include attention deficit hyperactivity disorder, dyspraxia, dyslexia and autism. There is considerable co-morbidity of these disorders and their identification often presents difficulties to those making a diagnosis. This is especially difficult when a multidisciplinary approach is not adopted. All of these disorders have been reported as associated with fatty acid abnormalities ranging from genetic abnormalities in the enzymes involved in phospholipid metabolism to symptoms reportedly improved following dietary supplementation with long chain fatty acids. Ward PE Prostaglandins Leukot Essent Fatty Acids 2000 Jul-Aug;63(1-2):65-8.

Powell, Phelan. Tom Cruise / Phelan Powell; introduction by James Scott Brady. Philadelphia [Pa.]: Chelsea House Publishers, c1999. Description: 110 p.: ill.; 24 cm. ISBN: 079104940X (hardcover) 0791049418 (pbk.) Summary: Follows the life and career of the popular actor, focusing on his struggle with dyslexia, his starring roles in such movies as "Risky Business," "Top Gun," and "Jerry Maguire," and his involvement in the Church of Scientology. LC Classification: PN2287.C685 P68 1999 Dewey Class No.: 791.43/028/092 B 21

Pray that it is not a neurologic problem. Crawford D J Child Neurol 1995 Jan;10 Suppl 1:S108-9.

Pre-attentive processing of auditory patterns in dyslexic human subjects. Abstract: It has been hypothesized that auditory temporal processing plays a major role in the aetiology of dyslexia. Event-related brain potentials (mismatch negativity, MMN) of auditory temporal processing were assessed in 15 dyslectic adults and 20 controls. A complex tonal pattern was used where the difference between standard and deviant stimuli was the temporal, not the frequency structure. Dyslexics had a significantly smaller MMN in the time window of 225-600 ms. Schulte-Korne G Deimel W Bartling J Remschmidt H Neurosci Lett 1999 Nov 26;276(1):41-4.

Precursors of literacy delay among children at genetic risk of dyslexia. Abstract: This paper reports the literacy skills of 63 children selected as being at genetic risk of dyslexia compared with 34 children from families reporting no history of reading impairment. Fifty-seven per cent of the at-risk group were delayed in literacy development at 6 years compared with only 12% of controls. The "unimpaired" at-risk group were not statistically different from controls on most cognitive and language measures at 45 months, whereas the literacy-delayed group showed significantly slower speech and language development, although they did not differ from controls in nonverbal ability Gallagher A Frith U Snowling MJ J Child Psychol Psychiatry 2000 Feb;41(2):203-13.

Predicting dyslexia at 8 years of age using neonatal brain responses. Abstract: Auditory event-related potentials recorded at birth to speech and nonspeech syllables from six scalp electrodes discriminated between newborn infants who 8 years later would be characterized as dyslexic, poor, or normal readers. These findings indicate that reading problems can be identified and possible interventions undertaken up to 9 years earlier than is currently possible. Molfese DL Brain Lang 2000 May;72(3):238-45.

Prediction and qualitative assessment of five- and six-year-old children's reading: a longitudinal study. Abstract: This paper describes a longitudinal study comparing the power of two screening batteries (that of Clay, 1979, and that of a set of tests of phonological awareness and sound-to-letter correspondence knowledge) to identify, in the first term at school, children at risk of failing to learn to read successfully. A single test from one of the batteries is shown to provide an adequate screening procedure. Stuart M Br J Educ Psychol 1995 Sep;65 (Pt 3):287-96.

Predictive accuracy of the wide range assessment of memory and learning in children with attention deficit hyperactivity disorder and reading difficulties. Abstract: The predictive accuracy of the Wide Range Assessment of Memory and Learning (WRAML; Sheslow & Adams, 1990) over and above more standardized diagnostic tools in children with attention deficit hyperactivity disorder (ADHD) and reading disabilities (RD) was examined. Fifty-three children with ADHD, 63 with RD, 63 with ADHD-RD, and 112 normal comparison children were administered the WRAML, the Wechsler Intelligence Scale for Children-Third Edition (WISC-III; Wechsler, 1991), the Achenbach (1991) Child Behavior Checklist (CBCL), and the Woodcock-Johnson Psycho-Educational Battery-Revised (WJ-R; Woodcock & Johnson, 1989). Dewey D Kaplan BJ Crawford SG Fisher GC Dev Neuropsychol 2001;19(2):173-89.

Predictors of cognitive test patterns in autism families. Abstract: In a case-control study of cognitive performance, tests of intelligence, reading, spelling, and pragmatic language were administered to the parents and siblings of 90 community-ascertained probands with autism (AU group) and to the parents and siblings of 40 similarly ascertained probands with trisomy 21 Down syndrome (DS group). The two samples were comparable for age and parents' education; both groups were well-educated and had above-average intelligence. AU parents scored slightly but significantly lower on the WAIS-R Full Scale and Performance IQ, on two subtests (Picture Arrangement and Picture Completion), and on the Word Attack Test (reading nonsense words) from the Woodcock-Johnson battery. Folstein SE Santangelo SL Gilman SE Piven J Landa R Lainhart J Hein J Wzorek M J Child Psychol Psychiatry 1999 Oct;40(7):1117-28.

Preliminary evidence of widespread morphological variations of the brain in dyslexia. Abstract: The MR images of 16 men with dyslexia and 14 control subjects were compared using a voxel-based analysis. Evidence of decreases in gray matter in dyslexic subjects, most notably in the left temporal lobe and bilaterally in the temporoparietooccipital juncture, but in the frontal lobe, caudate, thalamus, and cerebellum, was found. Widely distributed morphologic differences affecting several brain regions may contribute to the deficits associated with dyslexia. Brown WE Eliez S Menon V Rumsey JM White CD Reiss AL Neurology 2001 Mar 27;56(6):781-3.

Prescribing ritalin in combined modality management of hyperactivity with attention deficit Abstract: Attention Deficit Hyperactivity Disorder (ADHD) is a relatively frequent affection that can generate severe problems (school, social, professional) if no take in charge is done. Treatment of ADHD is generally multifactorial; it can associate medical treatment, comportemental and analytical psychotherapies, reeducation of associated disorders (orthophony, psychomotor reeducation) and educative approach. Methylphenidate, considered as therapeutic reference, is a central nervous system stimulant. Bricard C Boidein F Encephale 2001 Sep-Oct;27(5):435-43.

Preserved implicit reading and the recovery of explicit reading in a pure alexic Abstract:

We described a 55-year-old, right-handed, university-educated Japanese man who showed pure alexia after an infarction in the territory of the left posterior cerebral artery. Damage to the corpus callosum was limited to the most caudal part of the splenium. In the early days of his illness, he demonstrated the inability to read aloud on either Kana (Japanese syllabograms) or Kanji (Japanese morphograms). Hashimoto R Tanaka Y Rinsho Shinkeigaku 1996 Mar;36(3):456-61.

Preserved insight in an artist with extrapersonal spatial neglect. Abstract: Several reports of cases of experienced artists showing neglect after a brain lesion can be gleaned from the literature. The analysis of their drawings might provide better insight into the symptoms of neglect than that of non-artists's production. However, most of these reports are anedoctal. We describe in some detail the case of neglect of a distinguished artist, the internationally known Federico Fellini (FF), whom we followed-up for two months after his right parietal stroke. Cantagallo A Della Sala S Cortex 1998 Apr;34(2):163-89.

Preserved semantic access in neglect dyslexia. Abstract: The aim of this study was to investigate the preservation of semantic access in patients with severe neglect dyslexia for words and non-words. Patients were given the following tasks: (1) reading aloud letter strings (first basic reading task), (2) making semantic decisions (categorial and inferential judgements), (3) making semantic decisions and reading the letter strings immediately afterwards (semantic-reading tasks), (4) reading letter strings again (final basic reading tasks) and (5) auditory control tasks. Ladavas E Shallice T Zanella MT Neuropsychologia 1997 Mar;35(3):257-70.

Preserved semantic priming effect in alexia. Abstract: BH, a left-handed patient with alexia and nonfluent aphasia, was presented with a lexical-decision task in which words and pronounceable pseudowords were preceded by semantically related or unrelated picture primes (Experiment 1). In Experiment 2, BH was given an explicit reading task using the word lists from Experiment 1. Performance on Experiment 2 disclosed severe reading deficits in both oral reading and semantic matching of the words to pictures. However, in Experiment 1, BH demonstrated a significant semantic priming effect, responding more accurately and more quickly to words preceded by related primes than by unrelated primes. Mimura M Goodglass H Milberg W Brain Lang 1996 Sep;54(3):434-46.

Pretty in pink... King NJ Redox Rep 2000;5(1):11-3.

Prevalence of dyslexia among Texas prison inmates. Abstract: Approximately 80% of prison inmates are reported to be functionally illiterate. We hypothesized that poor single word decoding (the chief feature of dyslexia) accounts for a significant percentage of that rate. We studied 253 subjects selected randomly from more than 130,000 Texas prison inmates. Among them, we conducted a cross-sectional sample survey of recently admitted Texas inmates, beginning with social and educational background and followed by an educational test battery that included measures of word attack skill and reading comprehension. Moody KC Holzer CE 3rd Roman MJ Paulsen KA Freeman DH Haynes M James TN Tex Med 2000 Jun;96(6):69-75.

Primary progressive aphasia: a patient with stress assignment impairment in reading aloud. Abstract: Surface dyslexia is a pattern of reading impairment which has been seldom described in Italian native speakers. We report the case of a female Italian patient, RM, suffering from primary progressive aphasia (PPA) of the fluent type, who presented stress assignment errors in reading aloud. In Italian these errors are considered to be strongly suggestive of surface dyslexia. We studied RM's reading performance in light of existing cognitive models on reading. Since the first assessment, she presented multi-level impairment involving pre-semantic, lexical-semantic and post-semantic stages. Galante E Tralli A Zuffi M Avanzi S Neurol Sci 2000 Feb;21(1):39-48.

Processing of palindromes in neglect dyslexia. Abstract: We report an investigation into the processing of symmetrical lexical stimuli by a patient with moderate visual neglect. This subject's neglect dyslexia was significantly less pronounced when presented with symmetrical lexical stimuli (palindromes) than with matched non-symmetrical words. We discuss the hypothesis that symmetry facilitates processing. Shillcock RC Kelly ML Monaghan P Neuroreport 1998 Sep 14;9(13):3081-3.

Processing speed in children with attention deficit/hyperactivity disorder, inattentive type. Abstract: Attention Deficit Hyperactivity Disorder (ADHD) is among the most common and most often reconceptualized neurobehavioral disorders of childhood. In the most recent DSM-IV, a primarily inattentive subtype of ADHD (AD) has again been identified. Weiler MD Bernstein JH Bellinger DC Waber DP Neuropsychol Dev Cogn Sect C Child Neuropsychol 2000 Sep;6(3):218-34.

Profiles of cognitive performance associated with reading disability in temporal lobe epilepsy. Abstract: 92 patients with temporal lobe epilepsy (TLE) were classified into reading deficient (RD; N = 41) and non-reading deficient (no-RD; N = 51) groups. A cutoff of 80 was used to further classify patients as having low average or better (AVG: IQ > 79) or below average (LOW: 69 < IQ < 80) intellectual ability. Differences between RD-AVG and no-RD-AVG patients in profiles of performance on cognitive tests were specific to verbal and non-verbal memory and verbal abilities, but not visuoconstructional and executive abilities. RD-LOW patients exhibited globally reduced abilities. Breier JI Fletcher JM

Wheless JW Clark A Cass J Constantinou JE J Clin Exp Neuropsychol 2000 Dec;22(6):804-16.

Progressive severity of left unilateral apraxia in 2 cases of Alzheimer disease Abstract: Two patients presented with progressive left unilateral motor apraxia and progressive visuo-spatial difficulties, including constructional apraxia, dressing apraxia, spatial dysgraphia and dyslexia, spatial acalculia and neglect of the left side, without significant changes in the other cognitive functions. In both patients, radiological tests demonstrated cortical atrophy, more marked in the retrorolandic areas. A diagnosis of Alzheimer's disease was made in the first patient by cortical biopsy and in the second patient by post-mortem examination. Ceccaldi M Poncet M Gambarelli D Guinot H Bille J Rev Neurol (Paris) 1995 Apr;151(4):240-6.

Progressive ventral posterior cortical degeneration presenting as alexia for music and words. Abstract: Patients with posterior cortical atrophy may have dorsal visual system (occipital-parietal) dysfunction (optic ataxia, visuospatial disorientation, and simultanagnosia), ventral visual system (occipital-temporal) dysfunction (pure alexia, prosopagnosia, visual anomia, and agnosia), or both. We report a professional musician with ventral system dysfunction whose first symptom was alexia for music. Subsequently, she developed pure alexia for words but had preserved sorting of words. Beversdorf DQ Heilman KM Neurology 1998 Mar;50(3):657-9.

Prolonged attentional dwell time in dyslexic adults. Abstract: Dyslexic adults have been shown to be slow in processing rapid sequences of stimuli in all sensory modalities. We now demonstrate, by means of an attentional blink task, that the attentional dwell time is prolonged by approximately 30% in dyslexic adults compared with normal readers. Thus a target captures attentional resources for considerably longer time in dyslexics than control subjects. The observed prolongation could significantly contribute to the sluggish temporal processing of dyslexic adults. Hari R Valta M Uutela K Neurosci Lett 1999 Aug 27;271(3):202-4.

Prosopagnosia and alexia without object agnosia. Abstract: Following a trauma causing bilateral posterior brain damage, a patient complained of dyslexia and prosopagnosia, but not object agnosia. On testing she showed intact recognition of object drawings, even when it was assessed with perceptually demanding tasks such as Ghent's overlapping figures and Street completion test. This pattern of deficit is inconsistent with Farah's (1990) prediction that the simultaneous occurrence of alexia and prosopagnosia is invariably associated with object agnosia. De Renzi E di Pellegrino G Cortex 1998 Jun;34(3):403-15.

Pseudoname learning by German-speaking children with dyslexia: evidence for a phonological learning deficit. Abstract: In 2 experiments, German-speaking dyslexic children (9-year-olds) showed impaired learning of new phonological forms (pseudonames) in a variety of visual-verbal learning tasks. The dyslexic deficit was found when phonological retrieval cues were provided and when the to-be-learned pseudonames were presented in spoken as well as printed form. However, the dyslexic children showed no name-learning deficit when short, familiar words were used and they had no difficulty with immediate repetition of the pseudowords. Mayringer H Wimmer H J Exp Child Psychol 2000 Feb;75(2):116-33.

Psychiatric comorbidity in children and adolescents with reading disability. Abstract: This study investigated the association between reading disability (RD) and internalizing and externalizing psychopathology in a large community sample of twins with (N = 209) and without RD (N = 192). The primary goals were to clarify the relation between RD and comorbid psychopathology, to test for gender differences in the behavioral correlates of RD, and to test if common familial influences contributed to the association between RD and other disorders. Results indicated that individuals with RD exhibited significantly higher rates of all internalizing and externalizing disorders than individuals without RD. Willcutt EG Pennington BF J Child Psychol Psychiatry 2000 Nov;41(8):1039-48.

Psychoactive substance use: some associated characteristics. Abstract: A questionnaire designed to assess the prevalence of psychoactive substance use and its relation with: (a) central nervous system risk factors, (b) associated disorders (allergies, migraine-type headaches, developmental dyslexia history, smoking, suicide attempt, and sleep disorders), and (c) cognitive-type symptoms, was given to a general population sample of 1,879 university students (mean age = 24.0) from Bogota (Colombia, South America). A prevalence of 3.4% of self-reported psychoactive substance use was found. Ardila A Bateman JR Addict Behav 1995 Jul-Aug;20(4):549-54.

Psychologie cognitive de la lecture / Michel Fayol... [et al.]. Edition Information: 1re éd. Paris: Presses universitaires de France, c1992. Fayol, Michel, 1947- Description: 288 p.; 22 cm. ISBN: 2130446248 LC Classification: BF456.R2 P8 1992 Dewey Class No.: 418/.4/019 21

Psychophysical evidence for a general temporal processing deficit in children with dyslexia. Abstract: The hypothesis of a general (i.e. cross-modal) temporal processing deficit in dyslexia was tested by examining rapid processing in both the auditory and the visual system in the same children with dyslexia. Participants were 10- to 12-year-old dyslexic readers and age-matched normal reading controls. Psychophysical thresholds were estimated for auditory gap and visual double flash detection, using a two-interval, two-alternative forced-choice paradigm. Significant group differences were found for the auditory and the visual test. Van Ingelghem M van Wieringen A Wouters J

Vandenbussche E Onghena P Ghesquiere P Neuroreport 2001 Nov 16;12(16):3603-7.

Psychophysical evidence for a magnocellular pathway deficit in dyslexia. Abstract: The relationship between reading ability and psychophysical performance was examined to test the hypothesis that dyslexia is associated with a deficit in the magnocellular (M) pathway. Speed discrimination thresholds and contrast detection thresholds were measured under conditions (low mean luminance, low spatial frequency, high temporal frequency) for which psychophysical performance presumably depends on M pathway integrity. Dyslexic subjects had higher psychophysical thresholds than controls in both the speed discrimination and contrast detection tasks, but only the differences in speed thresholds were statistically significant. Demb JB Boynton GM Best M Heeger DJ Vision Res 1998 Jun;38(11):1555-9.

Psychophysical sensitivity and physiological response to amplitude modulation in adult dyslexic listeners. Abstract: This study reports two experiments conducted to assess the sensitivity of dyslexic listeners to amplitude modulation (AM) of acoustic stimuli. The smallest detectable depth of AM of white noise was measured as a function of modulation frequency. Dyslexic listeners had significantly higher thresholds of AM depth than did matched control listeners. We recorded the scalp potential evoked by AM of white noise (the amplitude modulation following response, AMFR). Dyslexic listeners had significantly smaller AMFRs than did matched control listeners. Menell P McAnally KI Stein JF J Speech Lang Hear Res 1999 Aug;42(4):797-803.

Pumfrey, Peter D. (Peter David) Specific learning difficulties (dyslexia): challenges and responses / a national inquiry coordinated and written by Peter D. Pumfrey and Rea Reason with a working group of educational psychologists. Windsor, Berkshire, UK: NFER-Nelson, 1991. Reason, Rea. Description: 338 p.: 1 facsim.; 24 cm. ISBN: 0700512683 0700512675 (pbk.) LC Classification: LB1050.5.P93 1991 Dewey Class No.: 371.91/44 20

Pupils with special needs: a Scottish perspective. Abstract: The distinction between ordinary and special schooling in Scotland was effectively erased by the Education (Scotland) Act of 1981. This Act recognizes that any pupil who requires extra support to succeed in a regular classroom is a child who has special education needs. Presently, all pupils who, for whatever reason, do not cope successfully at school are collectively referred to as children with learning difficulties. The term "learning difficulties" reflects a broader spectrum of problems than those characteristically found in the category of learning disabilities used in the United States. Morris L Watt J Wheatley P J Learn Disabil 1995 Aug-Sep;28(7):386-90.

Pure alexia and word-meaning deafness in a patient with multiple sclerosis. Abstract: To describe pure alexia and auditory comprehension problems in a young woman with multiple sclerosis (MS Pure alexia is unusual in MS and to our knowledge only 1 other case has been reported (in Japanese). Memory impairments and slowed information processing are probably the most frequent cognitive sequelae of the disease and, consequently, the literature is biased toward the study of those cognitive domains. However, given the wide distribution of sclerotic plaques in MS, it could be argued that we should expect some variability of cognitive changes in MS. Striking deficits as seen in this patient should make us more sensitive to this possibility. Jonsdottir MK Magnusson T Kjartansson O Arch Neurol 1998 Nov;55(11):1473-4.

Pure alexia could not be a disconnection syndrome. Benito-Leon J Sanchez-Suarez C Diaz-Guzman J Martinez-Salio A Neurology 1997 Jul;49(1):305-6.

Pure alexia due to a fusiform gyrus lesion Abstract: We present a patient with pure alexia following a hemorrhagic infarction in the left fusiform gyrus. The symptom began with alexia preferentially disturbed for kana, but during the course of recovery slight agraphia for kanji became pronounced. In the earlier phase, alexia was more severe than agraphia and he could write kanji that he could not read. Furthermore, kinesthetic reading was effective. Takada T Sakurai Y Takeuchil S Sakuta M Rinsho Shinkeigaku 1998 Feb;38(2):154-6.

Pure alexia from a posterior occipital lesion. Abstract: The authors report a patient with pure alexia (letter-by-letter reading) selectively impaired for kana (Japanese phonograms), cerebral achromatopsia, and right lower quadrantanopsia after hemorrhage in the left posterior occipital lobe, mainly under the lateral occipital gyri. The patient could not recognize some single-character kana, nor could he discriminate between two shapes of a similar size. The authors believe that the posterior occipital lobe, including the lateral occipital gyri, is specialized to recognize kana characters in this patient. Sakurai Y Ichikawa Y Mannen T Neurology 2001 Mar 27;56(6):778-81.

Pure alexia: clinical-pathologic evidence for a lateralized visual language association cortex. Abstract: Traditional views of pure alexia have held that the disorder results from a disconnection between the secondary visual cortices of both hemispheres and the angular gyrus of the dominant hemisphere. Evidence has accumulated, however, suggesting the importance of the posterior inferior temporal area in visual language processing. We describe clinical-pathological support for the presence of a lateralized visual language association area residing in the dominant posterior inferior temporal lobe. Beversdorf DQ Ratcliffe NR Rhodes CH Reeves AG Clin Neuropathol 1997 Nov-Dec;16(6):328-31.

Pure alexia: presentation of a case Abstract: Therefore, we confirm the cliniconeurophysiologic diagnosis of a pure alexia without agraphia, by means of this non-invasive method studying cerebral cognitive process. Caceres-Toledo M Marquez-Fernandez M Perez-Nellar J Caceres-Toledo O Rev Neurol 1998 Apr;26(152):615-8.

Pure alexia: presentation of three cases and review of the literature Abstract: Pure alexia is a syndrome characterized by the inability to read aloud in the absence of agraphia or apnasia In the review of the literature, the disorder and the contributions of various authors, from Deperine in 1892 to the present day, are considered in detail. Garcia-Hernandez I Gil-Saladie D Delgado M Martinell M Ugarte A Narberhaus B Rev Neurol 1997 Jun;25(142):863-9.

Pure somaesthetic alexia: somaesthetic-verbal disconnection for letters. Abstract: We studied a patient who manifested a bilateral reading disorder through the somaesthetic modality, without deficit of elementary tactile sensation or tactile object naming, due to a left parietal infarct. Detailed investigation established the following points. (i) The patient showed normal function on elementary somaesthetic examination, normal function on high level tactile perception, except for minimal impairment of the right hand on the two-point discrimination test, and normal latencies on the somatosensory evoked potential in both hands. (ii) Fukatsu R Fujii T + Brain 1998 May;121 (Pt 5):843-50.

Pure word deafness after cerebral hemorrhage in the left temporal lobe: a case report Abstract: We report a patient with pure word deafness after subcortical hemorrhage in the left temporal lobe. Repetition and auditory comprehension were severely impaired, while reading and visual comprehension of the same material were almost normal. He did not show hearing loss, but speech discrimination and melody recognition was poor. On the speech discrimination test, his score was low especially in the right ear. The threshold on the directional hearing test was mildly elevated. There was no temporal summation by click sounds Ohnaka K Sakurai Y Fuse S Shimpo T Kaga K Rinsho Shinkeigaku 1995 Mar;35(3):290-5.

Purtell, Thelma C. Can't read, can't write, can't takl [sic] too good either; how to recognize and overcome dyslexia in your child [by] Louise Clarke. New York, Walker [1973] Description: xvi, 280 p. illus. 24 cm. ISBN: 0802703925 LC Classification: RJ496.A5 P87 1973 Dewey Class No.: 618.9/28/553

Quantitative trait locus for reading disability on chromosome 6p is pleiotropic for attention-deficit/hyperactivity disorder. Abstract: Comorbidity is pervasive among both adult and child psychiatric disorders; however, the etiological mechanisms underlying the majority of comorbidities are unknown. This study used genetic linkage analysis to assess the etiology of comorbidity between reading disability (RD) and attention-deficit hyperactivity disorder (ADHD), two common childhood disorders that frequently co-occur. Sibling pairs (N = 85) were ascertained initially because at least one individual in each pair exhibited a history of reading difficulties. Willcutt EG Pennington BF Smith SD Cardon LR Gayan J Knopik VS Olson RK DeFries JC Am J Med Genet 2002 Apr 8;114(3):260-8.

Quantitative trait locus for reading disability: correction. Cardon LR Smith SD Fulker DW Kimberling WJ Pennington BF DeFries JC Science 1995 Jun 16;268(5217):1553.

Quantitative-trait locus for specific language and reading deficits on chromosome 6p. Abstract: Reading disability (RD), or dyslexia, is a complex cognitive disorder manifested by difficulties in learning to read, in otherwise normal individuals. Individuals with RD manifest deficits in several reading and language skills.

Previous research has suggested the existence of a quantitative-trait locus (QTL) for RD on the short arm of chromosome 6. In the present study, RD subjects' performance in several measures of word recognition and component skills of orthographic coding, phonological decoding, and phoneme awareness were individually subjected to QTL analysis, with a new sample of 126 sib pairs, by means of a multipoint mapping method and eight informative DNA markers on chromosome 6 (D6S461, D6S276, D6S105, D6S306, D6S258, D6S439, D6S291, and D6S1019). Gayan J Smith SD Cherny SS Cardon LR Fulker DW Brower AM Olson RK Pennington BF DeFries JC Am J Hum Genet 1999 Jan;64(1):157-64.

Radigk, Werner. Lesenlernen ohne Versagen?: ein Grundschulversuch zum Problem d. Legasthenie / [Werner Radigk, unter Mitarb. von Rosemarie Knebel u. Uwe Bruns]. Hannover; Dortmund; Darmstadt; Berlin: Schroedel, 1978. Knebel, Rosemarie, joint author. Bruns, Uwe, joint author. Description: 180 p.: ill.; 19 cm. ISBN: 350700772X: LC Classification: LB1050.5.R32 National Bib. No.: GFR78-A43

Rainov, Vasil G. Za psikhosemantichnata spetsifika na ezikovoto vuzpriiatie / Vasil Rainov. Variant Title on leaf facing t.p.: Psychosemantics and language perception Sofiia: Akademichno izd-vo "Prof. Marin Drinov", 1998. Description: 94 p.; 20 cm. ISBN: 9544304959 LC Classification: P37.R27 1998 Other System No.: (DLC) 99237207

Randomised controlled trial of the effect of coloured overlays on the rate of reading of people with specific learning difficulties. Abstract: A randomised controlled trial has demonstrated that, for selected children with reading difficulties, individually prescribed coloured filters reduce symptoms of asthenopia. In the present study, we investigate the effect of individually prescribed coloured overlays on the rate of reading. Subjects were 33 children and adults who: had consulted a specific learning difficulties clinic; had received treatment to normalise any conventional optometric and orthoptic anomalies; and subsequently reported symptomatic relief from coloured filters. Bouldoukian J Wilkins AJ Evans BJ Ophthalmic Physiol Opt 2002 Jan;22(1):55-60.

Rapid auditory processing and phonological ability in normal readers and readers with dyslexia. Abstract: According to a prominent theory, the phonological difficulties in dyslexia are caused by an underlying general impairment in the ability to process sequences of rapidly presented, brief sounds. Two studies examined this theory by exploring the relationships between rapid auditory processing and phonological processing in a sample of 82 normally reading children (Study 1) and by comparing 17 children with dyslexia to chronological-age and reading-age control participants on these tasks (Study 2 Marshall CM Snowling MJ Bailey PJ J Speech Lang Hear Res 2001 Aug;44(4):925-40.

Rapid automatized naming in children referred for evaluation of heterogeneous learning problems: how specific are naming speed deficits to reading disability? Abstract: Because the Rapid Automatized Naming (RAN) test reliably predicts reading skill, it is typically viewed as a diagnostic indicator of risk for reading disability (RD). Since most of the work on naming speed has been undertaken within the framework of reading research, however, the extent to which poor RAN is specifically associated with RD or with learning impairment (LI) in general is uncertain. We tested the hypothesis that slow naming speed is specific to RD. Participants were 188 children (ages 7 to 11) referred for evaluation of learning problems. Waber DP Wolff PH Forbes PW Weiler MD Neuropsychol Dev Cogn Sect C Child Neuropsychol 2000 Dec;6(4):251-61.

Rapid naming deficits in children and adolescents with reading disabilities and attention deficit hyperactivity disorder. Abstract: Seventy-one children in three groups (reading disabilities, ADHD without reading disabilities, and normal controls) were compared on their ability to rapidly name colors, letters, numbers, and objects (RAN Tasks) and alternating letters/numbers and letters/numbers/colors (RAS tasks). Children with reading disabilities were found to be slower on letter- and number-naming tasks and made more errors on all tasks than controls or children with ADHD. Semrud-Clikeman M Guy K Griffin JD Hynd GW Brain Lang 2000 Aug;74(1):70-83.

Rapid word identification in pure alexia is lexical but not semantic. Abstract: Following the notion that patients with pure alexia have access to two distinct reading strategies-letter-by-letter reading and semantic reading-a training program was devised to facilitate reading via semantics in a patient with pure alexia. Training utilized brief stimulus presentations and required category judgments rather than explicit word identification. The training was successful for trained words, but generalized poorly to untrained words. Additional studies involving oral reading of nouns and of functors resulted in improved reading of trained words. Friedman RB Lott SN Brain Lang 2000 May;72(3):219-37.

Rate of information segregation in developmentally dyslexic children. Abstract: Slowed processing of sequential perceptual information is related to developmental dyslexia. We investigated this unimodally and crossmodally in developmentally dyslexic children and controls ages 8-12 years. The participants judged whether two spatially separate trains of brief stimuli, presented at various stimulus onset asynchronies (SOA) in one or two senses, were synchronous or not. The stimulus trains consisted of light flashes in vision, clicks in audition, and indentations of the skin in the tactile sense. Laasonen M Tomma-Halme J Lahti-

Nuuttila P Service E Virsu V Brain Lang 2000 Oct 15;75(1):66-81.

Rawson, Margaret B. Developmental language disability; adult accomplishments of dyslexic boys [by] Margaret B. Rawson. Baltimore, Johns Hopkins Press [1968] Description: xv, 127 p. illus. 24 cm. LC Classification: LB1050.R34 Dewey Class No.: 371.92

Rawson, Margaret B. Dyslexia over the lifespan: a fifty-five-year longitudinal study / Margaret B. Rawson. Cambridge, Mass.: Educators Pub. Services, 1995. Description: xxiii, 197 p.: ill.; 23 cm. ISBN: 0838816703   (pbk.)   LC Classification: RC394.W6   R28   1995 Dewey Class No.: 616.85/53 20

Re: Critical response to dyslexia, literacy and psychology   assessment.   Patterson   F Dyslexia 2001 Jul-Sep;7(3):175-7.

Re: Critical response to dyslexia, literacy and psychology   assessment.   Reason   R Dyslexia 2001 Jul-Sep;7(3):174.

Re: Knivsberg, A.-M.: urine peptide patterns in dyslexia. Pediatric Rehabilitation, 1: 25-33, 1997. Stanley O Pediatr Rehabil 1997 Oct-Dec;1(4):245.

Reading ability and processing in Duchenne muscular dystrophy and spinal muscular atrophy. Abstract: We analysed the reading abilities and processing of 21 children   with   Duchenne   muscular dystrophy (DMD), 11 matched children suffering from spinal muscular atrophy (SMA) and 42 children receiving normal education. The principal result observed was that the DMD children exhibited a reading age which was significantly lower than the SMA children compared with their chronological age. These learning disabilities were not related to a deficit in non-verbal performance intelligence, but psycholinguistic evaluation showed a deficit in verbal intelligence, especially in the Similarities and Arithmetic WISC-R subtests, in phonological abilities, oral word repetition, and in digit span score.

Billard C Gillet P Barthez M Hommet C Bertrand P Dev Med Child Neurol 1998 Jan;40(1):12-20.

Reading ability as an estimator of premorbid intelligence: does it remain stable in emergent dementia? Abstract: The 6-year stability of reading performance was investigated in subjects who were normal at baseline but suspect for dementia at follow-up (MMSE score < or = 23; n = 197), and in a cognitively intact control group (n = 117). The Dutch version of the National Adult Reading Test (DART) was used. The DART-based estimate of IQ appeared to be very stable in healthy elderly. In the "suspect" group, the decline after 6 years was about 3 IQ-points in subjects who were still not demented, minimally demented, or mildly demented. Reliability remained satisfactory in these subgroups. In cases with moderate and severe Schmand B Geerlings MI Jonker C Lindeboom J J Clin Exp Neuropsychol 1998 Feb;20(1):42-51.

Reading achievement by learning disabled students in resource and regular classes. Abstract: K-TEA Comprehensive Reading scores of 34 elementary boys in either resource rooms or regular settings were compared. The boys were identified as learning disabled in reading. They were pretested at the beginning of the school year and posttested at the end. Treatment was one year of daily instruction in reading provided by six teachers in resource setting and six teachers in regular settings. K-TEA Reading Decoding and Reading Comprehension scores, separately compared in 2 x 2 repeated-measures analysis of variance, were not significantly different. Goldman R Sapp GL Foster AS Percept Mot Skills 1998 Feb;86(1):192-4.

Reading   and   attention   disorders: neurobiological   correlates   /   edited   by Drake D. Duane. Baltimore, Md.: York Press, c1999. Duane, Drake D, 1936- Description: x, 253 p.: ill.; 23 cm. ISBN: 0912752556   LC   Classification: RC394.W6 R347 1999 Dewey Class No.: 616.85/53 21

Reading and dyslexia: visual and attentional processes / edited by John Everatt. London; New York: Routledge, 1999. Everatt, John. Description: xi, 212 p.: ill.; 24 cm. ISBN: 0415123275 (hbk) 0415206332 (pbk) LC Classification: LB1050.5.R362 1999 Dewey Class No.: 371.91/44 21

Reading and language in 9- to 12-year olds prenatally exposed to cigarettes and marijuana. Abstract: Facets of reading and language were examined in 131 9- to 12-year-old children for whom prenatal exposure to marijuana and cigarettes had been ascertained. The subjects were from a low-risk, predominantly middle class sample who are participants in an ongoing longitudinal study. Discriminant Function Analysis revealed a dose-dependent association that remained after controlling for potential confounds, between prenatal cigarette exposure and lower language and lower reading scores, particularly on auditory-related aspects of this latter measure. Fried PA Watkinson B Siegel LS Neurotoxicol Teratol 1997 May-Jun;19(3):171-83.

Reading and spelling disorders: clinical features and causes. Abstract: Developmental dyslexia (specific reading and specific spelling disorder) is thought to stem from specific features in cognitive processing strongly related to biological maturation of the central nervous system which interact with non-biological learning conditions. The specific learning disorder should not be accounted for by mental age, gross neurological deficits, emotional disturbances or inadequate schooling. As a clinical guideline, the child's level in reading and spelling must be significantly below that expected for the population of children of the same mental age. Warnke A Eur Child Adolesc Psychiatry 1999;8 Suppl 3:2-12.

Reading and writing difficulties do not always occur as the researcher expects. Abstract: Making a prognosis about reading and learning difficulties is a tricky business, even if a large array of relevant variables is taken into account. The present article discusses such an endeavour, on the basis of a longitudinal four-year study which started with an orthodox intervention on linguistic awareness. However, after initial success, new groups of reading, writing and math disabled children were identified in the course of years. Niemi P Poskiparta E Vauras M Maki H Scand J Psychol 1998 Sep;39(3):159-61.

Reading disabilities with and without behaviour problems at 7-8 years: prediction from longitudinal data from infancy to 6 years. Abstract: Seven-year-old children with reading disabilities (RD-only), behaviour problems (BP-only), both conditions (RD-BP) and neither condition (Comparison) were compared on indices including temperament and behaviour, gathered in five periods between infancy and 6 years of age. The RD-BP group differed clearly from the RD-only group from infancy onwards. This comorbid group was similar to the BP-only group, while the RD-only group was similar to the Comparison group, until school age. Sanson A Prior M Smart D J Child Psychol Psychiatry 1996 Jul;37(5):529-41.

Reading disabilities: genetic and neurological influences / edited by Bruce F. Pennington. Dordrecht; Boston: Kluwer Academic, c1991. Pennington, Bruce Franklin, 1946- Related Titles: [Reading and writing. Description: 252 p.: ill.; 25 cm. ISBN: 0792316061 (HB: alk. paper) LC Classification: RC394.W6 R38 1991 NLM Class No.: W1 NE342DG v.4 WL 340 R286 1992 Dewey Class No.: 616.85/53 20

Reading disabilities: the interaction of reading, language, and neuropsychological deficits / Donald G. Doehring... [et al.]. New York: Academic Press, 1981. Doehring, Donald G. Description: xiii, 280 p.: ill.; 23 cm. ISBN: 0122191803 LC Classification: LB1050.5.R384 NLM Class No.: WL 340.6 R287 Dewey Class No.: 372.4 19

Reading disability, attention deficit hyperactivity disorder, and the immune system.

Warren RP Odell JD Warren WL Burger RA Maciulis A Daniels WW Torres AR Science 1995 May 12;268(5212):786-8.

Reading disability: evidence for a genetic etiology. Abstract: A review of evidence for genetic influences on reading disabilities (RD) is presented, with focus on twin study design and sib-pair linkage techniques. DeFries-Fulker multiple regression analyses result in significant estimates of heritability for group deficits on several reading and language measures. Structural equation modeling techniques reveal the presence of significant common and independent genetic effects on individual differences on reading skills. Finally, linkage techniques confirm a candidate locus for RD on chromosome 6. Gayan J Olson RK Eur Child Adolesc Psychiatry 1999;8 Suppl 3:52-5.

Reading disorders: varieties and treatments / edited by R.N. Malatesha, P.G. Aaron; with a foreword by O.L. Zangwill. New York: Academic Press, 1982. Malatesha, R. N. Aaron, P. G. Description: xxvi, 510 p.: ill.; 24 cm. ISBN: 0124663206 LC Classification: RC394.W6 R4 1982 Dewey Class No.: 616.85/53 19

Reading epilepsy: report of five new cases and further considerations on the pathophysiology. Abstract: Five new cases of reading epilepsy (RE) are reported. This is an epilepsy syndrome belonging to the group of idiopathic localization-related epilepsies. They all have some interesting features which contribute to the understanding of the pathomechanism and nosology of this specific type of reflex epilepsy. In our first patient the precipitating effect of texts in unknown languages depended upon phonematic intricacy. With our second case, changes of script within the text (Latin to Greek) increased the precipitating effect. Wolf P Mayer T Reker M Seizure 1998 Aug;7(4):271-9.

Reading errors following right hemisphere injection of sodium amobarbital. Abstract: The role of the nondominant hemisphere in reading is controversial. We characterized the reading errors made by 64 right-handed adults with complex partial seizures (half with seizure foci on the right and half on the left), after right hemisphere injection of sodium amobarbital. Subjects were presented with 20 six-word sentences and all were found to have speech associated with the left hemisphere only. A variety of reading errors occurred, most of which fell under the syndrome of "neglect dyslexia" including deletions and substitutions of whole words on the left side of a line of text as well as within-word neglect errors. Schwartz TH Ojemann GA Dodrill CB Brain Lang 1997 Jun 1;58(1):70-91.

Reading in Arabic orthography: the effect of vowels and context on reading accuracy of poor and skilled native Arabic readers in reading paragraphs, sentences, and isolated words. Abstract: This study investigated the effect of vowels and context on the reading accuracy of poor and skilled native Arabic readers in reading paragraphs, sentences, and words. Central to this study is the belief that reading theory today should consider additional variables, especially when explaining the reading process in Arabic orthography among poor and normal/skilled readers. This orthography has not been studied. Reading theory today is the sum of conclusions from studies conducted in Latin orthography. Abu-Rabia S J Psycholinguist Res 1997 Jul;26(4):465-82.

Reading lexically without semantics: evidence from patients with probable Alzheimer's disease. Abstract: Recent modifications of the lexical model of oral reading make the prediction that under conditions where sublexical reading processes alone cannot achieve the target pronunciation (i.e, when words have exceptional spellings or when sublexical processes are impaired), patients with severe semantic impairment should have more difficulty reading aloud semantically impaired words than semantically retained words. In a battery of lexical-semantic and reading tasks, two neurologically normal control subjects and two subjects with probable Alzheimer's disease (AD) and only moderate semantic impairment read aloud all words accurately Raymer AM Berndt RS J Int Neuropsychol Soc 1996 Jul;2(4):340-9.

Reading numbers in pure alexia: effects of the task and hemispheric specialization Abstract: Selective conservation of the ability to read Arabic numbers in patients unable to read words or even letters is a classical characteristic of pure alexia described by Dejerine (1982). We report our work on the capacity of two patients with pure typical alexia to process numbers. Our main finding was that these patients could count pairs of Arabic numbers correctly when the reading task was simple (example 2 4-->"two four") or when the task involved comparing sizes (example 2 4-->"four is bigger than two"). Cohen L Dehaene S Rev Neurol (Paris) 1995 Aug-Sep;151(8-9):480-5.

Reading of kana (phonetic symbols for syllables) in Japanese children with spastic diplegia and periventricular leukomalacia. Abstract: In 31 Japanese children with spastic diplegia and periventricular leukomalacia (PVL), the age at which they could read Hiragana (phonetic symbols for syllables) and psychometric data were examined. Reading of Hiragana was achieved between 2 and 8 years of age in all subjects except one. Four children could read Hiragana at 2 to 3 years of age, an age which is considered early among Japanese children. Performance IQs of the Wechsler Scale were lower than Verbal IQs in 18 of 19 children who were administered this test, and DQs of the cognitive adaptive (C-A) area of the K-form developmental test (a popular test in Japan) were lower than those of the language social area in all 12 children taking this test. Yokochi K Brain Dev 2000 Jan;22(1):13-5.

Reading problems and antisocial behaviour: developmental trends in comorbidity. Abstract: Samples of poor and normal readers were followed through adolescence and into early adulthood to assess continuities in the comorbidity between reading difficulties and disruptive behaviour problems. Reading-disabled boys showed high rates of inattentiveness in middle childhood, but no excess of teacher-rated behaviour problems at age 14 and no elevated rates of aggression, antisocial personality disorder or officially recorded offending in early adulthood. Increased risks of juvenile offending among specifically retarded-reading boys seemed associated with poor school attendance, rather than reading difficulties per se. Reading problems were associated with some increases in disruptive behaviour in their teens in girls. Maughan B Pickles A Hagell A Rutter M Yule W J Child Psychol Psychiatry 1996 May;37(4):405-18.

Reading skills in hyperlexia: a developmental perspective. Abstract: Hyperlexia is characterized by advanced word-recognition skills in individuals who otherwise have pronounced cognitive, social, and linguistic handicaps. Language, word recognition, and reading-comprehension skills are reviewed to clarify the nature and core deficits associated with the disorder. It is concluded that hyperlexia should be viewed as part of the normal variation in reading skills, which are themselves associated with individual differences in phonological, orthographic, and semantic processing, short-term memory, and print exposure. Nation K Psychol Bull 1999 May;125(3):338-55.

Reading speed in pure alexia. Abstract: This study investigated possible causes of differences in reading speed between two alexic patients who read words letter by letter. As both patients appeared to rely on serial left-to-right processing of letters within words, the difference in reading speed did not seem to be related to any differences in the extent to which the patients could recognize letters in words in parallel or 'ends-in'. Differences in reading speed seemed to be unrelated to the patients ability to identify individual letters since their letter recognition accuracy was very similar. Hanley JR Kay J Neuropsychologia 1996 Dec; 34 (12): 1165-74.

Reading too little into reading?: strategies in the rehabilitation of acquired dyslexia. Abstract: This paper examines four recent therapy studies, two involving deep dyslexic patients and two involving surface dyslexic patients. These studies illustrate that remediation of aspects of acquired dyslexia can have positive benefits for the patients concerned which often extend beyond an improvement in reading aloud. It is argued that, although it may not be immediately apparent, the remediation of acquired reading impairments (and even of reading aloud) can be of functional significance for an aphasic subject. Nickels L Eur J Disord Commun 1995;30(1):37-50.

Reading words and pseudowords: an eye movement study of developmental dyslexia. Abstract: The pattern of eye movements during reading was studied in 12 developmental dyslexics and in 10 age-matched controls. According to standard reading batteries, dyslexics showed marked reading slowness and prevalently used the sublexical procedure in reading. Eye movements were recorded while they read lists of short and long words or pseudowords. In normal readers, saccade amplitude increased with word length without a concomitant change in the number of saccades; in contrast, the number of saccades increased for long pseudowords. De Luca M Borrelli M Judica A Spinelli D Zoccolotti P Brain Lang 2002 Mar;80(3):617-26.

Reading-related wavelength and spatial frequency effects in visual spatial location. Abstract: Specific deficits in the processing of transient visual stimuli have been identified in reading-disabled children, and it has been shown that the filtering out of some medium to high spatial frequencies and some visible wavelengths impacts on their performance in a number of visual tasks. To assess further how these light diffusing and colour filtering manipulations might mediate visual processing, this study compared the letter-naming accuracy and visual spatial location judgements of eighteen poor readers with those made by eighteen good readers of the same age Solman RT Dain SJ Lim HS May JG Ophthalmic Physiol Opt 1995 Mar;15(2):125-32.

Readings in dyslexia. Portion of Dyslexia Guilford, Conn.: Special Learning Corp, [c1978- Description: v.: ill.; 28 cm. 1st ed.- Current Frequency: Annual LC Classification: LB1050.5.R395 Dewey Class No.: 371.91/4 19 Other System No.: (OCoLC)ocm06105184 Acquisition Source: Special Learning Corp, 42 Boston Post Rd, Guilford, CT 06437 Serial Record Entry: Readings in dyslexia. Guilford, Conn. 86-640822

Recall of morphologically complex forms is affected by memory task but not dyslexia. Abstract: The authors studied the effect of morphological complexity on working memory in list recall tasks with base words (boy), inflected words (boy + 's) and derived words (boy + hood) in a morphologically rich language: Finnish. Simple serial recall was compared to complex working memory tasks, combining word recall with sentence verification in 8-year-old normally reading participants, dyslexic children, and adults. The normally reading children performed better than dyslexic children on both memory tasks and a test of morphology. Base words were better recalled than morphologically complex words. Memory was better for derived than inflected words in simple but not complex span tasks. Service E Tujulin AM Brain Lang 2002 Apr-Jun;81(1-3):42-54.

Recovery from deep alexia to phonological alexia: points on a continuum. Abstract: Reports of five patients whose deep alexic reading all evolved into phonological alexia in a similar fashion point to the hypothesis that deep alexia and phonological alexia represent different points on the same continuum. This hypothesis is explored further through an examination of previously published case reports of eleven patients with phonological alexia. Data from these patients suggest that there is a predictable succession of symptoms which form a continuum of severity of phonological alexia, with deep alexia as its endpoint. Friedman RB Brain Lang 1996 Jan;52(1):114-28.

Red blood cell fatty acid compositions in a patient with autistic spectrum disorder: a characteristic abnormality in neurodevelopmental disorders? Abstract: The fatty acid compositions of red blood cell (RBC) phospholipids from a patient with autistic spectrum disorder (ASD) had reduced percentages of highly unsaturated fatty acids (HUFA) compared to control samples. The percentage of HUFA in the RBC from the autistic patient was dramatically reduced (up to 70%) when the sample was stored for 6 weeks at -20 degrees C. However, only minor HUFA reductions were recorded in control samples stored similarly, or when the autistic sample was stored at -80 degrees C. A similar instability in RBC HUFA compositions upon storage at -20 degrees C has been recorded in schizophrenic patients. Bell JG Sargent JR Tocher DR Dick JR Prostaglandins Leukot Essent Fatty Acids 2000 Jul-Aug;63(1-2):21-5.

Reduced cognitive inhibition in schizotypy. Abstract: The relationship between negative priming and the positive symptoms of schizotypy was investigated. It was hypothesized that high schizotypes would display less negative priming than low schizotypes. A further important aim of the study was to disentangle the modalities involved in negative priming performance, since a reduction in negative priming, as revealed by schizophrenics and schizotypes, might reflect a failure to actively inhibit irrelevant information (cognitive inhibition) as well as dyslexia or a general slowness in information processing. Results support the hypothesis that reduced cognitive inhibition may underlie positive schizotypal symptomatology. Moritz S Mass R Br J Clin Psychol 1997 Sep;36 (Pt 3):365-76.

Reflections on foreign language study for students with language learning problems: research, issues and challenges. Abstract: The study of foreign language (FL) learning for individuals who have found learning to read and write in their first language extremely problematic has been an under-researched area throughout the world. Since the 1980s, Leonore Ganschow and Richard Sparks have conducted pioneering research into the nature of difficulties, why they are encountered and how they can be minimized. Ganschow L Sparks RL Dyslexia 2000 Apr-Jun;6(2):87-100.

'Reflections on StudyScan'. Allane L Dyslexia 2001 Oct-Dec;7(4):247-8.

Reflections on StudyScan. De Montfort University, Lincoln, UK. Sanderson A Dyslexia 2000 Oct-Dec;6(4):284-90.

Reflections on visual evoked cortical potentials and selective attention: methodological and historical. Abstract: Details of research in which Russ Harter participated in his formative years are reviewed. Harter's participation in the early work on Visual Selective Attention (Eason, Harter & White, 1969) probably contributed most importantly to his career. While reviewing Russ's early experience with basic vision research and pioneer visual evoked potentials (VEPs), there is reference to extensive information regarding stimulus effects on VEPs (exogenous components of the ERP). There can be complex early and late waveforms and waveform changes with changes in certain stimulus conditions. White CT White CL Int J Neurosci 1995;80(1-4):13-30.

Refractory dyslexia: evidence of multiple task-specific phonological output stores. Abstract: We investigated the case of a patient whose reading was characterized by multiple phonemic paraphasic errors. An error analysis of a large corpus of reading responses (758 words, 86 nonwords) highlighted the preponderance of phonological errors which did not occur in his naming, repetition or spontaneous speech. His comprehension of the written word was relatively preserved, even for words he was unable to read aloud. We suggest that his impairment lies at the level of the phonological output store. Crutch SJ Warrington EK Brain 2001 Aug;124(Pt 8):1533-43.

Rehabilitation of a case of pure alexia: exploiting residual abilities. Abstract: We present a case study of a 43-year-old woman with chronic and stable pure alexia. Using a multiple baseline design we report the results of two different interventions to improve reading. First, a restitutive treatment approach using an implicit semantic access strategy was attempted. This approach was designed to exploit privileged access to lexical-semantic representations and met with little success. Maher LM Clayton MC Barrett AM Schober-Peterson D Gonzalez Rothi LJ J Int Neuropsychol Soc 1998 Nov;4(6):636-47.

Reid, Gavin, 1950- Dyslexia in adults: education and employment / Gavin Reid and Jane Kirk. Chichester; New York: John Wiley, c2001. Kirk, Jane. Description: xi, 244 p.: ill.; 25 cm. ISBN: 0471852058 (pbk.) LC Classification: HV1570.5.U6 R44 2001 Dewey Class No.: 362.1//968553086/0973 21

Reid, Gavin, 1950- Dyslexia: a practitioner's handbook/Gavin Reid. Chichester; New York: J. Wiley, c1998. Description: vii, 250 p.: ill.; 25 cm. ISBN: 0471973912 (pbk.: acid-free paper) LC Classification: LC4708.R45 1998 Dewey Class No.: 371.91/44 21 Electronic File Info. http://www.loc.gov/catdir/toc/onix 03/97017407.html

Reid, Jessie F, comp. Reading: problems and practices: a selection of papers edited with introductions by Jessie F. Reid. London, Ward Lock, 1972. Description: 415 p. illus. 23 cm. ISBN: 0706233441 0706231228 (pbk.) LC Classification:

RC394.W6 R44 NLM Class No.: WL340 R356r 1972 Dewey Class No.: 371.9/14 National Bib. No.: B72-30985

Relative hand skill predicts academic ability: global deficits at the point of hemispheric indecision. Abstract: Population variation in handedness (a correlate of cerebral dominance for language) is in part genetic and, it has been suggested, its persistence represents a balanced polymorphism with respect to cognitive ability. This hypothesis was tested in a sample of 12,770 individuals in a UK national cohort (the National Child Development Study) by assessing relative hand skill (in a square checking task) as a predictor of verbal, non-verbal, and mathematical ability and reading comprehension at the age of 11 years. Crow TJ Crow LR Done DJ Leask S Neuropsychologia 1998 Dec;36(12):1275-82.

Relearning after damage in connectionist networks: toward a theory of rehabilitation. Abstract: Connectionist modeling offers a useful computational framework for exploring the nature of normal and impaired cognitive processes. The current work extends the relevance of connectionist modeling in neuropsychology to address issues in cognitive rehabilitation: the degree and speed of recovery through retraining, the extent to which improvement on treated items generalizes to untreated items, and how treated items are selected to maximize this generalization. A network previously used to model impairments in mapping orthography to semantics is retrained after damage. Plaut DC Brain Lang 1996 Jan;52(1):25-82.

Research initiatives in learning disabilities: contributions from scientists supported by the National Institute of Child Health and Human Development. Abstract: The National Institute of Child Health and Human Development has been and will continue to be, responsive to the critical research needs in learning disabilities and related disorders. As an index of the heightened research activity in this arena, consider that National Institute of Child Health and Human Development's support for projects related to learning and language disabilities has increased from 1.75 million dollars in 1975 to over 15 million dollars in 1993--a cumulative total of approximately 80 million dollars. Lyon GR J Child Neurol 1995 Jan;10 Suppl 1:S120-6.

Response biases in oral reading: an account of the co-occurrence of surface dyslexia and semantic dementia. Abstract: This paper reports a case study of a subject (EP) with a progressive impairment of semantic memory and a coincident surface dyslexia. These two disorders frequently occur together, but their association is not readily explained within current models of reading. This study investigated two theories that offer different principled accounts of this association, the "semantic glue hypothesis" (Patterson & Hodges, 1992) and the "summation hypothesis" (Hillis & Caramazza, 1991) and found both hypotheses wanting. Funnell E Q J Exp Psychol A 1996 May;49(2):417-46.

Reversal of alexia in multiple sclerosis by weak electromagnetic fields. Abstract: The occurrence of cognitive deficits in patients with multiple sclerosis (MS) has been recognized since 1877 when Charcot first observed "enfeeblement of memory" in his patients. Cognitive deficits have been reported in almost 50% of patients with a relapsing-remitting course and in a significantly higher percentage of patients with a chronic progressive course leading to intellectual disability which is often severe enough to preclude employment Sandyk R Int J Neurosci 1995 Nov;83(1-2):69-79.

Richardson, Sylvia O. Doctors ask questions about dyslexia / Sylvia O.Richardson. Baltimore, MD: Orton Dyslexia Society, 1996. Description: 1 v.

Richardson, Ulla. Familial dyslexia and sound duration in the quantity distinctions of Finnish infants and adults / Ulla Richardson. Jyväskylä: University of Jyväskylä, 1998. Description: 211 p.: ill.; 25 cm. ISBN: 9513901750 LC Classification: PH151.R53 1998 Dewey Class No.: 494/.54116 21

Riezinger, Beate, 1966- Legasthenie-prävention: Fördermassnahmen im Schuleingangsbereich / Beate Riezinger. Frankfurt am Main; New York: P. Lang, c1998. Description: 146 p.; 21 cm. ISBN: 3631336233 LC Classification: LB1050.5.R55 1998

Right body side performance decrement in congenitally dyslexic children and left body side performance decrement in congenitally hyperactive children. Abstract: Simple and complex visuomotor performance of the right and left sides of the body was investigated in 37 children with left hemisphere lesions, 35 children with right hemisphere lesions, 53 developmentally dyslexic children, 29 developmentally hyperactive children, and 35 "normal" children who had endured a very mild head injury with no sequelae. BACKGROUND: Lateralized soft signs, EEG topography, metabolic brain imaging, and neuropsychological test profiles suggest a predominance of left hemisphere dysfunction in dyslexia and right hemisphere dysfunction in hyperactivity. We propose that (1) contralateral performance decrement results from a unilateral cortical lesion in children, and (2) developmental dyslexia may comprise a slight predominance of left hemisphere dysfunction and developmental hyperactivity of right hemisphere dysfunction. Universite du Quebec a Montreal, Departement de Psychologie, Canada. Braun.Claude@UQAM.CA Braun CM Archambault MA Daigneault S Larocque C Neuropsychiatry Neuropsychol Behav Neurol 2000 Apr; 13 (2): 89-100.

Role of auditory temporal processing for reading and spelling disability. Abstract: The role of auditory temporal processing in reading and spelling was investigated in a sample of 30 children and one of 31 adults, using a gap-detection task with nonspeech stimuli. There was no evidence for a relationship between reading and spelling disability (dyslexia) and the gap-detection threshold. The results were discussed regarding the relevance for the popular hypothesis of an auditory temporal processing deficit underlying dyslexia. Schulte-Korne G Deimel W Bartling J Remschmidt H Percept Mot Skills 1998 Jun;86(3 Pt 1):1043-7.

Rorby, Ginny. Dolphin sky / Ginny Rorby. New York: Putnam's Sons, c1996. Description: 246 p.: map; 22 cm. ISBN: 0399229051 Summary: Twelve-year-old Buddy, whose dyslexia makes things difficult for her both at home and at school, hopes to rescue the dolphins that are being held captive and mistreated at a swamp farm near her home in the Everglades. LC Classification: PZ7.O2915 Re 1996 Dewey Class No.: [Fic] 20

Rosenberg, Renate von. Legastenie, Ursachen und Auswege bei schulischem Versagen / Renate Dangschat [i. e. R. v. Rosenberg]. Dornburg-Frickhofen: Frankonius-Verlag, 1972. Description: 56 p.; 21 cm. ISBN: 387962013X: LC Classification: LB1050.5.R59 National Bib. No.: GFR75-A

Routes to reading: a report of a non-semantic reader with equivalent performance on regular and exception words. Abstract: This study reports the case of a stroke patient, EW, who had severely-impaired comprehension of written words but could read aloud regular and exception words, non-words and sentences flawlessly. EW's auditory comprehension was impaired. It is argued that these results support a three-route model of reading, where the phonological output lexicon can be activated directly from the orthographic input lexicon, as her reading performance did not conform to the pattern that would be expected from a combination of lexical-semantic and sublexical processing alone. Gerhand S Neuropsychologia 2001;39 (13): 1473-84.

Row blindness in Gestalt grouping and developmental dyslexia. Abstract: A classic Gestalt figure is a 4 x 4 array of items grouped by similarity into either rows or columns. We found that some people do not see rows ("row blindness"). Furthermore, row blindness correlates with difficulties processing written language-- more than half of the college-age dyslexics tested were row blind. Reading difficulties are probably not a cause of row blindness and forming rows by grouping is a part of reading, suggesting that row blindness might be one source of problems processing written language. Lewis JP Frick RW Neuropsychologia 1999 Mar;37(3):385-93.

Ruhfus, Sabine, 1949- Legasthenie und Rechtschreibreform: Möglichkeiten u. Grenzen e. Behebung legasthener Erscheinungsformen durch e. gezielte Reform d. dt. Rechtschreibung / Sabine Ruhfus. Frankfurt am Main; Bern; Cirencester/U.K.: Lang, 1980. Description: v, 271 p.; 21 cm. ISBN: 3820466711 LC Classification: LB1050.5.R83 National Bib. No.: GFR79-A

Ryden, Michael, 1960- Dyslexia: how would I cope? / Michael Ryden; foreword by Derek Copley. Edition Information: 3rd ed. London; Bristol, Pa.: Jessica Kingsley Publishers, 1997. Description: 64 p.: ill.; 22 cm. ISBN: 185302385X LC Classification: LB1050.5.R93 1997 Dewey Class No.: 371.91/44 21

Ryden, Michael, 1960- Dyslexia: how would I cope? / Michael Ryden; with an introduction by Derek Copley. London: Jessica Kingsley Publishers, 1989. Description: 64 p.: ill.; 22 cm. ISBN: 1853020265 LC Classification: LB1050.5.R93 1989 Dewey Class No.: 371.91/44 20

Sagmiller, Girard J. Dyslexia, my life: one man's story of his life with a learning disability: an autobiography / by Girard J. Sagmiller, with Gigi Lane. Waverly, IA: G & R Pub. Co, c1995. Lane, Gigi.

Description: vi, 120 p.: ill.; 22 cm. ISBN: 0964308711 LC Classification: MLCS 97/02808 (R)

Sagripanti, Nazzareno. Disprattognosie e disturbi dell'apprendimento scolastico in età evolutiva / Nazzareno Sagripanti. Macerata: Tip. S. Giuseppe, [1975?] Description: 65 p.: ill.; 24 cm. LC Classification: LC4704.S23 National Bib. No.: It77-Feb

Sampling strategies for model free linkage analyses of quantitative traits: implications for sib pair studies of reading and spelling disabilities to minimize the total study cost. Abstract: One approach to establish linkage is based on allele sharing methods for sib pairs. In recent years the use of selected sib pairs to increase power for mapping quantitative traits in humans has been discussed intensively. In this paper the different basic principles for sib pair sampling proposed in the literature are made evident. Implications for ascertainment schemes of sib pairs to minimize the total study cost in linkage analyses on reading and spelling disabilities are discussed. Ziegler A Eur Child Adolesc Psychiatry 1999;8 Suppl 3:35-9.

Sanders, Marion. Understanding dyslexia and the reading process: a guide for educators and parents / Marion Sanders. Boston: Allyn and Bacon, c2001. Description: xiv, 210 p.; 23 cm. ISBN: 0205309070 (pbk.) LC Classification: LB1050.5.S224 2001 Dewey Class No.: 371.91/44 21

Sanders, Pete. Dyslexia / Pete Sanders and Steve Myers; illustrated by Mike Lacy and Liz Sawyer. Uniform [Dyslexia & associated difficulties Spine What do you know about dyslexia Brookfield, Conn.: Copper Beech Books, 1999. Myers, Steve. Lacy, Mike, ill. Description: 32 p.: col. ill.; 28 cm. ISBN: 0761309152 (lib. bdg.) Summary: Examines the nature, symptoms, effects, and diagnosis of dyslexia and the specialized help available for those with this condition. LC Classification: RJ496.A5 S26 1999 Dewey

Class No.: 616.85/53 21 Other System No.: (DLC) 98044971

Saqmiller, Girard J. Dyslexia, my life: one man's story of his life with a learning disability / Girard J. Sagmiller, Gigi Lane. Waverly, IA: Doubting Thomas Pub, 1996. Description: p. cm. ISBN: 0964308711 (pbk.) LC Classification: 9601 BOOK NOT YET IN LC

Sargent, Dave, 1941- What every teacher and parent should know about dyslexia / by Dave Sargent & Laura Tirella. Prairie Grove, AR: Ozark Pub, c1996. Tirella, Laura. Description: vii, 91 p.; 29 cm. ISBN: 1567631282 (cloth: alk. paper) 1567631274 (paper: alk. paper) LC Classification: LB1050.5.S227 1996 Dewey Class No.: 371.91/44 20

Sartori, Giuseppe. La lettura: processi normali e dislessia. Bologna: Mulino, c1984. Description: 285 p.: ill.; 22 cm. ISBN: 8815006672: LC Classification: LB1050.S18 1984

Savage, John F, 1938- Dyslexia: understanding reading problems / John F. Savage. New York: J. Messner, c1985. Description: 90 p.: ill.; 22 cm. ISBN: 0671542893 Summary: Describes the characteristics of dyslexia, its causes, how it affects children, and how these children can learn to read. LC Classification: RJ496.A5 S28 1985 Dewey Class No.: 618.92/8553 19

Scalp potentials evoked by amplitude-modulated tones in dyslexia. Abstract: We recorded the far-field EEG potential evoked by amplitude modulation of acoustic stimuli (the amplitude modulation following response, AMFR) in adults with developmental dyslexia and in a matched control group of adults with no history of reading problems. The mean AMFR recorded from participants with dyslexia was significantly smaller than that recorded from members of the control group. McAnally KI Stein JF J Speech Lang Hear Res 1997 Aug;40(4):939-45.

Schenk-Danzinger, Lotte. Handbuch der Legasthenie im Kindesalter / von Lotte Schenk-Danzinger, unter Mitarb. von W. Böck... [et al.]. Edition Information: 3, durchges. u. erw. Aufl. Weinheim; Basel: Beltz, 1975. Description: xxiii, 599 p.: ill.; 22 cm. ISBN: 340720101X LC Classification: RJ496.A5 S33 1975 National Bib. No.: GFR75-A

Schenk-Danzinger, Lotte. Legasthenie und Linkshändigkeit / Lotte Schenk-Danzinger. Wien; München: Jugend & Volk; Wien: Österr. Bundesverl, c1974. Description: 22, [4] p.; 30 cm. ISBN: 3714159207: LC Classification: LB1050.5.S284 National Bib. No.: Au74-22-154 Series:

Schizophrenia: the illness that made us human. Abstract: Any hypotheses concerning the origins of humans must explain many things. Among these are: 1, the growth in brain size around two million years ago; 2, the presence of subcutaneous fat; 3, the near absence of change or cultural progress for around 2 million years after the brain grew in size; 4, the cultural explosion which began somewhere between fifty thousand and one hundred thousand years ago with the emergence of art, music, religion and warfare; 5, the further cultural explosion around ten thousand to fifteen thousand years ago which developed with the emergence of agriculture and which has continued since. Horrobin DF Med Hypotheses 1998 Apr;50(4):269-88.

Schlee, Jörg. Legasthenieforschung am Ende? / Jörg Schlee. Edition Information: 1. Aufl. München; Berlin; Wien: Urban und Schwarzenberg, 1976. Description: ix, 180 p.: 16 ill.; 21 cm. ISBN: 3541401710: LC Classification: LB1050.5.S323 National Bib. No.: GFR76-A

Schlieper, Anne. The best fight / Anne Schlieper; illustrations by Mary Beth Schwark. Morton Grove, Ill.: A. Whitman, c1995. Schwark, Mary Beth, ill. Description: 63 p.: ill.; 20 cm. ISBN: 0807506621 Summary: Fifth-grader

Jamie, who goes to a special class because he has difficulty reading, thinks he's dumb until the school principal helps him realize that he also has many talents. LC Classification: PZ7.S34714 Be 19954 Dewey Class No.: [Fic] 20

School maladjustment common among children with very low birth weight Special attention and support are required during school start Abstract: Children of very low birth weight (VLBW), defined as less than 1500 g, and normal birth weight controls (NBW) were enrolled in a long-term follow-up study. Five of 86 surviving VLBW children had a neurological handicap. Seventy VLBW children and 72 NBW children were re-examined at the age of nine, which entailed a neurological examination, a non-verbal intelligence test and a test for reading ability, mathematical skills and vocabulary. Their behavior was rated regarding hyperactivity, social behavior and fine and motor skills. Finnstrom O Leijon I Samuelsson S Bylund B Cervin T Gaddlin PO Mard S Sandstedt P Warngard O Lakartidningen 2000 Aug 9;97(32-33):3492-5, 3498.

Scotopic sensitivity in dyslexia and requirements for DHA supplementation. Abstract: Much interest is shown in reduced scotopic sensitivity in dyslexia and the possible role of docosahexaenoic-acid deficiency as a causative factor. However, we found that significant decreases in scotopic sensitivity are not a general characteristic of dyslexia, which may cast doubt on the value of DHA supplementation. Greatrex JC Drasdo N Dresser K Lancet 2000 Apr 22;355(9213):1429-30.

Scotopic sensitivity/Irlen syndrome and the use of coloured filters: a long-term placebo controlled and masked study of reading achievement and perception of ability. Abstract: This study investigated the effects of using coloured filters on reading speed, accuracy, and comprehension as well as on perception of academic ability. A double-masked, placebo-controlled crossover design was used, with subjects being assessed over a period of 20 mo. There were three treatment groups (Placebo filters, Blue filters, and Optimal filters) involving 113 subjects with "reading difficulties", ranging in age from 9.2 yr. to 13.1 yr. and with an average discrepancy between chronological age and reading age of 1.8 yr. Robinson GL Foreman PJ Percept Mot Skills 1999 Aug;89(1):83-113.

Scotopic sensitivity/Irlen syndrome and the use of coloured filters: a long-term placebo-controlled study of reading strategies using analysis of miscue. Abstract: This study investigated the long-term effects of using coloured filters on the frequency and type of errors in oral reading. A double-masked, placebo-controlled crossover experimental design was used, with subjects being assessed over a period of 20 months. There were three experimental groups (Placebo tints, Blue tints, and Diagnosed tints) involving 113 subjects with reading difficulties, ranging in age from 9.2 yr. to 13.1 yr. The 35 controls (ranging in age from 9.4 yr. to 12.9 yr.) had reading difficulties but did not require coloured filters. Robinson GL Foreman PJ Percept Mot Skills 1999 Feb;88(1):35-52.

Search for letter identity and location by disabled readers. Abstract: Reading-disabled boys, reading- and age-matched controls, and adults searched letter arrays for the identity or location of a probe letter. Response time (RT) and accuracy were examined as a function of the temporal relation between probe and array letters (probe first, simultaneous, array first), and array size (1-5 letters). Although disabled readers closely resembled age controls in RT, their accuracy differed significantly when large letter arrays were tested. Enns JT Bryson SE Roes C Can J Exp Psychol 1995 Sep;49(3):357-67.

Segregation analysis of phenotypic components of learning disabilities. I. Nonword memory and digit span. Abstract: Dyslexia is a common and complex disorder with evidence for a genetic component. Multiple loci (i.e, quantitative-trait loci [QTLs]) are likely to be involved, but the number is unknown. Diagnosis is complicated by the lack of a standard protocol, and many diagnostic measures have been proposed as understanding of the component processes has evolved. One or more genes may, in turn, influence these measures. Wijsman EM Peterson D Leutenegger AL Thomson JB Goddard KA Hsu L

Selected problems with ocular accommodation in children and youth Abstract: This paper intends to present some accommodative disturbances which cause difficulties in reading and should be differentiated from dyslexia. The work describes the way of evaluation of accommodative convergence to accommodation rate (AC/A ratio). Clinical forms of two types of nonrefractive accommodative convergence excess connected with high AC/A ratio, namely hyperkinetic and hypoaccommodative, are presented. In hyperkinetic type, disturbances of ocular movements coordination during reading prevail. Patients with hypoaccommodation disorders suffer from youth presbyopia. Kubatko-Zielinska A Krzystkowa KM Klin Oczna 1996;98(6):459-61.

Selective deficit in processing double letters. Abstract: This paper reports a patient with a selective difficulty in spelling words and pseudowords with geminate (double) consonants. In all writing tasks, deletions of a geminate consonant occurred ten times more often than deletions of a consonant in a non-geminate cluster. In addition, the probability of substituting both geminate consonants was indistinguishable from the probability of substituting one consonant in a non-geminate cluster; and, the probability of substituting only one geminate consonant was close to zero, and significantly lower than the probability of substituting one consonant in a non-geminate cluster. Miceli G Benvegnu B CapasJournalR Caramazza A Cortex 1995 Mar;31(1):161-71.

Selective deficits of vibrotactile sensitivity in dyslexic readers. Abstract: Developmental dyslexia is a disability of literacy skill that has been associated with sensory processing deficits, primarily for the detection of dynamic auditory and visual stimuli. Here we examined whether analogous deficits extend into the domain of somatosensory perception. Detection thresholds for each of three frequencies of vibration were obtained for 11 readers with a prior history of dyslexia and 14 similarly aged adult controls. Stoodley CJ Talcott JB Carter EL Witton C Stein JF Neurosci Lett 2000 Dec 1;295(1-2):13-6.

Selective disorders of reading? Abstract: Over the past few decades, refined cognitive architectures with highly specific components have been proposed to explain apparently selective disorders of reading, resulting from brain disease or injury, in previously literate adults. Recent analysis of the more general linguistic and cognitive abilities supported by neural systems damaged in the various forms of alexia favours a rather different view of reading and the kinds of models sufficient to account for its acquisition, skilled performance and disruption. Patterson K Ralph MA Curr Opin Neurobiol 1999 Apr;9(2):235-9.

Selective impairment in manipulating Arabic numerals. Abstract: This paper describes an acalculic patient (B.A.L.) with an unusual selective deficit in manipulating arabic numerals. The patient was unimpaired in reading aloud letters, words and written number names but unable to read aloud single arabic numerals. Furthermore, his ability to produce the next number in the sequence and his ability to produce answers to simple addition and subtraction was relatively spared when the stimuli were presented as number names but impaired when the stimuli were presented as arabic numerals. Cipolotti L Warrington EK Butterworth B Cortex 1995 Mar;31(1):73-86.

Selective language aphasia from herpes simplex encephalitis. Abstract: We report the case of a 16-year-old right-handed Chinese/English bilingual patient who developed herpes simplex encephalitis involving the left temporal lobe, with resultant aphasia. His native language was Mandarin, but he had received extensive training in English for 6 years after moving to the United States and was fluent in English. One week after admission, he could not speak, comprehend, repeat, name, read, or write in English, but he had relative preservation of most of these facilities in Mandarin. Ku A Lachmann EA Nagler W Pediatr Neurol 1996 Sep;15(2):169-71.

Selective predictive value of rapid automatized naming in poor readers. Abstract: This study considers the differential predictive value of rapid naming tests for various aspects of later reading, where the differential is between nondisabled and poor readers. Two large-N longitudinal samples of students who have been evaluated from third through eighth grades are studied: (a) a randomly accessed, normally distributed group including students with varying degrees of reading ability (N = 154), and (b) a group of poor readers whose single-word reading in third grade is at or below the population 10th percentile (N = 64). Meyer MS Wood FB Hart J Learn Disabil 1998 Mar-Apr; 31(2):106-17.

Selective uppercase dysgraphia with loss of visual imagery of letter forms: a window on the organization of graphomotor patterns. Abstract: We report a patient who, after a left parieto-occipital lesion, showed alexia and selective dysgraphia for uppercase letters. He showed preserved oral spelling, associated with handwriting impairment in all written production; spontaneous writing, writing to dictation, real words, pseudowords, and single letters were affected. The great majority of errors were well-formed letter substitutions: most of them were located on the first position of each word, which the patient always wrote in uppercase (as he used to do before his illness). Del GrosJournalDestreri N Farina E Alberoni

M Pomati S Nichelli P Mariani C Brain Lang 2000 Feb 15;71(3):353-72.

Self-reported reading problems in parents of twins with reading difficulties. Abstract: Parents of 323 twin pairs with reading disability (RD) reported significantly more problems learning to read (16% of mothers and 33% of fathers) than parents of 309 twin pairs without reading difficulties (6% of mothers and 9% of fathers). These rates of self-reported reading problems in parents of twins are highly similar to those previously obtained in parents of non-twin children with RD and controls, suggesting that the etiology of reading deficits in twin and non-twin children may be highly similar. Davis CJ Knopik VS Wadsworth SJ DeFries JC Twin Res 2000 Jun;3(2):88-91.

Selikowitz, Mark. Dyslexia and other learning difficulties: the facts / Mark Selikowitz. Edition Information: 2nd ed. Oxford; New York: Oxford University Press, 1998. Description: x, 159 p.: ill.; 20 cm. ISBN: 0192626612 LC Classification: RJ506.L4 S45 1998 Dewey Class No.: 618.92/85889 21

Selikowitz, Mark. Dyslexia and other learning difficulties: the facts / Mark Selikowitz. Oxford; New York: Oxford University Press, 1993. Description: vi, 130 p.: ill.; 23 cm. ISBN: 0192622994: 0192623001 (pbk.): LC Classification: RJ506.L4 S45 1993 Dewey Class No.: 618.92/85889 20

Semantic and phonological coding in poor and normal readers. Abstract: Three studies were conducted evaluating semantic and phonological coding deficits as alternative explanations of reading disability. In the first study, poor and normal readers in second and sixth grade were compared on various tests evaluating semantic development as well as on tests evaluating rapid naming and pseudoword decoding as independent measures of phonological coding ability. In a second study, the same subjects were given verbal memory and visual-verbal learning tasks using high and low meaning words as verbal stimuli and

Chinese ideographs as visual stimuli Vellutino FR Scanlon DM Spearing D J Exp Child Psychol 1995 Feb;59(1):76-123.

Semantic capacities of the right hemisphere as seen in two cases of pure word blindness. Abstract: Two patients with pure alexia were studied with tachistoscopically presented stimuli to examine factors influencing their ability to distinguish words from nonwords and to derive semantic information at exposures too brief for explicit letter identification. Both patients had profound right hemianopia and computerized tomography (CT) evidence of splenial destruction. Both patients were successful in making word/nonword decisions for high-frequency, but not low-frequency, words Goodglass H Lindfield KC Alexander MP J Psycholinguist Res 2000 Jul;29(4):399-422.

Semantic cortical activation in dyslexic readers. Abstract: The combined temporal and spatial resolution of MEG (magnetoencephalography) was used to study whether the same brain areas are similarly engaged in reading comprehension in normal and developmentally dyslexic adults. To extract a semantically sensitive stage of brain activation we manipulated the appropriateness of sentence-ending words to the preceding sentence context. Sentences, presented visually one word at a time, either ended with a word that was (1) expected, (2) semantically appropriate but unexpected, (3) semantically anomalous but sharing the initial letters with the expected word, or (4) both semantically and orthographically inappropriate to the sentence context J Cogn Neurosci 1999 Sep;11(5):535-50.

Semantic information is used by a deep dyslexic to parse compounds. Abstract: We report a case study of a 48 year-old patient, J.O, who was tested 20 years after the removal of a tumor in the left temporal-parietal region. This surgery and subsequent radiation resulted in right side paralysis and numerous language problems. Tests of J.O.'s single word reading abilities indicate that she could be classified as a deep dyslexic with over 16% of her errors in word naming having a clear semantic relationship with the target word (Coltheart, 1980). We examined her ability to read compound words aloud and following Libben (1993) we provide evidence that J.O. is a second case in which there is obligatory access of morphological constituents of compound words. McEwen S Westbury C Buchanan L Libben G Brain Cogn 2001 Jun-Jul;46(1-2):201-5.

Semantic memory and reading abilities: a case report. Abstract: We document the unexpected dissociation of preserved reading skills in a patient with severely impaired semantic memory. The common co-occurrence between impairment of word meaning and surface dyslexia has not been observed. The patient (hereafter called DRN) had marked naming and word comprehension difficulties. A strong word frequency effect was observed on tests of word comprehension but was absent in a test of word reading. DRN's ability to read both regular and exception words that he failed to comprehend was remarkably well preserved. Cipolotti L Warrington EK J Int Neuropsychol Soc 1995 Jan;1(1):104-10.

Seminario Latinoamericano sobre Dislexia, 3d, Montevideo, 1967. Dislexia escolar. Montevideo: O.E.A, Instituto Interamericano del Niño, 1968. Interamerican Children's Institute. Sociedad de Dislexia del Uruguay. Description: 264 p.: ill.; 24 cm. LC Classification: LB1050.5.S38 1967 Dewey Class No.: 371.91/4

Sense and nonsense with respect to the gene for dyslexia Abstract: Genetic studies recently reported linkages between two chromosomal regions and two phenotypes of dyslexia. These findings should not be taken to mean that the gene for dyslexia has been discovered. It is argued that a gene for dyslexia is improbable. The difficulty in learning to read is of a multidimensional nature, of which the features are not yet unequivocally known. Deficits and strategies of the child learning to read still have to be disentangled and environmental as well as biological variables define the condition. Furthermore, as reading is a rather novel acquisition of mankind, an evolutionary explanation seems rather questionable. Jennekens-Schinkel A Ned Tijdschr Geneeskd 1998 Nov 7;142(45):2445-7.

Sensitivity to dynamic auditory and visual stimuli predicts nonword reading ability in both dyslexic and normal readers. Abstract: Developmental dyslexia is a specific disorder of reading and spelling that affects 3-9% of school-age children and adults. Contrary to the view that it results solely from deficits in processes specific to linguistic analysis, current research has shown that deficits in more basic auditory or visual skills may contribute to the reading difficulties of dyslexic individuals. These results further implicate neuronal mechanisms that are specialised for detecting stimulus timing and change as being dysfunctional in many dyslexic individuals. The dissociation observed in the performance of dyslexic individuals on different auditory tasks suggests a sub-modality division similar to that already described in the visual system. These dynamic tests may provide a non-linguistic means of identifying children at risk of reading failure. Witton C Talcott JB Hansen PC Richardson AJ Griffiths TD Rees A Stein JF Green GG Curr Biol 1998 Jul 2;8(14):791-7.

Sequencing, expression analysis, and mapping of three unique human tropomodulin genes and their mouse orthologs. Abstract: Tropomodulin (TMOD) is the actin-capping protein for the slow-growing end of filamentous actin, and a neuronal-specific isoform, neuronal tropomodulin (NTMOD), is the major binding protein to brain tropomyosin in rat. The Drosophila TMOD homolog, Sanpodo, alters sibling cell fate determination, Journalwe used a cross-species approach to identify additional TMOD family members that may play a critical role in this process. We characterized the human and mouse orthologs to rat NTMOD (TMOD2 and Tmod2, respectively) as well as two novel tropomodulin family members (TMOD3, Tmod3 and TMOD4, Tmod4). (Cox PR Zoghbi HY Genomics 2000 Jan 1;63(1):97-107.

Serial recall of poor readers in two presentation modalities: combined effects of phonological similarity and word length. Abstract: Immediate ordered memory for words in poor readers was compared with that of two control groups of normal readers, matched on chronological age and reading age, respectively. The groups were equated for basal memory capacity. Phonological similarity and word length were simultaneously manipulated. Items were presented either auditorily (spoken words) or visually (their corresponding drawings). Irausquin RS de Gelder B J Exp Child Psychol 1997 Jun;65(3):342-69.

Sex differences in dyslexia / edited by Alice Ansara... [et al.]. Towson, Md.: Orton Dyslexia Society, 1981. Ansara, Alice. Orton Dyslexia Society. Description: xviii, 196 p.: ill.; 23 cm. LC Classification: RC394.W6 S49 1981 Dewey Class No.: 616.85/53 19

Sex differences in intelligence. Implications for education. Abstract: Sex differences in intelligence is among the most politically volatile topics in contemporary psychology. Although no single finding has unanimous support, conclusions from multiple studies suggest that females, on average, score higher on tasks that require rapid access to and use of phonological and semantic information in long-term memory, production and comprehension of complex prose, fine motor skills, and perceptual speed. Males, on average, score higher on tasks that require transformations in visual-spatial working memory, motor skills involved in aiming, spatiotemporal responding, and fluid reasoning, especially in abstract mathematical and scientific domains.

Halpern DF Am Psychol 1997 Oct;52(10):1091-102.

Seymour, Philip H. K. (Philip Herschel Kean), 1938- Cognitive analysis of dyslexia / Philip H.K. Seymour. London; New York: Routledge & Kegan Paul, 1986. Description: xi, 265 p.: ill.; 25 cm. ISBN: 0710098413: LC Classification: RJ496.A5 S49 1986 Dewey Class No.: 616.85/53 19

Silverstein, Alvin. Dyslexia / Alvin Silverstein, Virginia Silverstein, and Laura Silverstein Nunn. New York: F. Watts, c2001. Silverstein, Virginia B. Nunn, Laura Silverstein. Description: 48 p.: col. ill.; 24 cm. ISBN: 0531118622 LC Classification: RC394.W6 S54 2001 Dewey Class No.: 616.85/53 21

Simpson, Eileen B. Reversals: a personal account of victory over dyslexia / Eileen Simpson. Boston: Houghton Mifflin, 1979. Description: ix, 246 p.; 22 cm. ISBN: 0395275164: LC Classification: RC394.W6 S55 Dewey Class No.: 616.8/553/09

Simpson, Eileen B. Reversals: a personal account of victory over dyslexia / Eileen Simpson; with a new preface by the author. Edition Information: Rev. ed. New York: Noonday Press, 1991. Description: xiii, 246 p.; 22 cm. ISBN: 0374523169 LC Classification: RC394.W6 S55 1991b Dewey Class No.: 362.1/968553/0092 B 21

Simpson, Eileen B. Reversals: a personal account of victory over dyslexia / Eileen Simpson; with a new preface by the author. Edition Information: Rev. ed. New York: Noonday Press, 1991. Description: xiii, 240 p.; 22 cm. ISBN: 0374523169: LC Classification: RC394.W6 S55 1991 Dewey Class No.: 362.1/968553/0092 B 20

Simultaneous activation of reading mechanisms: evidence from a case of deep dyslexia. Abstract: We report the performance of LC, a deep dyslexic. We investigated extensively her errors according to serial cognitive neuropsychological models of oral reading. Initial evaluation of her reading suggested impaired access to the phonological output lexicon (POL). Impaired grapheme-to-phoneme conversion (GPC) and semantic errors in reading suggested that LC read via an impoverished semantic route. However, a serial model of oral reading could not explain error differences in reading, picture naming, spontaneous speech, and repetition. Southwood MH Chatterjee A Brain Lang 1999 Mar;67(1):1-29.

Simultaneous pattern electroretinogram and visual evoked potential recordings in dyslexic children. Abstract: To help clarify the conflicting evidence of neurophysiologic abnormalities in children with reading problems (dyslexia), we examined pattern electroretinograms and visual evoked potentials to stimulation with checks of 24', 49' and 180', each at 5%, 42% and 100% contrast, in a group of dyslexic children and a group of normal (i.e, normally reading) children. Neurophysiologic difference between the groups was restricted to the visual evoked potential, which showed a significant prolongation of the P100 wave in dyslexic children at the highest contrast (100%) and the smallest checks (24'). Brecelj J Strucl M Raic V Doc Ophthalmol 1997-98;94(4):355-64.

Slowly progressive alexia. Mendez MF J Neuropsychiatry Clin Neurosci 2002 Winter;14(1):84.

Sluggish auditory processing in dyslexics is not due to persistence in sensory memory. Abstract: The hypothesis that dyslexics show prolonged audible persistence was tested by an event-related brain response technique and rejected in favour of an attentional explanation. Loveless N Koivikko H Neuroreport 2000 Jun 26;11(9):1903-6.

Small wonder. Interview by Alison Whyte. Wigan W Nurs Times 2001 May 31-Jun 6;97(22):28.

Smith, Neil, 1966- Yes I can!: struggles from childhood to the NFL / by Neil Smith with Brad Hamann; design and illustrations by Jerry Hirt. Lenexa, KS: Addax Pub. Group; Kansas City, MO: Distributed to the trade by Andrews McMeel Pub, c1998. Hamann, Brad. Hirt, Jerry, ill. Description: 40 p.: col. ill.; 27 cm. ISBN: 1886110638 Summary: Tells the story of the Denver Bronco's fight to overcome dyslexia, graduate from high school, and become a successful NFL player. LC Classification: GV939.S637 A3 1998 Dewey Class No.: 796.332/092 B 21

Smook, Marian. De spelling van bastaardwoorden: strategieën, oefeningen, woordenlijsten: voor dyslectici / Marian Smook. Amsterdam: Swets & Zeitlinger, c1993. Description: 108 p.; 17 cm. ISBN: 9026513267 LC Classification: PF143.S58 1993

Snowling, Margaret J. Dyslexia / Margaret J. Snowling. Edition Information: 2nd ed. Malden, MA: Blackwell Publishers, 2000. Description: xiv, 253 p.; 24 cm. ISBN: 0631221441 (alk. paper) 0631205748 (alk. paper) LC Classification: RJ496.A5 S65 2000 Dewey Class No.: 618.92/8553 21

Snowling, Margaret J. Dyslexia: a cognitive developmental perspective / Margaret Snowling. Oxford, UK; Cambridge, Mass, USA: B. Blackwell, 1990. Description: 162 p.: ill.; 22 cm. ISBN: 0631144331 (pbk.): 0631144323: LC Classification: RJ496.A5 S65 1987 NLM Class No.: WL 340.6 S674d Dewey Class No.: 618.92/8553 19

Socio-economic differences in foundation-level literacy. Abstract: The foundation literacy skills of children from differing socio-economic backgrounds were investigated in a cross-sectional study. The children were aged between 4 and 8 years and attended Nursery or Primary 1, 2 or 3 classes. Low socioeconomic status (SES) was associated with impairments for chronological age in letter knowledge as well as in both logographic and alphabetic foundation components. There was an effect on metaphonological++ skill. However, once the SES groups were equated for reading age, high and low SES performance was indistinguishable. Duncan LG Seymour PH Br J Psychol 2000 May;91 (Pt 2):145-66.

Some remarks on the magnocellular deficit theory of dyslexia. Skottun BC Vision Res 1997 Apr;37(7):965-6.

Sources of priming in text rereading: intact implicit memory for new associations in older adults and in patients with Alzheimer's disease. Abstract: The contributions of text meaning, new between-word associations, and single-word repetition to priming in text rereading in younger and older adults, and in patients with Alzheimer's disease. (AD), were assessed in Experiment 1. Explicit recognition memory for text was assessed. Equivalent single-word and between-word priming was observed for all groups, even though patients with AD showed impaired explicit memory for individual words in the text. Monti Psychol Aging 1997 Sep;12(3):536-47.

Spafford, Carol Sullivan. Dyslexia: research and resource guide / Carol Sullivan Spafford, George S. Grosser. Boston: Allyn and Bacon, c1996. Grosser, George S. Description: xi, 340 p.: ill.; 25 cm. ISBN: 0205159079 LC Classification: LB1050.5.S63 1996 Dewey Class No.: 371.91/44 20

Spatial cognition in children. II. Visuospatial and constructional skills in developmental reading disability. Abstract: Cognitive models for developmental dyslexia are nowadays centered on the hypothesis of a specific deficit within the phonologic module of the language system. To ascertain whether defects of spatial cognition are associated with developmental reading disability, we investigated a sample of 43 school children (aged 8-9 years) found to be reading impaired during a wide screening survey for developmental dyslexia in the province of Naples, Italy. After one year

all children were tested again and only 9/43 still presented reading impairment, while the remaining had achieved a variable range of spontaneous recovery. Del Giudice E Trojano L Fragassi NA Posteraro S Crisanti AF Tanzarella P Marino A Grossi D Brain Dev 2000 Sep;22(6):368-72.

Spatio-temporal contrast sensitivity, coherent motion, and visible persistence in developmental dyslexia. Abstract: Three experiments measured spatio-temporal contrast sensitivity, coherent motion, and visible persistence in a single group of children with developmental dyslexia and a matched control group. The findings were consistent with a transient channel disorder in the dyslexic group which showed a reduction in contrast sensitivity at low spatial frequencies, a significant reduction in sensitivity for coherent motion, and a significantly longer duration of visible persistence. Slaghuis WL Ryan JF Vision Res 1999 Feb;39(3):651-68.

Spatiotemporal visual function in tinted lens wearers. Abstract: Tinted lenses have been widely publicized as a successful new treatment for reading disorders and visual stress in children. The present study was designed to investigate a variety of visual deficits reported by children who experience high levels of visual stress and perceptual distortions when reading (Meares-Irlen syndrome; MIS) and to assess the improvements in visual comfort they report when tinted lenses are worn Under thorough psychophysical investigation, these results revealed no significant difference in visual function between subject group, and this finding is consistent with the absence of any effect of the tinted lenses in the group with MIS. Simmers AJ Bex PJ Smith FK Wilkins AJ Invest Ophthalmol Vis Sci 2001 Mar;42(3):879-84.

Speaker's Symposium on Language Disabilities, Austin, Tex, 1966. Proceedings. [Austin? 1966?] Description: 48 p. ports. 27 cm. LC Classification:

RJ496.L35 S63 1966 Dewey Class No.: 618.92/8552 19

Special educational needs in East Surrey from a school doctor's point of view. Bisazza P J R Soc Health 1999 Mar;119(1):50-1.

Specific developmental disorders. The language-learning continuum. Abstract: The goal of this article is to inform and educate those who work with children who present with language-learning disorders about phonologic processing deficits, because this area has been shown to have a significant impact on children and adults who exhibit reading disabilities. Mental health professionals who work with children with reading problems need to be aware of what is known about this source of reading disorders and the implications of this knowledge for prevention and treatment. Swank LK Child Adolesc Psychiatr Clin N Am 1999 Jan;8(1):89-112, vi.

Specific learning disabilities: a neuropsychological perspective. Abstract: A dispersion in cognitive abilities is expected in normal populations. Specific learning disabilities would represent an extreme polarity in a continuum of normal cognitive dispersion. Three propositions relative to learning disabilities are advanced in the present paper. First, specific learning disabilities are expected to be found for diverse cognitive functions, even though some of these specific learning disorders have yet to be described in scientific literature. Ardila A Int J Neurosci 1997 Feb;89(3-4):189-205.

Specific reading difficulty or decompensated heterophoria? Abstract: This case report illustrates the importance of both an educational psychology and optometric assessment in the management of reading difficulties. Only after these have been concluded can the aetiology of the reading difficulty be determined and the correct course of treatment instigated. Rundstrom MM Eperjesi F Ophthalmic Physiol Opt 1995 Mar;15(2):157-9.

Specific reading disability: a multiplanar view. Abstract: In the past three decades a revolution has altered the way society approaches people with disabilities. Social changes resulted in a significant increase in fundamental and applied research that seeks to improve the lives of people with disabilities by facilitating better understanding of the mechanisms, manifestations, prevention, and treatment of functional impairment. Specific Reading Disability (SRD) has benefited from this revolution. Shapiro BK Ment Retard Dev Disabil Res Rev 2001;7(1):13-20.

Specific reading disability: a view of the spectrum / edited by Bruce K. Shapiro, Pasquale J. Accardo, and Arnold J. Capute. Timonium, Md.: York Press, 1998. Shapiro, Bruce K. Accardo, Pasquale J. Capute, Arnold J, 1923- Description: x, 267 p.: ill.; 23 cm. ISBN: 0912752459 (pbk.) LC Classification: RC394.W6 S64 1998 Dewey Class No.: 616.85/53 21

Speech and language in the laboratory, school, and clinic / James F. Kavanagh and Winifred Strange, editors. Cambridge: MIT Press, c1978. Kavanagh, James F. Strange, Winifred. National Institute of Child Health and Human Development (U.S.) Description: xviii, 511 p.: ill.; 24 cm. ISBN: 0262110652 LC Classification: RJ496.S7 S63 Dewey Class No.: 618.9/28/55

Speech perception deficit in dyslexic adults as measured by mismatch negativity (MMN). Abstract: Deficits in phonological processing are known to play a major role in the aetiology of dyslexia, and speech perception is a prerequisite condition for phonological processing. Significant group differences between dyslexics and controls have been found in the categorical perception of synthetic speech stimuli. In a previous work, we have demonstrated that these group differences are already present at an early pre-attentive stage of signal processing in dyslexic children: the late component of the MMN elicited by passive speech perception was attenuated in comparison to a control group. Schulte-Korne G Deimel W Bartling J Remschmidt H Int J Psychophysiol 2001 Feb;40(1):77-87.

Speech perception in children with specific reading difficulties (dyslexia). Abstract: Many experimental studies over the last two decades have suggested that groups of children who suffer significant delay in reading show a weakness in phoneme discrimination and identification. In order to look further at the relation between type of reading deficit, auditory acuity, and speech discrimination, a group of 13 children with specific reading difficulty (SRD), 12 chronological-age controls, and 12 reading-age controls were tested on a battery of speech-perceptual, psychoacoustic, and reading tests. Adlard A Hazan V Q J Exp Psychol A 1998 Feb;51(1):153-77.

Speech perception, lexicality, and reading skill. Abstract: This study examined the interaction between speech perception and lexical information among a group of 7-year-old children, of which 26 were poor readers and 36 were good readers. The children's performance was examined on tasks assessing reading skill, phonological awareness, pseudoword repetition, and phoneme identification. Although good readers showed clearly defined categorical perception in the phoneme identification task for both the /bif/-/pif/ and the /bis/-/pis/ continua, the category boundary for /bif/-/pif/ was at longer VOTs than the boundary for /bis/-/pis/, which characterizes the classic lexicality effect. Chiappe P Chiappe DL Siegel LS J Exp Child Psychol 2001 Sep;80(1):58-74.

Speech-language pathology and dysphagia in multiple sclerosis. Abstract: Dysarthria occurs in approximately 40% of all patients with MS. When speech and voice disturbances do occur, they usually present as a spastic-ataxic dysarthria with disorders of voice intensity, voice quality, articulation, and intonation. While language disturbances such as aphasia, auditory agnosia, anomia, dysgraphia, and dyslexia are very rare in MS, cognitive deficits and swallowing disorders are common. Treating dysarthria, dysphagia, and cognitive deficits in MS patients is effective for reestablishing functional daily activities. Merson RM Rolnick MI Phys Med Rehabil Clin N Am 1998 Aug;9(3):631-41.

Spell check. Cobley R Parry R Nurs Times 1997 Apr 16-22;93(16):38-40.

Spoken language correlates of reading impairments acquired in childhood. Abstract: This study reports the reading difficulties of five children following unilateral left hemisphere stroke sustained either before or during the early stages of literacy acquisition. Although each of the children experienced a period of disturbed language processing in the initial stages postonset, at the time of testing none of the children were considered to be clinically aphasic. Yet, on a standardized test of oral reading each of the children achieved a reading age that lagged behind chronological age and marked reading impairments were disclosed in four of the five children Pitchford NJ Brain Lang 2000 Apr;72(2):129-49.

Sprenger-Charolles, Liliane. Lire: lecture et écriture, acquisition et troubles du développement / Liliane Sprenger-Charolles, Séverine Casalis. Edition Information: 1re éd. Paris: Presses universitaires de France, c1996. Casalis, Séverine. Description: 258 p.: ill.; 22 cm. ISBN: 2130477054 LC Classification: LB1050.S67 1996

Stability of gaze control in dyslexia. Abstract: The neurobiological basis of saccade control has at least three components: fixation, reflexes, voluntary control. It was found in earlier studies that the voluntary component of saccade is specifically impaired in dyslexics as compared with controls of the same age. In this study, we searched for evidence of fixation instability by analyzing the eye movements of 99 control subjects and 262 dyslexics (age 7-17 years) performing an overlap prosaccade and a gap antisaccade task. Fischer B Hartnegg K Strabismus 2000 Jun;8(2):119-22.

Steltzer, Saskia. Wenn die Wörter tanzen: Legasthenie und Schule / Saskia Steltzer. Edition Information: 1. Aufl. Krenzlingen: Ariston, c1998. Description: 237 p.: ill.; 22 cm. ISBN: 3720520390 LC Classification: LB1050.5.S75 1998

Stewart, J. I. M. (John Innes Mackintosh), 1906- Parlour 4 and other stories / by J.I.M. Stewart. London: V. Gollancz, 1986. Related Titles: Parlour four and other stories. Description: 184 p.; 23 cm. ISBN: 0575037350: LC Classification: PR6037.T466 P37 1986b Dewey Class No.: 823/.912 19

Stewart, J. I. M. (John Innes Mackintosh), 1906- Parlour 4 and other stories / J.I.M. Stewart. Edition Information: 1st American ed. New York: Norton, 1986. Related Titles: Parlour four and other stories. Parlor 4 and other stories. Description: 184 p.; 22 cm. LC Classification: PR6037.T466 P37 1986 Dewey Class No.: 823/.912 19

Stimulus characteristics within directives: effects on accuracy of task completion. Abstract: Three experiments were conducted in an outpatient setting with young children who had been referred for treatment of noncompliant behavior and who had coexisting receptive language or receptive vocabulary difficulties. Experiment 1 studied differential responding of the participants to a brief hierarchical directive analysis (least-to-most complex stimulus prompts) to identify directives that functioned as discriminative stimuli for accurate responding. Experiment 1 identified distinct patterns of accurate responding relative to manipulation of directive stimulus characteristics. Richman DM Wacker DP Cooper-Brown LJ Kayser K Crosland K Stephens TJ Asmus J J Appl Behav Anal 2001 Fall;34(3):289-312.

Stimulus-specific neglect in a deep dyslexic patient. Abstract: We report a patient (B.V.) who appears to suffer from two dyslexic disorders. First, B.V. showed a severe impairment in reading aloud nonwords (e.g, reading TREST as TREE), in addition to making several semantic errors when reading aloud words (e.g, reading ILL as SICK) and in picture naming (e.g, responding KNIFE to a picture of a FORK). These results suggest that B.V. suffers from deep dyslexia. Second, B.V. showed an impairment in reading the final letters of both words and nonwords (e.g, reading SHOWN as SHORT and reading PROGE as PROOF. Siakaluk PD Buchanan L Brain Cogn 2001 Jun-Jul;46(1-2):268-71.

Stockdale, Carol. The source for solving reading problems / Carol Stockdale, Carol Possin. East Moline, IL: LinguiSystems, c2001. Possin, Carol. Stockdale, Carol. For parents and professionals. Solving reading problems. Description: 164 p.: ill. (some col.); 28 cm. ISBN: 0760604045 LC Classification: RC394.W6 S76 1984 Dewey Class No.: 616.85/53 19

Stone, Rhonda. The light barrier: a color solution to your child's light-based reading difficulties / Rhonda Stone. Edition Information: 1st ed. New York: St. Martin's Press, 2002. Projected Pub. Date: 0210 Description: p. cm. ISBN: 0312304056 LC Classification: RC394.W6 S765 2002 Dewey Class No.: 618.92/8553 21

Stordy, B. Jacqueline. The LCP solution: the remarkable nutritional treatment for ADHD, dyslexia, and dyspraxia / B. Jacqueline Stordy and Malcolm J. Nicholl. Edition Information: 1st ed. New York: Ballantine Books, c2000. Nicholl, Malcolm J. Description: xii, 339 p.: ill.; 21 cm. ISBN: 0345438728 (pbk.) LC Classification: RC394.L37 S76 2000 Dewey Class No.: 616.85/8890654 21

Stowe, Cynthia. How to reach & teach students with dyslexia / Cynthia M. Stowe. Variant How to reach and teach students with dyslexia Subtitle on cover: Practical strategies and activities for helping students with dyslexia West Nyack, N.Y.: Center for Applied Research in Education, c2000. Description: xxviii, 337 p.: ill.; 28 cm. ISBN: 0130135712 LC Classification: LC4708.S86 2000 Dewey Class No.: 371.91/44 21

Structural imaging in dyslexia: the planum temporale. Abstract: The search for a neurobiological substrate for dyslexia has focused on anomalous planum symmetry. The results of imaging studies of the planum have been inconsistent, perhaps due to diagnostic uncertainty, technical differences in measurement criteria, and inadequate control of handedness, sex, and cognitive ability. Although structural imaging studies have not clarified the neurobiology of reading disability, converging evidence suggests that variation in asymmetry of the planum temporale does have functional significance. Eckert MA Leonard CM Ment Retard Dev Disabil Res Rev 2000;6(3):198-206.

Subcortical mechanisms in language: lexical-semantic mechanisms and the thalamus. Abstract: Four previously published cases of dominant thalamic lesion in which the author has participated are reviewed to gain a better understanding of thalamic participation in lexical-semantic functions. Naming deficits in two cases support Nadeau and Crosson's (1997) hypothesis of a selective engagement mechanism involving the frontal lobes, inferior thalamic peduncle, nucleus reticularis, and other thalamic nuclei, possibly the centromedian nucleus. Crosson B Brain Cogn 1999 Jul;40(2):414-38.

Subtle symptoms associated with self-reported mild head injury. Abstract: We conducted a survey on the relationship between mild head injury incidence and a variety of psychological and educational symptoms in a sample of 1,345 high school and 2,321 university students. Once figures were adjusted to represent a 50:50 gender ratio, 30% to 37% of subjects reported having experienced a head injury incident, with 12% to 15% of the total group of subjects reporting such an incident with loss of consciousness. We found significant relationships between the incidence of such mild head injury and gender, sleep difficulties, social difficulties, handedness pattern, and diagnoses of attention deficit, depression, and speech, language, and reading disorders. Segalowitz SJ Lawson S J Learn Disabil 1995 May;28(5):309-19.

Successive signal representation in noise in dyslexics. Nagarajan S Clin Neurophysiol 2002 Apr;113(4):459-61.

Sulcal/gyral pattern morphology of the perisylvian language region in developmental dyslexia. Abstract: Two systems for classification of morphology of the perisylvian cortical area have been suggested, that of Steinmetz et al. (1990) and that of Witelson and Kigar (1992). This study examines whether the variations in placement of these convolutions in the language cortex are related to diagnosis of dyslexia in a clinic-referred sample of 55 children ages 8 to 12 years. Additionally, the systems are compared to determine their relationship to neurolinguistic performance. Hiemenz JR Hynd GW Brain Lang 2000 Aug;74(1):113-33.

Supportive evidence for the DYX3 dyslexia susceptibility gene in Canadian families. Petryshen TL Kaplan BJ Hughes ML Tzenova J Field LL J Med Genet 2002 Feb;39(2):125-6.

Surface dyslexia in nonfluent progressive aphasia. Abstract: This article presents the case of a 59-year-old male, JH, with a 6-year history of primary progressive aphasia (PPA), a disorder characterized by isolated language deterioration with relative preservation of other cognitive abilities. JH shows typical features of surface dyslexia, a reading disorder exemplified by the selective preservation of phonological reading. One recent theory is that surface dyslexia in individuals with PPA results from a loss of semantic knowledge. Watt S Jokel R Behrmann M Brain Lang 1997 Feb 1;56(2):211-33.

Surgical treatment of anterior callosal tumors. Abstract: Thirteen patients with neoplasm of anterior corpus callosum have undergone our observation during the last two years. Thus, no severe neuropsychological deficits developed after surgical treatment of anterior callosal tumors. D'Angelo V Napolitano M Gorgoglione L Scarabino T Latino R Simone P Bisceglia M J Neurosurg Sci 1997 Mar;41(1):117-22.

Susceptibility loci for distinct components of developmental dyslexia on chromosomes 6 and 15. Abstract: Six extended dyslexic families with at least four affected individuals were genotyped with markers in three chromosomal regions: 6p23-p21.3, 15pter-qter, and 16pter-qter. Five theoretically derived phenotypes were used in the linkage analyses: (1) phonological awareness; (2) phonological decoding; (3) rapid automatized naming; (4) single-word reading; and (5) discrepancy between intelligence and reading performance, an empirically derived, commonly used phenotype. Grigorenko EL Wood FB Meyer MS Hart Am J Hum Genet 1997 Jan;60(1):27-39.

Syntactic processing of Hebrew sentences in normal and dyslexic readers: electrophysiological evidence.Abstract: The authors examined differences in brain activity as measured by amplitudes and latencies of event-related potential (ERP) components in Hebrew-speaking adult dyslexic and normal readers. The participants were measured while processing words' syntactic functions during reading of sentences with subject-verb-object syntactic order. The results suggested that among dyslexic and normal readers, N100 and P300 ERP components were sensitive to certain constituents of syntactic analysis for target words in accordance with their grammatical roles. Breznitz Z Leikin M J Genet Psychol 2000 Sep;161(3):359-80.

Systematic identification and intervention for reading difficulty: case studies of children with EAL. Abstract: Literacy underpins education. There is now very widespread concern over standards of literacy for children from multi-cultural backgrounds, who are learning English as a second or subsequent language, and who may have special educational needs. Research evidence suggests that the earlier children's difficulties can be identified, the more effective (and cost-effective) intervention will be, provided that the intervention is tailored to the child's abilities and skills. Fawcett AJ Lynch L Dyslexia 2000 Jan-Mar;6(1):57-71.

Tactile perception in developmental dyslexia: a psychophysical study using gratings. Abstract: Multiple sensory abnormalities have been reported in individuals with developmental dyslexia, especially in the visual and auditory systems. We used gratings of alternating ridges and grooves to investigate tactile perception in this disorder using two tasks: spatial acuity-dependent discrimination of grating orientation and discrimination of gratings varying in ridge width. Compared to age-matched normal subjects, dyslexics were significantly impaired on grating orientation discrimination, with mean thresholds that were nearly twice normal. Grant AC Zangaladze A Thiagarajah MC Sathian K Neuropsychologia 1999 Sep;37(10):1201-11.

Task-specificity and similarities in processing numbers and words: available data and future directions. Denes G Signorini M Brain Lang 2000 Jan;71(1):56-8.

Teaching reading to disabled readers with language disorders: a controlled evaluation of synthetic speech feedback. Abstract: In a long-term study two groups of language and reading impaired students (N = 15 + 15) were reading with the aid of segmented speech-feedback in a computerized program. One group received feedback that was simultaneously segmented visually and auditorily into syllables, the other received feedback by letter names. In both groups subjects were expected to synthesize segments into words and to compare their synthesis to whole word feed-back subsequently provided by the computer. Elbro C Rasmussen I Spelling B Scand J Psychol 1996 Jun;37(2):140-55.

Temple, Robin. Dyslexia: practical and easy-to-follow advice / Robin Temple. Shaftesbury, Dorset; Boston, Mass: Element, 1998. Projected Pub. Date: 9811 Description: p. cm. ISBN: 1862043140 (pbk.: alk. paper) LC Classification: RJ496.A5 T45 1998 Dewey Class No.: 618.92/8553 21

Temporal and spatial processing in reading disabled and normal children. Abstract: The ability to process temporal and spatial visual stimuli was studied to investigate the role these functions play in the reading process. Previous studies of this type have often been confounded by memory involvement, or did not take into account the evidence which suggests a visual transient deficient in some dyslexics. Normal (n = 39), reading disabled (n = 26), and backward reading children (n=12) were compared on a visual computer game, which consisted of a temporal and a analogous spatial dot counting task. Reading disabled children performed significantly worse than normal children on the Temporal Dot Task, but were only mildly impaired on the Spatial Dot Task, Backward readers were not significantly better than the reading disabled group on either task, suggesting that poor poor visual temporal processing is not specific to dyslexia. Eden GF Stein JF Wood HM Wood FB Cortex 1995 Sep;31(3):451-68.

Temporal information processing in the nervous system: special reference to dyslexia and dysphasia / [editors] Paula Tallal... [et al.]. New York, N.Y.: New York Academy of Sciences, 1993. Tallal, Paula, 1947- Description: ix, 442 p.: ill.; 24 cm. ISBN: 0897667859 (cloth: alk. paper) 0897667867 (paper: alk. paper) LC Classification: Q11.N5 vol. 682 RC423 NLM Class No.: W1 AN626YL v.682

1993 WL 340.5 T288 1992 Dewey Class No.: 500 s 616.85/5 20

Temporal inhibition in character identification. Abstract: Models of information processing tasks such as character identification often do not consider the nature of the initial sensory representation from which task-relevant information is extracted. An important component of this representation is temporal inhibition, in which the response to a stimulus may inhibit, or in some cases facilitate, processing of subsequent stimuli. Three experiments demonstrate the existence of temporal inhibitory processes in information processing tasks such as character identification and digit recall Busey TA Percept Psychophys 1998 Nov;60(8):1285-304.

Temporal lobe asymmetry and dyslexia: an in vivo study using MRI. Abstract: Three measures of the right and left temporal lobes were taken with magnetic resonance imaging (MRI) in groups of dyslexics (N = 17), retarded readers (N = 6), and normal controls (N = 12). The most pronounced differences among the groups were found with measures on coronal slices of the cross sectional area of the temporal cortex with subcortical white matter--in particular lateral to insula. While most of the normal and the retarded readers (13 of 18) had left asymmetry (left area larger than right), most of the dyslexics (14 of 17) had symmetry or right asymmetry. Dalby MA Elbro C Stodkilde-Jorgensen H Brain Lang 1998 Mar;62(1):51-69.

Temporal processing and phonological impairment in dyslexia: effect of phoneme lengthening on order judgment of two consonants. Abstract: The evidence of supporting phonological deficit as a cause of developmental dyslexia has been accumulating rapidly over the past 2 decades, yet the exact mechanisms underlying this deficit remain controversial. Some authors assume that a temporal processing deficit is the source of the phonological disorder observed in dyslexic children. Others maintain that the phonological deficit in dyslexia is basically linguistic, not acoustic, in nature Rey V De Martino S Espesser R Habib M Brain Lang 2002 Mar;80(3):576-91.

Temporal processing deficits in remediation-resistant reading-impaired children. Abstract: There is considerable interest in whether a deficit in temporal processing underlies specific learning and language disabilities in school-aged children. This view is particularly controversial in the area of developmental reading problems. The temporal-processing hypothesis was tested in a sample of normal children, 9-11 years of age, and in a sample of age-matched children with reading impairments, by assessing temporal-order discrimination. Five different binary temporal-order tasks were evaluated in the auditory and visual sensory modalities. Cacace AT McFarland DJ Ouimet JR Schrieber EJ Marro P Audiol Neurootol 2000 Mar-Apr;5(2):83-97.

Test construction, analysis and trial of the Heidelberg Sound Discrimination Test for measuring auditory-kinesthetic perceptual discrimination acuity Abstract: The provisional trial was carried out in a sample of 133 second- and 139 fourth-graders from the Heidelberg area. The HD-LT was subjected to an item selection, test criteria were ascertained and temporary percentile norms for the second and fourth grades were established. High item difficulty resulted for both grades, i.e. the test was relatively easy. Test criteria were generally satisfactory. Significant correlations were found in both grades between the HD-LT and the children's spelling ability. Dierks A Seibert A Brunner M Korkel B Haffner J Strehlow U Parzer P Resch F Z Kinder Jugendpsychiatr Psychother 1999 Feb;27(1):29-36.

Testing the direct-access model: GOD does not prime DOG. Abstract: In three repetition priming experiments that employed identical (e.g, DOG-DOG) and reversed repetitions (e.g, GOD-DOG), it was found that relative to controls (e.g, DOG-DOG),

GOD-type words did not prime DOG-type words. Also, neither DUT-type nor TUD-type nonwords primed DUT-type nonwords. In Experiments 1 and 2, these results occurred using both long- and short-term repetition priming conditions, respectively. In Experiment 3, the word results held under conditions of short-term priming coupled with stimulus misorientation. Huntsman Percept Psychophys 1998 Oct;60(7):1128-40.

Testosterone and dyslexia. Abstract: Geschwind, Behan and Galaburda have presented empirical research which indicates an association between left-handedness, immune disorders, and learning difficulties. Moreover, they have presented an hypothesis that purports to explain these associations, i.e. the 'testosterone hypothesis'. This article seeks to show that their hypothesis cannot explain: (a) which types and degrees of the conditions will appear, (b) why these conditions appear more often in males than in females, and (c) why these conditions seem to run in families. Tonnessen FE Pediatr Rehabil 1997 Jan-Mar;1(1):51-7.

Test-retest reliability of colored filter testing. Abstract: This article evaluates the reliability of colored filter testing procedures. Properly chosen colored filters, with the tint being specific to each patient, are said to be effective in the treatment of dyslexia. We investigated the test-retest reliability of colored filter testing in relationship to two specific symptom levels using a forced-choice test procedure. This research was to evaluate test-retest reliability, not the validity of colored filter testing. Woerz M Maples WC J Learn Disabil 1997 Mar-Apr;30(2):214-21.

Text comprehension training for disabled readers: an evaluation of reciprocal teaching and text analysis training programs. Abstract: We are particularly grateful to Dr. Annemarie Sullivan Palincsar for her helpful advice and generosity in sharing materials, procedures, and sample dialogues for use in the version of Reciprocal Teaching used in the present study. This research was supported by an operating grant to the first author from the Ontario Mental Health Foundation. We gratefully acknowledge the contributions of Janet Hinchley and Karen Steinbach in assisting with data collection and Nancy Benson, Carolyn Kroeber, and Karen Steinbach in assisting with data analysis. Lovett MW Borden SL Warren-Chaplin PM Lacerenza L DeLuca T Giovinazzo R Brain Lang 1996 Sep;54(3):447-80.

The "temporal processing deficit" hypothesis in dyslexia: new experimental evidence. Abstract: The notion that developmental dyslexia may result from a general, nonspecific, defect in perceiving rapidly changing auditory signals is a current subject of debate (so-called "temporal processing deficit" hypothesis). Thirteen phonological dyslexics (age 10-13 years) and 10 controls matched for chronological and reading age were compared on a temporal order judgment (TOJ) task using the succession of two consonants (/p/-/s/) within a cluster. De Martino S Espesser R Rey V Habib M Brain Cogn 2001 Jun-Jul;46(1-2):104-8.

The /O/ in OVER is different from the /O/ in OTTER: phonological effects in children with and without dyslexia. Abstract: First-letter naming was used to investigate the role of phonology in printed word perception in children with and without dyslexia. In 2 experiments, all children showed faster first-letter-naming times in a congruent condition than in an incongruent condition, which suggests that phonology is a fundamental constraint in the printed word perception of readers of all levels and all skills. An explanation in terms of a recurrent network put forward by G. C. Van Orden and S. D. Goldinger (1996) is discussed to account for the apparent paradox in the reading behavior of readers with dyslexia, that is, that in first-letter naming, dyslexic readers appear to show phonological congruity effects, whereas in pseudoword reading, their phonological knowledge appears to be deficient or absent. Bosman AM van Leerdam M de Gelder B Dev Psychol 2000 Nov;36(6):817-25.

The angular gyrus in developmental dyslexia: task-specific differences in functional connectivity within posterior cortex. Abstract: Converging evidence from neuroimaging studies of developmental dyslexia reveals dysfunction at posterior brain regions centered in and around the angular gyrus in the left hemisphere. We examined functional connectivity (covariance) between the angular gyrus and related occipital and temporal lobe sites, across a series of print tasks that systematically varied demands on phonological assembly. Results indicate that for dyslexic readers a disruption in functional connectivity in the language-dominant left hemisphere is confined to those tasks that make explicit demands on assembly. Pugh KR Mencl WE Shaywitz BA Shaywitz SE Fulbright RK Constable RT Skudlarski P Marchione KE Jenner AR Fletcher JM Liberman AM Shankweiler DP Katz L Lacadie C Gore JC Psychol Sci 2000 Jan;11(1):51-6.

The application of cognitive event-related brain potentials (ERPs) in language-impaired individuals: review and case studies. Abstract: There is a substantial body of basic research that has utilized ERPs to investigate the neurological basis of cognition. This research has, in turn, led to the development of practical applications of cognitive ERPs in patient populations. In particular, recent work has focused on the development of ERP-based assessment measures for the neuropsychological assessment of dyslexia and language impairments secondary to stroke. This review describes the innovative assessment methods program (IAMP), an initiative to utilize ERPs for a neuropsychological assessment of patients who cannot be evaluated by traditional methods. Connolly JF D'Arcy RC Lynn Newman R Kemps R Int J Psychophysiol 2000 Oct;38(1):55-70.

The assessment of learning disabilities: preschool through adulthood / edited by Larry B. Silver. Austin: Pro-Ed, [1991?], c1989. Silver, Larry B. National Institute of Dyslexia (U.S.) Description: x, 180 p.: ill.; 23 cm. ISBN: 089079393X LC Classification: LC4705.A84 1991 Dewey Class No.: 371.9/0973 20

The Assessment of learning disabilities: preschool through adulthood / edited by Larry B. Silver. Boston: Little Brown, c1989. Silver, Larry B. National Institute of Dyslexia (U.S.) Description: x, 180 p.; 23 cm. ISBN: 0316791121 LC Classification: LC4705.A84 1989 Dewey Class No.: 371.9/0973 19

The association of reading disability, behavioral disorders, and language impairment among second-grade children. Abstract: Children with language impairment (LI) have been shown to be at risk for reading disability (RD) and behavior disorder (BD). Previous research has not determined the specific pattern of these conditions associated with LI. This study sought to determine if the behavior disorder and reading problems represented different outcomes or if these conditions occurred together when found with LI. A group of 581 second-grade children, including 164 children with LI, were examined for spoken language, reading, and behavior disorder. Patton JE Yarbrough DB Thursby D Percept Mot Skills 2000 Apr;90(2):577-8.

The caudal infrasylvian surface in dyslexia: novel magnetic resonance imaging-based findings. Abstract: To detect anatomic abnormalities of auditory association cortex in dyslexia by measuring the area of the perisylvian region known as the caudal infrasylvian surface(s) (cIS) in dyslexic and control subjects. The gross anatomic organization of this region is different in dyslexic subjects, and elucidation of the precise nature of these differences may be aided by surface modeling techniques. Green RL Hutsler JJ Loftus WC Tramo MJ Thomas CE Silberfarb AW Nordgren

RE Nordgren RA Gazzaniga MS Neurology 1999 Sep 22;53(5):974-81.

The cerebellum and dyslexia: perpetrator or innocent bystander? Zeffiro T Eden G Trends Neurosci 2001 Sep;24(9):512-3.

The child's route into reading and what can go wrong. Abstract: Two strands of linguistic development critically important for successful reading acquisition are outlined. One of these ontogenetic roots concerns phonological development and projects onto word decoding. The other root concerns the development of vocabulary and syntax projecting onto reading comprehension. Language development starts very early in infancy when the child learns to categorize the speech sounds according to the pattern typical of the mother tongue. Equipped with these sound categories the child is ready to learn to understand and to use new words. Lundberg I Dyslexia 2002 Jan-Mar;8(1):1-13.

The colored lenses controversy. Hunt L Insight 2000 Oct-Dec;25(4):128-9.

The compositionality of lexical semantic representations: clues from semantic errors in object naming. Abstract: We present evidence that semantic errors in object naming can arise not only from impairment to the semantic system but from damage to input and output processes. Although each of these levels of disruption can result in similar types of semantic errors in object naming, they have different types of consequences for performance on other lexical tasks, such as comprehension and naming to definition. We show that the analysis of the co-occurrence of semantic errors in naming with different patterns of performance in other lexical processing tasks can be used to localise the source of semantic errors in the naming process. Hillis AE Caramzza A Memory 1995 Sep-Dec;3(3-4):333-58.

The continuum of deep/surface dyslexia. Abstract: A right-handed male sustained traumatic brain injury which resulted in anomia, dyslexia and agraphia. The most severe CT (computed tomography)-identified brain damage was located in the right parieto-temporal lobe. In the first months following the injury, the pattern of reading errors was similar to that associated with deep dyslexia. However, nonlexical derivation of phonology from print was not abolished. As the patient's ability to associate letter patterns with sounds improved, oral reading improved. Nolan KA Volpe BT Burton J Psycholinguist Res 1997 Jul;26(4):413-24.

The contribution of attentional mechanisms to an irregularity effect at the graphemic buffer level. Abstract: This study analyzes acquired dysgraphia observed in a French-speaking woman. The results point to an impairment of the graphemic buffer, i.e, the processing stage where abstract orthographic representations are temporarily stored while planning the written production. However, the spelling errors were more frequent in the irregular than in the regular words. A qualitative analysis of the errors in the irregular misspelled words showed that, in general, these were not "regularization" errors, but rather the same characteristics as the phonologically implausible errors found in the regular words, such as letters substitutions, deletions, additions, and transpositions. Annoni JM Lemay MA de Mattos Pimenta MA Lecours AR Brain Lang 1998 Jun 1;63(1):64-78.

The definition of dyslexia. Thomson M Dyslexia 2002 Jan-Mar;8(1):53-4.

The development of spelling procedures in French-speaking, normal and reading-disabled children: effects of frequency and lexicality. Abstract: The spelling procedures of normal and reading-disabled French-speaking children matched for reading level were examined. Subjects had to spell frequent and infrequent words containing either inconsistent nondominant graphemes (e.g, /s/ spelled "c" as in "cigarette," the dominant spelling for /s/ being "s") or consistent context-dependent graphemes (e.g, /g/ followed by "i"-->"gu") as well as pseudo-words including inconsistent graphemes presented in different phonological contexts (e.g, /s/ can be spelled "s" or "c" if the following vowel is /i/, but "c" is incorrect if the following vowel is /y/). Alegria J Mousty P J Exp Child Psychol 1996 Nov;63(2):312-38.

The differentiation of semantic dementia and frontal lobe dementia (temporal and frontal variants of frontotemporal dementia) from early Alzheimer's disease: a comparative neuropsychological study. Abstract: The authors compared age-matched groups of patients with the frontal and temporal lobe variants of frontotemporal dementia (FTD; dementia of frontal type [DFT] and semantic dementia), early Alzheimer's disease (AD), and normal controls (n = 9 per group) on a comprehensive neuropsychological battery. A distinct profile emerged for each group: Those with AD showed a severe deficit in episodic memory with more subtle, but significant, impairments in semantic memory and visuospatial skills; patients with semantic dementia showed the previously documented picture of isolated, but profound, semantic memory breakdown with anomia and surface dyslexia but were indistinguishable from the AD group on a test of story recall; and the DFT group were the least impaired and showed mild deficits in episodic memory and verbal fluency but normal semantic memory. Hodges JR Patterson K Ward R Garrard P Bak T Perry R Gregory C Neuropsychology 1999 Jan;13(1):31-40.

The dyslexia ecosystem. Abstract: It is all too easy, in everyday interactions in dyslexia, to see the interactions in a semi-adversarial fashion--parents competing to get more support for children, researchers competing to get more support for their theories, schools trying to get more money for their programmes. Such a set of analyses may be described as 'zero-sum'. If one party gains, the other one loses. If, by contrast, one views the dyslexia community as a complex, inter-dependent 'ecosystem', a much more positive view emerges. Nicolson RI Dyslexia 2002 Apr-Jun;8(2):55-66.

The effect of contrast on reading speed in dyslexia. Abstract: Contrast coding has been reported to differ between dyslexic and normal readers. Dyslexic readers require higher levels of contrast to detect sinewave gratings for certain spatiotemporal conditions, and dyslexic readers show faster visual search at low contrast. We investigated whether these differences in early contrast coding generalize to reading performance by measuring reading speed as a function of text contrast for dyslexic children and adults and for age-matched controls. O'Brien BA Mansfield JS Legge GE Vision Res 2000;40(14):1921-35.

The effects of spatial filtering and contrast reduction on visual search times in good and poor readers. Abstract: Recent experiments with reading disabled children have shown that image blurring (produced with frosted acetate overlays) results in an immediate benefit in search performance, eye movement pattern and reading comprehension. This suggests that the contrast and spatial frequency content of visual stimuli are important factors for these children. In the present experiment, spatial frequency filtering and contrast reduction were employed to determine whether either of these factors contrissbutes to the beneficial effects observed. Letter arrays were spatially filtered to produce low pass (< 3.5 c/deg) and high pass (> 7.0 c/deg) images Vision Res 1995 Jan;35(2):285-91.

The efficacy of kinesthetic reading treatment for pure alexia. Abstract: This paper presents an effective treatment for pure alexia by a type of single-case design, which we termed a "material-control single-case design" [Sugishita et al, Neuropsychologia, Vol. 31, 559-569, 1993]. Two patients with pure alexia were treated using kinesthetic reading (reading by tracing or copying the outline of each letter with the patient's finger). The results

clearly demonstrated that both patients significantly improved their reading and copying performances. Their recovery of reading performance arose from improvement in copying. Seki K Yajima M Sugishita M Neuropsychologia 1995 May;33(5):595-609.

The Emergence of language: development and evolution: readings from Scientific American magazine / edited by William S.-Y. Wang. New York: W.H. Freeman, c1991. Wang, William S.-Y, 1933- Related Titles: [Scientific American. Description: xiv, 182 p.: ill. (some col.), maps (some col.); 24 cm. ISBN: 0716721465: LC Classification: P106.E45 1991 Dewey Class No.: 400 20

The evaluation of aphasic deficits for the definition of a targetted logotherapeutic treatment Abstract: The Aachener Aphasie Test (AAT) is the major German test for the diagnosis of aphasic disorders. The test is easy to use and is valid and reliable for the diagnosis of aphasia and its severity and to evaluate the recovery of the aphasic disorder after language rehabilitation. The AAT is, however, not sufficient to define cognitively sound logotherapeutic treatment. The use of tasks which are based on cognitive functional models allows the identification of specific processing levels that have been damaged by a cerebral lesion, and the definition of a focussed rehabilitation plan. Bazzini A Pezzoni F Zonca G Guarnaschelli C Zelaschi F Luzzatti C G Ital Med Lav Ergon 1997 Apr-Jun;19(2):29-35.

The evolution of alexia and simultanagnosia in posterior cortical atrophy. Abstract: Early alexia and higher visual impairments characterize Posterior cortical atrophy (PCA), a progressive dementing syndrome most often caused by Alzheimer disease. Posterior cortical atrophy is rare, and the nature of the visual impairments in PCA are unclear. The authors observed two patients who had an insidiously progressive reading difficulty characterized by letter-by-letter reading and otherwise intact cognitive functions.

Over time, these patients developed "ventral simultanagnosia" with preserved detection of multiple stimuli but inability to interpret whole scenes Mendez MF Cherrier MM Neuropsychiatry Neuropsychol Behav Neurol 1998 Apr;11(2):76-82.

The eye movements of pure alexic patients during reading and nonreading tasks. Abstract: We compared the eye-movements of two patients who read letter-by-letter (LBL) following a left occipital lobe lesion with those of normal control subjects and of hemianopic patients in two tasks: a nonreading visual search task and a text reading task. Whereas the LBL readers exhibited similar eye-movement patterns to those of the other two groups on the nonreading task, their eye movements differed significantly during reading, as reflected in the disproportionate increase in the number and duration of fixations per word and in the regressive saccades per word. Behrmann M Shomstein SS Black SE Barton JJ Neuropsychologia 2001;39(9):983-1002.

The familial incidence of symptoms of scotopic sensitivity/Irlen syndrome: comparison of referred and mass-screened groups. Abstract: The familial incidence of Scotopic Sensitivity/Irlen Syndrome was investigated in two samples. One sample involved parents and siblings of 126 children identified with symptoms who had been referred for screening. The other sample involved parents and siblings of 33 children who had been identified with symptoms through mass screening of all children in Grades 3 to 6 at two local schools. Two different samples were taken to investigate the possibility of parental referral bias. Robinson GL Foreman PJ Dear KB Percept Mot Skills 2000 Dec;91(3 Pt 1):707-24.

The familial incidence of symptoms of Scotopic Sensitivity/Irlen syndrome. Abstract: The familial incidence of Scotopic Sensitivity/Irlen Syndrome was investigated using parents of 751 children identified with symptoms. Children were identified by methods independent of their parents' symptoms or lack of symptoms. For these children, there was an 84% chance of either one or both parents showing similar symptoms, with similar numbers of mothers identified with symptoms as fathers. The data suggest that Scotopic Sensitivity/Irlen Syndrome may be a genetically based deficit in visual processing, but the simplest genetic models do not appear to fit. Robinson GL Foreman PJ Dear KB Percept Mot Skills 1996 Dec;83(3 Pt 1):1043-55.

The F-L test for determining alternating central scotoma Abstract: Based on their experiences several authors consider an alternating central scotoma as the main reason for reading difficulties due to dyslexia. Thus undisturbed reading seems not to demand perfect orthophoria. On the other hand a rapidly alternating central scotoma may be considered as an important factor causing reading difficulties. Safra D Klin Monatsbl Augenheilkd 1995 May;206(5):365-6.

The functional anatomy of single-word reading in patients with hemianopic and pure alexia. Abstract: We investigated single-word reading in normal subjects and patients with alexia following a left occipital infarct, using PET. The most posterior brain region to show a lateralized response was at the left occipitotemporal junction, in the inferior temporal gyrus. This region was activated when normal subjects, patients with hemianopic alexia and patients with an incomplete right homonymous hemianopia, but no reading deficit, viewed single words presented at increasing rates. Leff AP Crewes H Plant GT Scott SK Kennard C Wise RJ Brain 2001 Mar;124(Pt 3):510-21.

The genetic basis of cognition. Abstract: The molecular characterization of single-gene disorders or chromosomal abnormalities that result in a cognitive abnormality (predominantly mental retardation) and of the genetic variants responsible for variation in intellectual abilities (such as

IQ, language impairment and dyslexia) is expected to provide new insights into the biology of human cognitive processes. To date this hope has not been realized. Success in finding mutations that give rise to mental retardation has not been matched by advances in our understanding of how genes influence cognition. Flint J Brain 1999 Nov;122 (Pt 11):2015-32.

The genetics of children's oral reading performance. Abstract: Measures of reading achievement and verbal ability have been shown to be heritable. Additionally, recent evidence has been suggestive of a major gene effect on reading disability and for problem reading in a sample of normal readers. We report on the etiology of individual differences in oral reading performance, the Slosson Oral Reading Test (SORT), for which biometrical analyses have not been reported in the literature previously. Reynolds CA Hewitt JK Erickson MT Silberg JL Rutter M Simonoff E Meyer J Eaves LJ J Child Psychol Psychiatry 1996 May;37(4):425-34.

The genetics of cognitive abilities and disabilities. Plomin R DeFries JC Sci Am 1998 May;278(5):62-9.

The gradient of visual attention in developmental dyslexia. Abstract: This study investigated the gradient of visual attention in 21 children, 11 children with specific reading disorder (SRD) or dyslexia and 10 children with normal reading skills. We recorded reaction times (RTs) at the onset of a small point along the horizontal axis in the two visual fields. In 70% of the cases the target appeared inside a circle acting as focusing cue and in 30% of the cases it appeared outside, allowing us to study the distribution of attentional resources outside the selected area. Normally reading children showed a normal symmetric distribution of attention. Facoetti A Molteni M Neuropsychologia 2001;39(4):352-7.

The human genome--chromosome 15 Abstract: The Prader-Willi syndrome (PWS) with Angelman's syndrome form a pair known above all due to problems of genetic imprinting and uniparental disomy. Both phenomena drew attention to the importance of control of expression of different alleles and their genetic origin. The causes of the two syndromes have not been elucidated unequivocally Journalfar. In case of the PWS, at least, there is the possibility of a gene of the protein carrier of a small nuclear ribonucleic acid described as SNRPN. Brdicka R Cas Lek Cesk 1995 Aug 2;134(15):484-6.

The impact of genomics on mammalian neurobiology. Abstract: The benefit of genomics lies in the speeding up of research efforts in other fields of biology, including neurobiology. Through accelerated progress in positional cloning and genetic mapping, genomics has forced us to confront at a much faster pace the difficult problem of defining gene function. Elucidation of the function of identified disease genes and other genes expressed in the Central nervous system has to await conceptual developments in other fields. Hochgeschwender U Brennan MB Bioessays 1999 Feb;21(2):157-63.

The impact of orthographic consistency on dyslexia: a German-English comparison. Abstract: We examined reading and phonological processing abilities in English and German dyslexic children, each compared with two control groups matched for reading level (8 years) and age (10-12 years). We hypothesised that the same underlying phonological processing deficit would exist in both language groups, but that there would be differences in the severity of written language impairments, due to differences in orthographic consistency. Landerl K Wimmer H Frith U Cognition 1997 Jun;63(3):315-34.

The impact of ratee's disability on performance judgments and choice as partner: the role of disability-job fit stereotypes and interdependence of rewards. Abstract: An experiment assessed the impact of disability-job fit stereotypes and reward interdependence on personnel judgments about persons with disabilities. Students (N = 87) evaluated 3 confederates. The experiment varied disability of the target confederate (dyslexia vs. nondisabled), task, and dependence of rater rewards on partner performance. Two disability-task combinations represented stereotypical poor fit and good fit. Dependent variables were performance evaluations, performance expectations, and ranking of target as a partner. Colella A DeNisi AS Varma A J Appl Psychol 1998 Feb;83(1):102-11.

The impact of semantic memory impairment on spelling: evidence from semantic dementia. Abstract: We assessed spelling and reading abilities in 14 patients with semantic dementia (with varying degrees of semantic impairment) and 24 matched controls, using spelling-to-dictation and single-word reading tests which manipulated regularity of the correspondences between spelling and sound, and word frequency. All of the patients exhibited spelling and reading deficits, except at the very earliest stages of disease. Longitudinal study of seven of the patients revealed further deterioration in spelling, reading, and semantic memory. Graham NL Patterson K Hodges JR Neuropsychologia 2000;38(2):143-63.

The importance of interdisciplinary staff in the diagnosis of developmental dyslexia: case report Abstract: We describe the work of the interdisciplinary staff of FCM/UNICAMP for the diagnosis of developmental dyslexia, evaluating a 9 years old boy from the second year of a first grade public school. The procedure consisted of four stages: 1) Interview with the mother (anamnesis); 2) neuropsychological evaluation; 3) specific evaluation for reading and writing skills; 4) complementary exams. The results revealed that the child presented normal intelligence, normal auditory and visual function but difficulties in reading specific test, in auditory short-term memory (specially in auditory sequences), and in phonological conscience, as well as

slowness, lack of concentration, slight neurological signs and hypoperfusion of the mesial portion of the temporal lobe. Pestun MS Ciasca S Goncalves VM Arq Neuropsiquiatr 2002 Jun;60(2-A):328-32.

The influence of color on transient system activity: implications for dyslexia research. Abstract: Metacontrast and apparent motion experiments designed to utilize transient system resources were adopted to investigate the proposal that transient system activity is differentially influenced by different colored stimuli. The results generally showed no effect of color on transient system activity in either adults or children. However, the predicted pattern of results was demonstrated when contrast rather than color was manipulated in a final metacontrast experiment. Pammer K Lovegrove W Percept Psychophys 2001 Apr;63(3):490-500.

The influence of different diagnostic approaches on familial aggregation of spelling disability. Abstract: The influence of different diagnostic approaches on familial aggregation of spelling disability was investigated in three studies. In the first study, in a sample of 32 dyslexic children and their families, we found significantly increased rates of spelling-disabled sibs and parents by applying the IQ-discrepancy criterion. There was no evidence for the assumption that IQ-discrepancy and low achievement criteria define different subgroups of spelling disorder regarding familial aggregation. Remschmidt H Hennighausen K Schulte-Korne G Deimel W Warnke A Eur Child Adolesc Psychiatry 1999;8 Suppl 3:13-20.

The interaction of multiple routes in oral reading: evidence from dissociations in naming and oral reading in phonological dyslexia. Abstract: During oral reading we hypothesized that lexical representations are activated and selected for output by the simultaneous activation of the semantic, the direct lexical orthography to phonology, and the sublexical grapheme-to-phoneme conversion (GPC) routes (Southwood & Chatterjee, 1999). Serial models of reading argue that the semantic route governs oral reading with minimal influence from the nonlexical direct route and the sublexical GPC route. Southwood MH Chatterjee A Brain Lang 2000 Mar;72(1):14-39.

The interface between ophthalmology and optometric vision therapy. Press LJ Binocul Vis Strabismus Q 2002 Summer;17(2):81.

The lateralizing value of ictal clinical symptoms in uniregional temporal lobe epilepsy. Abstract: In order to assess the lateralizing value of several ictal and postictal clinical symptoms in temporal lobe epilepsy (TLE), we analyzed 89 seizures of 20 left dominant patients with intractable left (n = 9) versus right (n = 11) TLE who had undergone successful anterior temporal lobectomy. In left TLE, movement arrest at seizure onset, postictal dysphasia > 120 s and postictal dyslexia > 180 s were the most typical findings and associated with a sensitivity of 94, 94, and 100%, respectively. The highest specificity of 100% each was evident for contralateral versions of eyes and head and dystonic posturing. Steinhoff BJ Schindler M Herrendorf G Kurth C Bittermann HJ Paulus W Eur Neurol 1998;39(2):72-9.

The legacy of Jan Kappers. Bakker DJ J Learn Disabil 1997 Jan-Feb;30(1):99.

The magnocellular deficit hypothesis in dyslexia: a review of reported evidence. Abstract: Many reports suggest that the majority of dyslexic children have a measurable disorder of the fast processing pathway of the visual system. This pathway is believed to extend from the retina to the occipital and parietal areas of the brain, and is referred to as the magnocellular (M) or transient pathway. Evidence in support of the magnocellular deficit theory comes from several sources, but is not totally consistent. Histological studies have revealed shrinkage and disorganisation of M cells in the lateral geniculate nucleus of dyslexic subjects.

Greatrex JC Drasdo N Ophthalmic Physiol Opt 1995 Sep;15(5):501-6.

The magnocellular deficit theory of dyslexia. Skottun BC Trends Neurosci 1997 Sep;20(9):397-8.

The magnocellular deficit theory of dyslexia: the evidence from contrast sensitivity. Abstract: A number of authors have made the claim that dyslexia is the result of a deficit in the magnocellular part of the visual system. Most of the evidence cited in support of this claim is from contrast sensitivity studies. The present review surveys this evidence. The result of this survey shows that the support for the magnocellular deficit theory is equivocal. Skottun BC Vision Res 2000;40(1):111-27.

The magnocellular theory of developmental dyslexia. PG - 12-36Abstract: Low literacy is termed 'developmental dyslexia' when reading is significantly behind that expected from the intelligence quotient (IQ) in the presence of other symptoms--incoordination, left-right confusions, poor sequencing--that characterize it as a neurological syndrome. 5-10% of children, particularly boys, are found to be dyslexic. Reading requires the acquisition of good orthographic skills for recognising the visual form of words which allows one to access their meaning directly Stein J Dyslexia 2001 Jan-Mar;7(1):12-36.

The Marshall Cavendish encyclopedia of health / [editor-in-chief, Angela Sheehan]. Edition Information: Rev. ed. New York: M. Cavendish, c1995. Royston, Angela. Marshall Cavendish Corporation. Description: 14 v.: ill. (chiefly col.); 28 cm. ISBN: 1854352032 (set) LC Classification: RA776.9.M37 1995 Dewey Class No.: 610/.3 20

The mismatch negativity in evaluating central auditory dysfunction in dyslexia. Abstract: The mismatch negativity (MMN), a brain response elicited by a discriminable change in any repetitive aspect of auditory stimulation even in the absence of attention, has been widely used in both basic and clinical research during recent years. The fact that the MMN reflects the accuracy of auditory discrimination and that it can be obtained even from unattentive subjects makes it an especially attractive tool for studying various central auditory-system dysfunctions both in adults and children. Kujala T Naatanen R Neurosci Biobehav Rev 2001 Aug;25(6):535-43.

The more you know the less you can tell: inhibitory effects of visuo-semantic activation on modality specific visual misnaming. Abstract: WH, a 77-years old right-handed psychoanalyst, displayed modality specific visual misnaming as a sequel of an embolic stroke in the left posterior cerebral artery. WH's errors in visual object naming consisted mainly of semantic paraphasias and perseverations. His verbalizations during testing sometimes manifested a conflict between correct responses and perseverations. Analysis of the stream of information from visual perception via semantics to phonology suggested incomplete access from vision to semantics as the source of errors. Goldenberg G Karlbauer F Cortex 1998 Sep;34(4):471-91.

The neurobiology of reading difficulties. Stein J Prostaglandins Leukot Essent Fatty Acids 2000 Jul-Aug;63(1-2):109-16.

The neurological basis of developmental dyslexia: an overview and working hypothesis. Abstract: Five to ten per cent of school-age children fail to learn to read in spite of normal intelligence, adequate environment and educational opportunities. Thus defined, developmental dyslexia (hereafter referred to as dyslexia) is usually considered of constitutional origin, but its actual mechanisms are still mysterious and currently remain the subject of intense research endeavour in various neuroscientific areas and along several theoretical frameworks. Habib M Brain 2000 Dec;123 Pt 12:2373-99.

The neurology of dyslexia Abstract: Developmental dyslexia is a heterogeneous disorder in which the prominent manifestation is a discrepancy between reading achievement and intelligence. There is no serious auditory, visual, psychiatric, social or educational factor that could be responsible of the discrepancy. Males are more often affected than females. It is a pervasive condition but with adequate help and spontaneous compensation, reading ability may improve. Neuroimaging, mainly MRI, allows to demonstrate in two thirds, an absence of the usual symmetry of the planum temporale favoring the left side. Holguin-Acosta J Rev Neurol 1997 May;25(141):739-43.

The neuroprotective effects of MK-801 on the induction of microgyria by freezing injury to the newborn rat neocortex. Abstract: Four-layered microgyria is associated with many developmental disorders, including mental retardation, epilepsy, and developmental dyslexia. Freezing lesions to the newborn rodent neocortex result in the formation of four-layered microgyria. Previous research had suggested this type of injury acts as an hypoxic/ischemic event to the developing cortical plate. The current study examines the effectiveness of the non-competitive N-methyl-D-aspartate receptor antagonist dizocilpine (MK-801) in protecting against freezing injury to the newborn rat cortical plate. Rosen GD Sigel EA Sherman GF Galaburda AM Neuroscience 1995 Nov;69(1):107-14.

The nonword reading deficit in developmental dyslexia: evidence from children learning to read German. Abstract: This study examined whether dyslexic children learning to read German show the same nonword reading deficit, which is characteristic of dyslexic children learning to read English (Rack, Olson, & Snowling, 1992), a deficit which is taken as evidence for a phonological impairment underlying dyslexia. Because the German writing system, in contrast to English, exhibits comparatively simple and straightforward grapheme-phoneme correspondences, the generality of the nonword reading deficit across different alphabetic systems seemed questionable. Wimmer H J Exp Child Psychol 1996 Feb;61(1):80-90.

The other side of the error term: aging and development as model systems in cognitive neuroscience / Naftali Raz, editor. New York: Elsevier, 1998. Projected Pub. Date: 9803 Raz, Naftali. Description: p. cm. ISBN: 0444825223 LC Classification: QP360.5.O86 1998 Dewey Class No.: 612.8/2 21

The overstimulated state of dyslexia: perception, knowledge, and learning. Abstract: Dyslexia is far more than a learning disorder; it has significant impact on personality organization. While dyslexia usually begins to manifest most clearly in early latency when the challenge of learning to read is at its height, often the dyslexic child's ego development and functioning has already been adversely affected. The literature from neuropsychology suggests that dyslexia is a subtle language-processing disorder that affects emotional, cognitive, and social development. Arkowitz SW J Am Psychoanal Assoc 2000;48(4):1491-520.

The pattern of neurological sequelae of childhood cerebral malaria among survivors in Calabar, Nigeria. Abstract: To determine the pattern and long term outcome of neurological complications following cerebral malaria (CM) in a group of Nigerian children treated in Calabar. Although short lived, neurological sequelae of CM appear common among these Nigerian children. This problem could significantly add to the burden of childhood disability in Nigeria. Early diagnosis, use of appropriate drugs and large scale malaria control programmes can prevent malady. Meremikwu MM Asindi AA Ezedinachi E Cent Afr J Med 1997 Aug;43(8):231-4.

The persistence of rapid naming problems in children with reading disabilities: a nine-year follow-up. Abstract: In this study 9 children (6 boys, 3 girls) with reading disabilities and specific difficulties in rapid serial naming were followed from age 9 years to age 18 years. This group was taken from an earlier study sample of 82 third-grade children with learning disabilities. Tests of rapid serial naming, reading and spelling, general intelligence, articulation speed, and word fluency were administered to the subjects and to a matched control group (n = 10) in the initial study (at age 9) and in the present follow-up study (at age 18 Korhonen TT J Learn Disabil 1995 Apr;28(4):232-9.

The planum temporale: a systematic, quantitative review of its structural, functional and clinical significance. Abstract: The planum temporale (PT) is a triangular area situated on the superior temporal gyrus (STG), which has enjoyed a resurgence of interest across several disciplines, including neurology, psychiatry and psychology. Traditionally, the planum is thought to be larger on the left side of the brain in the majority of normal subjects [N. Geschwind, W. Levitsky, Human brain: left-right asymmetries in temporal speech regions, Science 161 (1968) 186-87.]. It coincides with part of Wernicke's area and it is believed to consist cytoarchitectonically of secondary auditory cortex. Consequently, it has long been thought to be intimately involved in language function Shapleske J Rossell SL Woodruff PW David AS Brain Res Brain Res Rev 1999 Jan;29(1):26-49.

The practical aspects of diagnosing and managing children with attention deficit hyperactivity disorder. Abstract: AD/HD is a behaviorally defined disorder with specific behavioral criteria. The most recent definitions decrease heterogeneity by defining subtypes although the current treatments tend to be more generic. The main well-established treatments are stimulant medication and behavior modification, which are most effective when used together. Wolraich ML Baumgaertel A Clin Pediatr (Phila) 1997 Sep;36(9):497-504.

The presence of a magnocellular defect depends on the type of dyslexia. Abstract: Previous studies have identified a magnocellular pathway defect in approximately 75% of dyslexics. Since these experiments have not classified dyslexia into subtypes, the purpose of this experiment was to determine if adult dyseidetic dyslexics or dysphoneidetic dyslexics suffer from a defect in the magnocellular pathway. Nine dyseidetic dyslexics, eight dysphoneidetic dyslexics, and nine normal readers participated in the experiment. Contrast sensitivity functions (CSF) were determined with vertically oriented sine wave gratings (0.5, 1.0, 2.0, 4.0, 8.0, 12.0 c/deg drifting at 1 and 10 Hz) by employing a two-alternative, forced-choice technique. Borsting E Ridder WH 3rd Dudeck K Kelley C Matsui L Motoyama J Vision Res 1996 Apr;36(7):1047-53.

The prevalence of dyslexia among art students. Abstract: It is widely held opinion that dyslexia is associated with remarkably artistic creativity. Speculations on different brain structures and brain functions have been proposed as an explanation. Very few objective studies have been reported that confirm the conjectures on the relationship between dyslexia and artistic creativity. Two studies are reported on the prevalence of dyslexia among university students-one group of art students and one group of students from non-art disciplines. Wolff U Lundberg I Dyslexia 2002 Jan-Mar;8(1):34-42.

The prevalence of optometric anomalies and symptoms in children receiving special tuition. Abstract: A case-control study was performed where 9 pupils receiving special tuition (ST-group) were compared with 36 controls. Six (66.7%) of the pupils in the ST-group were diagnosed as dyslexic. No significant correlation was revealed between receiving special tuition and having reduced visual function, nor between reduced visual function and number of visually related symptoms. Although the number of symptoms was not significantly greater in the ST-group, some of the symptoms were significantly more common in the ST-group, and none were significantly more common in the control group. Baraas RC Demberg A Ophthalmic Physiol Opt 1999 Jan;19(1):68-73.

The prevalence of reading and spelling difficulties among inmates of institutions for compulsory care of juvenile delinquents. Abstract: Recent studies have focused on reading and writing disabilities among inmates in prisons and at juvenile institutions. Some studies in Sweden have demonstrated that more than half of the delinquents have serious reading difficulties, and for immigrants the situation is even worse. However, these studies have focused on small groups. Furthermore, little attention has been paid to different types of reading and writing difficulties. The main purpose of this investigation was to estimate the prevalence of reading and writing disabilities in juvenile institutions. Svensson I Lundberg I Jacobson C Dyslexia 2001 Apr-Jun;7(2):62-76.

The production of semantic paralexias in a Spanish-speaking aphasic. Abstract: A case of a Spanish-speaking aphasic patient who produced a great number of semantic paralexias in reading aloud and who showed other symptoms consistent with the diagnosis of deep dyslexia is presented. In this study, (a) the production of semantic paralexias and the features of the deep dyslexia syndrome which have only recently begun to be studied in Spanish-speaking patients, are analyzed; and (b) the "obligatory character of phonological mediation in the reading of Ferreres AR Miravalles G Brain Lang 1995 May;49(2):153-72.

The public health office reports. Expert assessment of dyslexia--results of a survey Hoffmann D Gesundheitswesen 1997 Jun;59(6):418-20.

The ratio of 2nd to 4th digit length: a new predictor of disease predisposition?

Abstract: The ratio between the length of the 2nd and 4th digits is: (a) fixed in utero; (b) lower in men than in women; (c) negatively related to testosterone and sperm counts; and (d) positively related to oestrogen concentrations. Prenatal levels of testosterone and oestrogen have been implicated in infertility, autism, dyslexia, migraine, stammering, immune dysfunction, myocardial infarction and breast cancer. We suggest that 2D:4D ratio is predictive of these diseases and may be used in diagnosis, prognosis and in early life-style interventions which may delay the onset of disease or facilitate its early detection. Manning JT Bundred PE Med Hypotheses 2000 May;54(5):855-7.

The Reading brain: the biological basis of dyslexia / edited by Drake D. Duane and David B. Gray. Parkton, Md.: York Press, c1991. Duane, Drake D, 1936- Gray, David B. Orton Dyslexia Society. Meeting (1989: Dallas, Tex.) Description: xvi, 192 p.: ill.; 23 cm. ISBN: 0912752254 LC Classification: RC394.W6 R35 1991 Dewey Class No.: 616.85/53 20

The reading comprehension abilities of dyslexic students in higher education. Abstract: The reading comprehension abilities of a group of dyslexic university students were compared with those of non-dyslexic university students. A 655-word passage, followed by literal and inferential questions, was used to measure reading comprehension. The text was designed to be syntactically complex, yet place relatively modest demands on decoding skills. Although dyslexic students performed at a similar level to the non-dyslexic students on the literal questions, their performance on the inferential questions was poorer. Simmons F Singleton C Dyslexia 2000 Jul-Sep;6(3):178-92.

The relation of planum temporale asymmetry and morphology of the corpus callosum to handedness, gender, and dyslexia: a review of the evidence. Abstract: Asymmetry of the planum temporale in relation to handedness, gender, and dyslexia is reviewed. The frequency of rightward asymmetry is rather higher than are estimates of the proportion of right hemisphere speech representation in the general population. Conversely, the frequency of leftward asymmetry is lower than the proportion of the population with left hemisphere speech. Neuro-anatomic asymmetry may relate more to handedness than to language lateralization. Beaton AA Brain Lang 1997 Nov 15;60(2):255-322.

The relationship between language and reading. Preliminary results from a longitudinal investigation. Abstract: This longitudinal study investigated the relationship between language and reading from three perspectives. First, we examined the reading and writing outcomes of children identified with spoken language impairments (LIs). Second, the early language abilities of children identified as poor readers were investigated. Finally, reading and language abilities were treated as continuous variables and the developmental relationship between them was studied. Catts HW Fey ME Proctor-Williams K Logoped Phoniatr Vocol 2000;25(1):3-11.

The relationship between language-processing and visual-processing deficits in developmental dyslexia. Abstract: Some research on developmental dyslexia focuses on linguistic abnormalities such as poor reading of nonwords or poor reading of exception words. Other research focuses on visual abnormalities such as poor performance on psychophysical tasks believed to assess the functioning of the magnocellular and parvocellular layers of the lateral geniculate nucleus (LGN). Little is known about what the relationships are between these two types of abnormalities. Cestnick L Coltheart M Cognition 1999 Jul 30;71(3):231-55.

The representation of sublexical orthographic-phonologic correspondences: evidence from phonological dyslexia. Abstract: Although there is considerable evidence that grapheme and body units are involved in assembling phonology from print, there is little evidence supporting the involvement of syllabic representations. We provide evidence on this point from a phonological dyslexic patient (ML) who, as a result of brain damage, is relatively unable to read nonwords. ML was found to be able to perform tasks assumed to reflect processes involved in assembled phonology (i.e. segmentation, orthographic-phonologic conversion, and blending) when the units involved were syllables, but demonstrated considerable difficulty when they were onset, body, or phoneme units. Lesch MF Martin RC Q J Exp Psychol A 1998 Nov;51(4):905-38.

The role of analogies in learning to read. Abstract: A number of factors contribute to proficient word recognition, including phonological awareness and the ability to make orthographic analogies. The present study considered the relative contribution analogy abilities make toward early reading ability. Two analogy tasks and measures of phonological awareness, orthographic knowledge, visual memory, general language ability, and non-verbal intelligence were administered to 20 second grade good readers and 20 third and fourth grade poor readers. Kamhi AG Laing SP Logoped Phoniatr Vocol 2000;25(1):29-34.

The role of level of representation in the use of paired associate learning for rehabilitation of alexia. Abstract: Patients with phonological alexia (difficulty reading pseudowords) frequently have concomitant difficulty reading functor words and verbs compared with concrete nouns. The current study compares two techniques for helping two patients with phonological alexia regain the ability to read functors and verbs. One technique follows the approach of reorganization of function, while the other relies on the stimulation approach. Study 1, employing a reorganization approach, resulted in both patients increasing their reading accuracy from approximately 10 to 90% or greater Friedman RB Sample DM Lott SN Neuropsychologia 2002;40(2):223-34.

The role of phonological awareness, speech perception, and auditory temporal processing for dyslexia. Abstract: There is strong evidence that auditory processing plays a major role in the etiology of dyslexia. Auditory temporal processing of non-speech stimuli, speech perception, and phonological awareness have been shown to be influential in reading and spelling development. However, the relationship between these variables remains unclear. In order to analyze the influence of these three auditory processing levels on spelling, 19 dyslexic and 15 control children were examined. Schulte-Korne G Bartling J Remschmidt H Eur Child Adolesc Psychiatry 1999;8 Suppl 3:28-34.

The science of literacy: from the laboratory to the classroom. Tallal P Proc Natl Acad Sci U S A 2000 Mar 14;97(6):2402-4.

The sex ratios of families with a neurodevelopmentally disordered child. Abstract: It has been conjectured that mothers who give birth to neurodevelopmentally disordered (ND) children may have hormonal or immunological characteristics that bias them toward giving birth to male children. We examined this hypothesis in an epidemiological sample of 2,080 ND children drawn for the National Collaborative Perinatal Project (NCPP) who had one of nine kinds of NDs. No assumptions were made regarding the sex ratio of non-ND children since this could be computed from NCPP data for 11,213 families. Liederman J Flannery KA J Child Psychol Psychiatry 1995 Mar;36(3):511-7.

The simultaneous activation hypothesis: explaining recovery from deep to phonological dyslexia. Abstract: Deep dyslexia evolved into phonological dyslexia in one patient. Semantic errors resolved while phonological and derivational errors persisted in reading. Nonword reading improved but remained inferior to word reading. Despite a residual semantic deficit naming improved. The Simultaneous Activation Hypothesis explains recovery from deep to phonological dyslexia and the continued dissociation between reading and naming errors. Partial recovery to all three reading routes increased constraints for word selection at the phonological output lexicon (POL) improving word reading. Southwood MH Chatterjee A Brain Lang 2001 Jan;76(1):18-34.

The spatial distribution of visual attention in developmental dyslexia. Abstract: The present study investigated the spatial distribution of visual attention in dyslexic and normally reading children. The performances of the two groups were investigated using two different paradigms. In experiment 1 we analyzed the distribution of processing resources both inside and outside the focus of visual attention by simply recording reaction times to the detection of a white dot target projected at different eccentricities from the fovea. Facoetti A Paganoni P LorusJournalML Exp Brain Res 2000 Jun;132(4):531-8.

The structures of the WISC-R subtests: a comparison of the IQ-profiles of reading impaired and autistic subjects. Abstract: The present paper is an analysis of the WISC-R test profiles of reading impaired subjects and autistic subjects. It is argued that well-known classification systems such as Bannatyne's categories (1974) and Kaufman's factors (1975) cannot explain differences in the peaks and troughs across the two populations. A new classification system is then developed. The 11 different WISC-R subtests are characterised in terms of a combination of three modes of cognitive functioning: a knowledge mode (declarative-procedural), a processing mode (transformation-preservation of information), and a verbal-nonverbal mode (verbal-nonverbal-processing). Ottem E Scand J Psychol 1999 Mar;40(1):1-9.

The theory of an agnosic right shift gene in schizophrenia and autism. Abstract: The right shift (RS) theory (Annett, M, 1972. The distribution of manual asymmetry. Br. J. Psychol. 63, 343-358; Annett, M, 1985.

Left, Right, Hand and Brain: The Right Shift Theory. Lawrence Erlbaum, London) suggests that the typical pattern of human cerebral and manual asymmetries depends on a single gene (RS+) which impairs speech-related cortex of the right hemisphere. The theory offers solutions to several puzzles, including the distribution of handedness in families (Annett, M, 1978. A Single Gene Explanation of Right and Left Handedness and Brainedness. Lanchester Polytechnic, Coventry; Annett, M, 1996. Annett M Schizophr Res 1999 Oct 19;39(3):177-82.

The underachieving child. Abstract: Visual factors in specific learning difficulties (SpLD) are reviewed. People with SpLD fail to achieve at a level that is commensurate with their intelligence. The commonest SpLD is dyslexia, which usually results from phonological processing/decoding deficits. Additionally, there are several optometric correlates of SpLD which may, in some cases, contribute to the learning difficulty. Evans BJ Ophthalmic Physiol Opt 1998 Mar;18(2):153-9.

The use of orthographic and phonological strategies for the decoding of words in children with developmental dyslexia and average readers. Abstract: Children with developmental dyslexia are known to have problems with phonological awareness and, in particular, with phonological decoding. This study was aimed at determining the relationship between orthographic and phonological decoding strategies used by a group of children with developmental dyslexia and two groups of children who were average readers (matched on reading age and chronological age, respectively). The three groups of children, 12 in each, were presented with single words, either visually or orally. Martin F Pratt C Fraser J Dyslexia 2000 Oct-Dec;6(4):231-47.

The use of reaction time measures to evaluate nonword reading in primary progressive aphasia. Abstract: We reported on a subject with nonfluent primary progressive aphasia (PPA), NL, who demonstrated an impaired ability to make rhyme judgments (Dowhaniuk, Dixon, Roy, Black, & Square, in press). Our hypothesis was that these deficits represent a precursor to phonological alexia. However, no definitive evidence supported the existence of a phonological reading impairment as NL made relatively few errors reading nonwords. Dowhaniuk M Dixon M Roy E Black S Brain Cogn 2000 Jun-Aug;43(1-3):168-72.

The visual deficit theory of developmental dyslexia. Abstract: Dyslexia is an impairment in reading that can result from an abnormal developmental process in the case of developmental dyslexia or cerebral insult in the case of acquired dyslexia. It has long been known that the clinical manifestations of developmental dyslexia are varied. In addition to their reading difficulties, individuals with developmental dyslexia exhibit impairments in their ability to process the phonological features of written or spoken language. Recently, it has been demonstrated with a variety of experimental approaches that these individuals are impaired on a number of visual tasks involving visuomotor, visuospatial, and visual motion processing. Eden GF VanMeter JW Rumsey JM Zeffiro TA Neuroimage 1996 Dec;4(3 Pt 3):S108-17.

There's more to nursing than the three Rs. Wiles J Nurs Times 2001 Jul 5-11;97(27):19.

Theta band power changes in normal and dyslexic children. Abstract: Tonic and phasic (event-related) theta band power changes were analyzed in a sample of 8 dyslexic and 8 control children. Previous research with healthy subjects suggests that electroencephalograph (EEG) theta activity reflects the encoding of new information into working memory. The aim of the present study was to investigate whether the processing deficits of dyslexics are related to a reduced phasic theta response during reading Dyslexics

have a lack to encode pseudowords in visual working memory with a concomitant lack of frontal processing selectivity. The upper theta band shows a different pattern of results which can be best interpreted to reflect the effort during the encoding process. Klimesch W Doppelmayr M Wimmer H Schwaiger J Rohm D Gruber W Hutzler F Clin Neurophysiol 2001 Jul;112(7):1174-85.

Thompson, Lloyd J. Reading disability; developmental dyslexia, by Lloyd J. Thompson. With a foreword by Richard L. Masland. Springfield, Ill, Thomas [1966] Description: xxiii, 201 p. port. 24 cm. LC Classification: LB1050.5.T47 Dewey Class No.: 155.45

Thomson, Michael E. Developmental dyslexia / [Michael E.] Thomson. Edition Information: 3rd ed. London; Jersey City, NJ: Whurr, 1991. Description: xii, 307 p.: ill.; 24 cm. ISBN: 1870332709 LC Classification: RJ496.A5 T48 1991 Dewey Class No.: 618.92/8553 20

Thomson, Michael E. Developmental dyslexia: its nature, assessment, and remediation / Michael E. Thomson. London; Baltimore, Md, U.S.A.: E. Arnold, 1984. Description: viii, 277 p.: ill.; 24 cm. ISBN: 0713164131 (pbk.) LC Classification: RJ496.A5 T48 1984 Dewey Class No.: 618.92/855 19

Thomson, Michael E. Dyslexia: a teaching handbook / M.E. Thomson and E.J. Watkins; consultant in dyslexia, Margaret Snowling. Edition Information: 2nd ed. London: Whurr, 1998. Watkins, E. J. Description: xi, 252 p.: ill.; 24 cm. ISBN: 1861560397 LC Classification: LC4710.G7 T56 1998 Dewey Class No.: 371.91/44/0941 21 Other System No.: (OCoLC)38575401

Three-dimensional cortical morphometry of the planum temporale in childhood-onset schizophrenia. Abstract: Anomalous planum temporale asymmetry has been linked to both schizophrenia and dyslexia. The authors examined the planum temporale of adolescents with childhood-onset schizophrenia who had a high rate of prepsychotic language disorders These findings do not support anomalous planum temporale asymmetry as a basis for psychopathology in childhood-onset schizophrenia. Jacobsen LK Giedd JN Tanrikut C Brady DR Donohue BC Hamburger SD Kumra S Alaghband-Rad J Rumsey JM Rapoport JL Am J Psychiatry 1997 May;154(5):685-7.

Time estimation deficits in developmental dyslexia: evidence of cerebellar involvement. Abstract: In addition to their language-related difficulties, dyslexic children suffer problems in motor skill, balance, automatization and speeded performance. Given the recent evidence for cerebellar involvement in the acquisition of language fluency, these problems suggest cerebellar deficit. To test the hypothesis of cerebellar dysfunction in dyslexia, a time estimation task considered to be a sensitive index of cerebellar function was administered to matched groups of dyslexic and control children. Nicolson RI Fawcett AJ Dean P Proc R Soc Lond B Biol Sci 1995 Jan 23;259(1354):43-7.

To see but not to read; the magnocellular theory of dyslexia. Abstract: Developmental dyslexics often complain that small letters appear to blur and move around when they are trying to read. Anatomical, electrophysiological, psychophysical and brain-imaging studies have all contributed to elucidating the functional organization of these and other visual confusions. They emerge not from damage to a single visual relay but from abnormalities of the magnocellular component of the visual system, which is specialized for processing fast temporal information. Stein J Walsh V Trends Neurosci 1997 Apr;20(4):147-52.

Tod, Janet. Dyslexia / Janet Tod. London: D. Fulton Publishers, 2000. Description: viii, 104 p.: ill.; 30 cm. ISBN: 1853465232 LC Classification: RC394.W6T613 Dewey Class No.: 616.85/5

Toward a strong phonological theory of visual word recognition: true issues and false trails. Abstract: A strong phonological theory of reading is proposed and discussed. The first claim of this article is that current debates on word recognition are often based on different axioms regarding the cognitive structures of the mental lexicon rather than conflicting empirical evidence. These axioms lead to different interpretations of the same data. It is argued that once the implicit axioms of competing theories in visual word recognition are explicated, a strong phonological model presents a viable and coherent approach. Frost R Psychol Bull 1998 Jan;123(1):71-99.

Toward an integrated understanding of dyslexia: genetic, neurological, and cognitive mechanisms. Abstract: This paper reviews what is known about developmental dyslexia at three levels of analysis: cognitive, neurological, and genetic. It considers the difficult problem of establishing causal links between these levels of analysis, and argues that solving the gene-behavior problem is paradoxically easier than solving the brain-behavior problem. Pennington BF Dev Psychopathol 1999 Summer;11(3):629-54.

Trail Making Test in assessing children with reading disabilities: a test of executive functions or content information. Abstract: The speed of performance on Part A, Part B, and on an experimental version containing alphabetical series (Part A Alphabetic) of the Trail Making Test was studied with 19 children with reading disabilities and 34 controls from Grades 4 to 6. When the test was used in discriminant profile fashion, children with reading disabilities showed a deficit compared with control children on Part B relative to part A but did not relative to the new Part A Alphabetic. Narhi V Rasanen P Metsapelto RL Ahonen T Percept Mot Skills 1997 Jun;84(3 Pt 2):1355-62.

Training and transfer-of-learning effects in disabled and normal readers: evidence of specific deficits. Abstract: Two experiments were conducted to assess the specificity of training and transfer deficits in disabled readers, aged 7 to 9 years. Forty-eight children (reading disabled, age-matched normal controls, and reading-level-matched normal controls) participated in both a reading and a nonreading (music) acquisition paradigm. Children received instruction in grapheme-phoneme and symbol-note correspondence patterns, respectively. Posttraining tests (one day and one week) following rule training compared performance on trained exemplar items with performance on untrained transfer items. Benson NJ Lovett MW Kroeber CL J Exp Child Psychol 1997 Mar;64(3):343-66.

Trait and state EEG indices of information processing in developmental dyslexia. Abstract: L asymmetry in beta activity in the dyslexic group, again in both tasks. Theta activity did discriminate between the two tasks in the dyslexic group. In the phonological task, task-related frontal theta in the dyslexic group was significantly different from the control group, with the former showing an increase in amplitude and the latter a decrease. In the visual task, there was no significant difference between the dyslexic and the control group, with both showing a task-related decrease in amplitude. Rippon G Brunswick N Int J Psychophysiol 2000 Jun;36(3):251-65.

Transfer effects across contextual and linguistic boundaries: evidence from poor readers. Abstract: We report two experiments that are consistent with two hypotheses about poor, nonfluent readers: (1) fluency gains in text reading skill transfer across contextual and linguistic boundaries and (2) these fluency gains enable higher-order comprehension operations to function in the processing of text. We conclude that unlike the fluent reader, the nonfluent reader does not completely integrate the surface characteristics (words) of the text and the message of the text. Word-level representations remain free to support

transfer across various processing episodes Bourassa DC Levy BA Dowin S Casey A J Exp Child Psychol 1998 Oct;71(1):45-61.

Transfer of lexical information in adults with reading disorders. Abstract: This study was designed to test whether adults with reading disorders differ from adults with normal reading abilities in their interhemispheric transfer rates during a lexical decision task. Correlations of performance were completed between lexical decision vocal reaction times (msec.), interhemispheric reaction rates (RVF vocal reaction times-LVF vocal reaction times) and measures of decoding skills, including sight word decoding and phonological decoding for 20 adults with reading disorders and 20 with normal reading abilities. Walker MM Percept Mot Skills 2001 Aug;93(1):257-67.

Transient and sustained processing: effects of varying luminance and wavelength on reading comprehension. Abstract: Reading disability (RD) is a serious epidemiologic problem and may affect up to 15% to 20% of elementary school children. This study addresses whether the reading comprehension skills of children with RD improve as wavelength and contrast of light are altered. Our study suggests an association between wavelength of light, luminance, and reading performance. Blue filters were found to improve reading comprehension in poor readers. The results support the concept of a transient system deficit involving wavelength of light and reading performance. Solan HA Brannan JR Ficarra A Byne R J Am Optom Assoc 1997 Aug;68(8):503-10.

Transient deficit hypothesis and dyslexia: examination of whole-parts relationship, retinal sensitivity, and spatial and temporal frequencies. Abstract: A defect affecting the transient visual sub-system is believed to be one of the prime factors affecting reading disability. In this study, the transient deficit hypothesis was tested using the global precedence paradigm, examining retinal sensitivity, and comparing of patterns of responses to large versus small stimuli. Participants were three groups of dyslexic, chronologically age-matched, and reading age-matched children. The results revealed that although dyslexic individuals did not show any deficit in processing (a) wholes and parts (Experiment 1); (b) information in peripheral locations of the retina (Experiment 2); and (c) various sizes of the stimulus (Experiment 3); they showed a deficit in temporal processing of visual information. Keen AG Lovegrove WJ Vision Res 2000;40(6):705-15.

Transitory alexia without agraphia following head injury: letter to editor. Bhatoe HS Rohatgi S Neurol India 2002 Jun;50(2):226-8.

Treatment of a case of phonological alexia with agraphia using the Auditory Discrimination in Depth (ADD) program. Abstract: Phonological alexia and agraphia are acquired disorders characterized by an impaired ability to convert graphemes to phonemes (alexia) or phonemes to graphemes (agraphia). These disorders result in phonological errors typified by adding, omitting, shifting, or repeating phonemes in words during reading or graphemes when spelling. In developmental dyslexia, similar phonological errors are believed to result from deficient phonological awareness, an oral language skill that manifests itself in the ability to notice, think about, or manipulate the individual sounds in words. Conway TW Heilman P Rothi LJ Alexander AW Adair J Crosson BA Heilman KM J Int Neuropsychol Soc 1998 Nov;4(6):608-20.

Treatment of photosensitive epilepsy using coloured glasses. Abstract: A recently introduced optometric technique, colorimetry, enables the perceptual effects of ophthalmic tints to be evaluated subjectively, optimized, and then prescribed in tinted spectacles. The new technique is beneficial in reducing visual stress in patients with dyslexia and migraine. We describe an open trial designed to ascertain: (1) whether the colorimetry assessment, as it is now given, is safe for the investigation of photosensitive patients in optometry clinics where colorimetry equipment is most readily available, but where EEG control is not practical; (2) what proportion of patients with photosensitive epilepsy is likely to benefit to the extent already described in individual cases; (3) whether a tint selected by colorimetry could be shown to reduce the incidence of paroxysmal epileptiform EEG activity in response to flicker and patterns, thereby validating the subjective methods and corroborating the reported seizure reduction. Twenty-four females and nine males (aged 12-43 years) took part. Wilkins AJ Baker A Amin D Smith S Bradford J Zaiwalla Z Besag FM Binnie CD Fish D Seizure 1999 Dec;8(8):444-9.

Tuley, Ann Cashwell. Never too late to read: language skills for the adolescent with dyslexia: based on the work of Alice Ansara / Ann Cashwell Tuley; [foreword by Jeanne S. Chall]. Baltimore, Md.: York Press, c1998. Description: xv, 184 p.: ill.; 23 cm. ISBN: 0912752475 (pbk.) LC Classification: LB1050.5.T85 1998 Dewey Class No.: 371.91/44 21

Turner, Martin, 1948- Psychological assessment of dyslexia / Martin Turner; consultant in dyslexia, Margaret Snowling. San Diego: Singular Pub. Group, c1997. Snowling, Margaret J. Description: ix, 364 p.: ill.; 24 cm. ISBN: 1565937821 LC Classification: RC394.W6 T87 1997 Dewey Class No.: 616.85/53 21

Turner, Martin. The psychological assessment of dyslexia / Martin Turner. London: Whurr Publishers, 1996. Description: 200 p. ISBN: 1897635532:

Twin sibling differences in parental reports of ADHD, speech, reading and behaviour problems. Abstract: Differences between twins and siblings in behaviour problems were investigated in a non-selected sample of 1938 families with children aged 4-12 years. Families were sent a questionnaire based on DSM-III-R criteria for Attention Deficit Hyperactivity Disorder (ADHD), Oppositional Defiant Disorder (ODD), Conduct Disorder (CD) and Separation Anxiety (SA), which was validated by formal clinical interview. The questionnaire included measures of speech and reading problems. Levy F Hay D McLaughlin M Wood C Waldman I J Child Psychol Psychiatry 1996 Jul;37(5):569-78.

Twin study of the etiology of comorbidity between reading disability and attention-deficit/hyperactivity disorder. Abstract: This study utilized a sample of 313 eight-to sixteen-year-old same-sex twin pairs (183 monozygotic, 130 dizygotic) to assess the etiology of comorbidity between reading disability (RD) and attention-deficit/hyperactivity disorder (ADHD). RD was assessed by a discriminant function score based on the Peabody Individual Achievement Test, a standardized measure of academic achievement. The DSM-III version of the Diagnostic Interview for Children and Adolescents was used to assess symptoms of ADHD, and separate factor scores were computed for inattention and hyperactivity/impulsivity (hyp/imp). Willcutt EG Pennington BF DeFries JC Am J Med Genet 2000 Jun 12;96(3):293-301.

Two decades of research on learning disabilities in India. Abstract: This paper describes a range of research studies relating to learning disabilities in India during the last two decades. Attention is called to the existence of many different languages within India. Standardized and teacher-made tools have been developed for assessment and remediation purposes. The paper ends by making some suggestions for further research. Ramaa S Dyslexia 2000 Oct-Dec;6(4):268-83.

Two different readers in the same brain after a posterior callosal lesion. Abstract: Two different types of reading, one in each hemifield, were exhibited by a patient with a lesion of the posterior half of the corpus callosum. The patient read normally when words and non-words were presented to his right visual field. However, with left visual field presentations, the patient could not read non-words and vocalized real words very slowly, especially abstract words, inflected verbs and function words. He often replaced concrete words by semantic associates. Such an abnormal reading pattern is similar to that known as deep dyslexia. Michel F Henaff MA Intriligator J Neuroreport 1996 Feb 29;7(3):786-8.

Two translocations of chromosome 15q associated with dyslexia. Abstract: Developmental dyslexia is characterised by difficulties in learning to read. As reading is a complex cognitive process, multiple genes are expected to contribute to the pathogenesis of dyslexia. The genetics of dyslexia has been a target of molecular studies during recent years, but Journalfar no genes have been identified. However, a locus for dyslexia on chromosome 15q21 (DYX1) has been established in previous linkage studies. We have identified two families with balanced translocations involving the 15q21-q22 region Nopola-Hemmi J Taipale M Haltia T Lehesjoki AE Voutilainen A Kere J J Med Genet 2000 Oct;37(10):771-5.

Two types of phonological alexia. Abstract: It is hypothesized, on the basis of a lexical model of reading, that there are two different underlying causes of phonological alexia. It is predicted that these two types of phonological alexia will be accompanied by different sets of symptoms. Published cases of phonological alexia are examined for evidence in support of these predictions. Two distinct groups of phonological alexic patients are observed. These results support the notion of two types of phonological alexia. Friedman RB Cortex 1995 Jun;31(2):397-403.

Types of dyslexia and the shift to dextrality. Abstract: The prediction of the right shift theory that there are two types of dyslexia with different distributions of handedness was examined in a large cohort of school children. Dyslexics with poor phonology were less biased to dextrality than controls, while dyslexics without poor phonology tended to be more dextral than controls on measures of hand preference and hand skill. Relatives differed for handedness, as expected if phonological dyslexics were less likely than nonphonological dyslexics and controls to carry the hypothesized rs + gene. Annett M Eglinton E Smythe P J Child Psychol Psychiatry 1996 Feb;37(2):167-80.

Understanding childhood language disorders. Abstract: Developmental language disorders exist in 5% to 10% of preschoolers and have strong genetic implications. There are several variants of dysphasia: mixed receptive/expressive, expressive, or higher order language processing. Preschool children with pervasive developmental disorders are dysphasic as well as autistic. Some undergo a language and behavioral regression, most often as toddlers. The role of subclinical epilepsy in this regression is unknown because it is often ignored. Rapin I Curr Opin Pediatr 1998 Dec;10(6):561-6.

Understanding normal and impaired word reading: computational principles in quasi-regular domains. Abstract: A connectionist approach to processing in quasi-regular domains, as exemplified by English word reading, is developed. Networks using appropriately structured orthographic and phonological representations were trained to read both regular and exception words, and yet were able to read pronounceable nonwords as well as skilled readers. A mathematical analysis of a simplified system clarifies the close relationship of word frequency and spelling-sound consistency in influencing naming latencies. Plaut DC McClelland JL Seidenberg MS Patterson K Psychol Rev 1996 Jan;103(1):56-115.

Unidirectional dyslexia in a polyglot. Abstract: Alexia is usually seen after ischaemic insults to the dominant parietal lobe. A patient is described with a particular alexia to reading Hebrew (right to left), whereas no alexia was noted when reading in English. This deficit evolved after a hypertensive right occipitoparietal intracerebral haemorrhage, and resolved gradually over the ensuing year as the haematoma was resorbed. The deficit suggests the existence of a separate, language associated, neuronal network within the right hemisphere important to different language reading modes. Leker RR Biran I J Neurol Neurosurg Psychiatry 1999 Apr;66(4):517-9.

Unidirectional dyslexia in a polyglot. Mohamed MD Elsherbiny SM Goulding PJ J Neurol Neurosurg Psychiatry 2000 Apr;68(4):537.

Uniform [Dyslexia (Chichester, England) Dyslexia: the journal of the British Dyslexia Association. Dyslexia (Chichester, England. Print) Dyslexia (Chichester Engl, Print) Chichester, UK: Wiley, c1995- British Dyslexia Association. Description: v.: ill.; 25 cm. Vol. 1, no. 1 (May 1995)- Current Frequency: Two issues a year ISSN: 1076-9242 Cancel/Invalid LCCN: sn 94003681 CODEN: DYSLEO LC Classification: RC394.W6D952 NLM Class No.: W1 DY9895 Dewey Class No.: 616.85.53/005 21 Other System No.: (OCoLC)ocm30641425 Repro./Stock No.: John Wiley & Sons, Baffins Lane, Chichester, W. Sussex Po19 IUD, UK $70.00 Serial Record Entry: Dyslexia (Chichester, England) 96-642165

Uniform [Ouders over dyslexie. English. Parents on dyslexia / edited by Saskia van der Stoel; translated by G.D. Burton. Clevedon, Avon, England; Philadelphia: Multilingual Matters Ltd, c1990. Stoel, Saskia van der. Description: xv, 175 p.; 23 cm. ISBN: 1853590770 1853590762 (pbk.) LC Classification: RJ496.A5 O9313 1990 Dewey Class No.: 618.92/8553 20

United States. Secretary's (HEW) National Advisory Committee on Dyslexia and Related Reading Disorders. Reading disorders in the United States; report of the Secretary's (HEW) National Advisory Committee on Dyslexia and Related Reading Disorders. [Bethesda, Md.] 1969. Description: 90 p. maps. 26 cm. LC Classification: LB1050.5.U54 Dewey Class No.: 428.4/2

Universität Bayreuth. Lehrstuhl für Psychologie. Forschungsbericht / Kulturwissenschaftliche Fakultät der Universität Bayreuth, Lehrstuhl für Psychologie. [Bayreuth: UBT], 1979. Description: iv, 115 p.; 21 cm. LC Classification: RJ496.A5 U56 1979 National Bib. No.: GFR***

Unusual modality effects in less-skilled readers. Abstract: University students who were skilled or less-skilled readers were compared on tests of auditory information processing and immediate serial recall of auditory and visual digits. Reading skill was defined by performance on a pseudoword reading task. The good readers exhibited typical modality effects with higher recall of auditory than visual items from the last 3 serial positions. On the terminal list item, the less-skilled readers showed a modality effect comparable with that of the skilled readers, but on other list items the modality effect reversed and a visual superiority was obtained. Penney CG Godsell A J Exp Psychol Learn Mem Cogn 1999 Jan;25(1):284-9.

Update (National Institute of Dyslexia) Chevy Chase, MD. National Institute of Dyslexia Current Frequency: Irregular ISSN: 0896-2669 LC Classification: LB1050.5.V32 Dewey Class No.: 371.91/4

Varieties of developmental reading disorder: genetic and environmental influences. Abstract: There is widespread support for the notion that subgroups of dyslexics can be identified who differ in their reading profiles: Developmental phonological dyslexia is characterized by poor nonword reading, while developmental surface dyslexia is distinguished by a particular difficulty in reading irregular words.

However, there is much less agreement about how these subtypes, and particularly the surface dyslexic pattern, are to be accounted for within theoretical models of the reading system. Castles A Datta H Gayan J Olson RK J Exp Child Psychol 1999 Feb;72(2):73-94.

Vasek, Stefan. Aktuálne problémy detí s poruchami reci a cítania / [aut.] Stefan Vasek a kol. Edition Information: 1. vyd. Bratislava: SPN, 1979. Description: 322, [13] p.: ill.; 21 cm. LC Classification: RJ496.S7 V37

Vasquez, William R. An eagle named Bart / by William R. Vasquez. Middlebury, VT: P.S. Eriksson, c1990. Description: xii, 164 p, [16] p. of plates: ill.; 22 cm. ISBN: 0839719876: Summary: Describes the healing friendship which developed at a Maine wildlife refuge between a lonely dyslexic and a wounded bald eagle. LC Classification: QL85.V37 1990 Dewey Class No.: 636.6/869 20

Velle, Raymond. [from old catalog] Difficulties scolaires en français, en calcul et en mathématiques. Paris, les Éditions sociales françaises, 1969. Description: 195 p. illus. 24 cm. LC Classification: LB1050.5.V4

Vellutino, Frank R. Dyslexia: theory and research / Frank R. Vellutino. Cambridge, Mass.: MIT Press, c1979. Description: xv, 427 p.: ill.; 24 cm. ISBN: 0262220210 LC Classification: RC394.W6 V44 NLM Class No.: WM475.3 V442d Dewey Class No.: 616.8/553

Verbal and affective laterality effects in P-dyslexic, L-dyslexic and normal children. Abstract: Lateralization of verbal and affective processes was investigated in P-dyslexic, L-dyslexic and normal children with the aid of a dichotic listening task. The children were asked to detect either the presence of a specific target word or of words spoken in a specific emotional tone of voice. The number of correct responses and reaction time were recorded. For monitoring words, an overall right ear advantage was obtained. However, further tests showed no significant ear advantage for P-types, and a right ear advantage for L-types and controls. For emotions, an overall left ear advantage was obtained that was less robust than the word-effect. Patel TK Licht R Neuropsychol Dev Cogn Sect C Child Neuropsychol 2000 Sep;6(3):157-74.

Verbal and visual problems in reading disability. Abstract: Most individuals interested in reading disability favor the view that disordered language processing is the main cause of children's reading problems and that visual problems are seldom, if ever, responsible. Nevertheless, in a preliminary study (Eden, Stein, & Wood, 1993) we showed that visuospatial and oculomotor tests can be used to differentiate children with reading disabilities from nondisabled children. In the present study we investigated a larger sample of children to see if these findings held true. Using 93 children from the Bowman Gray Learning Disability Project (mean age = 11.3 years; 54 boys, 39 girls), we compared the phonological and visuospatial abilities of nondisabled children (children whose reading at fifth grade rated a Woodcock-Johnson reading standardized score between 85 and 115), and children with reading disability (whose reading standardized score was below 85 on the Woodcock-Johnson. Eden GF Stein JF Wood MH Wood FB J Learn Disabil 1995 May;28(5):272-90.

Vergence control across saccades in dyslexic adults. Abstract: Many aspects of vision have been investigated in developmental dyslexia. Some research suggests deficits in vergence control (e.g. Buzzelli, 1991, Optom. Vision Sci. 68, 842-846), although ability to control vergence across saccades has not yet been investigated. We have explored this question indirectly using Enright's (1996 Vision Res. 36, 307-312.) sequential stereopsis task. Moores E Frisby JP Buckley D Reynolds E Fawcett A Ophthalmic Physiol Opt 1998 Sep;18(5):452-62.

Vienne, Lucie de. [from old catalog] La dyslexie; Montréal, Leméac, 1972. Description: xv, 204 p.: ill.; 22 cm. LC Classification: RJ496.A5 V53

Violence exposure, trauma, and IQ and/or reading deficits among urban children. Abstract: Exposure to violence in childhood has been associated with lower school grades. However, the association between violence exposure and performance on standardized tests (such as IQ or academic achievement) in children is unknown. It is not known whether violence exposure itself or subsequent symptoms of trauma are primarily responsible for negative outcomes. In this study, exposure to violence and trauma-related distress in young children were associated with substantial decrements in IQ and reading achievement. Delaney-Black V Covington C Ondersma SJ Nordstrom-Klee B Templin T Ager J Janisse J Sokol RJ Arch Pediatr Adolesc Med 2002 Mar;156(3):280-5.

Vision and attention. II: Is visual attention a mechanism through which a deficient magnocellular pathway might cause reading disability? Abstract: Recent research in reading disability has discovered that at least some reading-disabled subjects have deficits in their magnocellular (M) visual pathways. However, the mechanism by which M pathway deficits affect reading has not been addressed. Abnormal attention has long been known to be associated with reading-disabled individuals, and new research in visual attention has determined that transient visual attention is dominated by M-stream inputs. Steinman SB Steinman BA Garzia RP Optom Vis Sci 1998 Sep;75(9):674-81.

Vision and learning to read. Croucher PH Clin Exp Optom 2002 Mar;85(2):112-3.

Vision and learning to read. Kaye G Clin Exp Optom 2002 Mar;85(2):111.

Vision and learning to read. McMonnies C Clin Exp Optom 2002 Mar;85(2):112.

Vision and reading / edited by Ralph P. Garzia. St. Louis: Mosby, c1996. Garzia, Ralph P. Description: xii, 322 p.: ill.; 24 cm. ISBN: 081513438X LC Classification: RC394.W6 V57 1995 Dewey Class No.: 617.7 20

Vision and visual dysfunction / general editor, John R. Cronly-Dillon. Boca Raton: CRC Press, 1991. Cronly-Dillon, J. Description: 17 v.: ill. (some col.); 26 cm. ISBN: 0849375002 (set) --LC Classification: QP474.V44 1991 NLM Class No.: WW 100 V831 Dewey Class No.: 612.8/4 20

Vision and visual dyslexia / edited by John F. Stein. Boca Raton: CRC Press, 1991. Stein, J. F. (John Frederick) Description: xiv, 285 p.: ill.; 26 cm. ISBN: 0849375134 LC Classification: QP474.V44 1991 vol. 13 RC394.W6 NLM Class No.: WW 100 V831 v. 13 Dewey Class No.: 612.8/4 s 616.85/53 20

Vision therapy for learning disabilities and dyslexia. Starr NB J Pediatr Health Care 2000 Jan-Feb;14(1):32-3.

Vision, its impact on learning / Robert M. Wold, editor. Seattle: Special Child Publications, c1978. Wold, Robert M. Description: 487 p.: ill.; 23 cm. ISBN: 0875620558: LC Classification: LC4704.V57 Dewey Class No.: 371.9/11

Vision, learning and dyslexia. A joint organizational policy statement of the American Academy of Optometry and the American Optometric Association. Abstract: 1. Vision problems can and often do interfere with learning. 2. People at risk for learning-related vision problems should be evaluated by an optometrist who provides diagnostic and management services in this area. 3. The goal of optometric intervention is to improve visual function and alleviate associated signs and symptoms. 4. Prompt remediation of learning-related vision problems enhances the ability of children and adults to perform to their full potential. 5. People with learning problems require help from many disciplines to meet the learning challenges they face. Optometric involvement constitutes one aspect of the multidisciplinary management approach required to prepare the individual for lifelong learning. J Am Optom Assoc 1997 May;68(5):284-6.

Vision, learning, and dyslexia. A joint organizational policy statement. American Academy of Optometry. American Optometric Association. Abstract: 1. Vision problems can and often do interfere with learning. 2. People at risk for learning-related vision problems should be evaluated by an optometrist who provides diagnostic and management services in this area. 3. The goal of optometric intervention is to improve visual function and alleviate associated signs and symptoms. 4. Prompt remediation of learning-related vision problems enhances the ability of children and adults to perform to their full potential. 5. People with learning problems require help from many disciplines to meet the learning challenges they face. Optom Vis Sci 1997 Oct;74(10):868-70.

Visual and language processing disorders are concurrent in dyslexia and continue into adulthood. Abstract: A recent study by Slaghuis. Lovegrove and Davidson (1994) found that visual and language processing differences were concurrent in a group of preadolescent dyslexic. In the present study, two experiments are reported that investigate the concurrence and continuity of visual and language processing differences in groups of young and adult dyslexics on a measure of visual processing and a measure of phonological coding. Slaghuis WL Twell AJ Kingston KR Cortex 1996 Sep;32(3):413-38.

Visual and visuomotor performance in dyslexic children. Abstract: The present study was designed to compare the performance of nine dyslexic boys and nine age- and IQ-matched controls on tasks which presumably tap visual functions dependent on the subcortical magnocellular (M) pathway (flicker sensitivity) and the cortical dorsal stream (stereoacuity, structure-from-motion, visuomotor control). Increasing evidence suggests that dyslexics experience impairments in M-system functioning. In keeping with previous work supporting this conclusion, dyslexic subjects in the present study were found to have reduced sensitivity to flicker relative to controls. Felmingham KL Jakobson LS Exp Brain Res 1995;106(3):467-74.

Visual complexity in letter-by-letter reading: "pure" alexia is not pure. Abstract: Standard accounts of pure alexia have favoured the view that this acquired disorder of reading arises from damage to a left posterior occipital cortex mechanism dedicated to the processing of alphanumeric symbols. We challenge these accounts in two experiments and demonstrate that patients with this reading deficit are impaired at object identification. In the first experiment, we show that a single subject, EL, who shows all the hallmark features of pure alexia, is impaired at picture identification across a large set of stimuli. Behrmann M Nelson J Sekuler EB Neuropsychologia 1998 Nov;36(11):1115-32.

Visual evoked potential abnormalities in dyslexic children. Abstract: Developmental reading disability (dyslexia) has traditionally been attributed to impaired linguistic skills. Recent psychophysical data suggest that dyslexia may be related to a visual perceptual deficit. A few visual evoked potential (VEP) studies have addressed this hypothesis, but their results are far from consistent. We submitted 9 dyslexic subjects and 9 age- and sex-matched normal controls to checkerboard pattern reversal VEPs. Romani A Conte S Callieco R Bergamaschi R Versino M Lanzi G Zambrino CA Cosi V Funct Neurol 2001 Jul-Sep;16(3):219-29.

Visual evoked potential evidence for magnocellular system deficit in dyslexia. Abstract: Some recent studies on dyslexia have suggested a selective abnormality in the magnocellular visual pathway. To verify this hypothesis, we investigated motion-onset visual evoked potentials (VEPs) (predominantly testing the magnocellular system) as well as pattern-reversal VEPs (presumably testing the parvocellular system) in 20 dyslexics and 16 controls (both groups with a mean age of 10.0 years. Kubova Z Kuba M Peregrin J Novakova V Physiol Res 1996;45(1):87-9.

Visual function, fatty acids and dyslexia. Abstract: There is mounting evidence that developmental dyslexia is a neurodevelopmental disorder which involves abnormalities of fatty acid metabolism, particularly with respect to certain long-chain highly unsaturated fatty acids (HUFAs). Psychophysical evidence strongly suggests that dyslexics may have visual deficits as well as phonological problems. Specifically, these visual deficits appear to be related to the magnocellular pathway, which is specialized for processing fast, rapidly-changing information about the visual scene. Taylor KE Richardson AJ Prostaglandins Leukot Essent Fatty Acids 2000 Jul-Aug;63(1-2):89-93.

Visual half-field contrast sensitivity in children with dyslexia. Abstract: We address the question whether left-hemispheric and/or right-hemispheric contrast thresholds differ between children with dyslexia and controls, and whether there are interhemispheric differences. In order to answer these questions we examined [1] thresholds for the detection of Contrast-Defined (CD) forms to left and right half-field stimulation, and [2] half-field pattern onset Evoked Potentials (EPs) as a function of stimulus contrast in 21 children with dyslexia of 8-15 years of age and in 17 age-matched healthy controls. Hollants-Gilhuijs M Spekreijse F Gijsberti-Hodenpijl M Karten Y Spekreijse H Doc Ophthalmol 1998-99;96(4):293-303.

Visual impairment and dyslexia in childhood. Abstract: Although visual screening programs seem to be more and more effective, we face new problems with visual dysfunction that are not always detected in the visual screening programs. Many children born prematurely develop cerebral visual impairment. These children suffer from a cognitive visual impairment, causing them to have problems with orientation and visual perception. Brain impairment seems to be relevant for the dyslexia syndrome, which continues to fascinate and puzzle many researchers. Ygge J Lennerstrand G Curr Opin Ophthalmol 1997 Oct;8(5):40-4.

Visual implicit memory deficit and developmental surface dyslexia: a case of early occipital damage. Abstract: This study reports the case of EBON, a fifteen-year-old right-handed female Swedish student, who suffered an early medial/dorsal occipital brain lesion and showed a clearly defined pattern of developmental surface dyslexia. EBON and 17 controls were examined with within and cross-modality (visual and auditory) word stem completion tasks together with tasks requiring free-recall and recognition for visually and auditory presented words. Compared to age-matched controls, EBON was found to show a significant deficit of visual priming following visual presentation, and a deficit approaching significance following auditory presentation. Samuelsson S Bogges TR Karlsson T Cortex 2000 Jun;36(3):365-76.

Visual localization in dyslexia. Abstract: Individuals with specific reading disability (SRD) may exhibit visual psychophysical abnormalities that include prolonged visual persistence, decreased luminance contrast sensitivity, lower flicker fusion thresholds, abnormal metacontrast masking, and lower motion detection sensitivity. These abnormalities could result from impairment of the magnocellular division of the visual afferent pathway to the cortex. The authors predicted that an impairment of this pathway would cause abnormalities in ability to localize visual stimuli. Graves RE Frerichs RJ Cook JA Neuropsychology 1999 Oct;13(4):575-81.

Visual motion activates V5 in dyslexics. Abstract: A recent functional magnetic resonance imaging (fMRI) study concluded that the motion-specific visual area V5 is not activated in dyslexic subjects. We report here opposing evidence based on whole-scalp neuromagnetic recordings. Apparent-motion stimuli elicited similar activation of V5 in both dyslexic and control subjects, with a trend for longer latencies in dyslexics. Both high- and low-contrast stimuli activated the V5 region in dyslexics. Vanni S Uusitalo MA Kiesila P Hari R Neuroreport 1997 May 27;8(8):1939-42.

Visual motion sensitivity in dyslexia: evidence for temporal and energy integration deficits. Abstract: In addition to poor literacy skills, developmental dyslexia has been associated with multisensory deficits for dynamic stimulus detection. In vision these deficits have been suggested to result from impaired sensitivity of cells within the retino-cortical magnocellular pathway and extrastriate areas in the dorsal stream to which they project. One consequence of such selectively reduced sensitivity is a difficulty in extracting motion coherence from dynamic noise, a deficit associated with both developmental dyslexia and persons with extrastriate, dorsal stream lesions. Talcott JB Hansen PC Assoku EL Stein JF Neuropsychologia 2000;38(7):935-43.

Visual paralexias in a Spanish-speaking patient with acquired dyslexia: a consequence of visual and semantic impairments? Abstract: We report the case of a Spanish patient SC who misread 55 per cent of the single words shown to her. SC's reading accuracy was affected by word imageability and frequency. Nonword reading was very poor. The majority of SC's errors to real-word targets bore a close visual similarity to the items that elicited them, but there was no indication of an effect of serial position on the probability that a letter from a target word would be incorporated into the error made to that word. SC made some visual errors in object naming and showed evidence of a general semantic impairment. Cuetos F Ellis AW Cortex 1999 Dec;35(5):661-74.

Visual processing and dyslexia. Abstract: Magnocellular-pathway deficits have been hypothesized to be responsible for the problems experienced by dyslexic individuals in reading. However, research has yet to provide a detailed account of the consequences of these deficits or to identify the behavioural link between them and reading disabilities. The aim of the present study was to determine the potential consequences of the magnocellular-pathway deficits for dyslexics in a comprehensive range of visual tasks. Everatt J Bradshaw MF Hibbard PB Perception 1999;28(2):243-54.

Visual search of good and poor readers: effects with targets having single and combined features. Abstract: This study examined differences between normal and poor readers in the visual-search strategy used to detect a target shape in a background of similar shapes. No differences between the two groups occur in search for simple features (Exps. 1 and 3) and conjunction of features (Exp. 2). However, the performance of the two groups differ on search tasks with multifeatured shapes, in which targets and nontargets differ in both the identity of features and their spatial relationship or in the spatial relationship of features alone. Casco C Prunetti E Percept Mot Skills 1996 Jun;82(3 Pt 2):1155-67.

Visual search performance in dyslexia. Abstract: According to the magnocellular theory of dyslexia, otherwise intelligent children may fail to learn to read because of abnormalities in the magnocellular layers of the lateral geniculate nucleus (mLGN). If this were the case, one would predict that dyslexic subjects who show a deficit on low-level psychophysical tasks which tax the magnocellular system would have deficits on higher-level visual tasks which do not rely on the properties of mLGN cells but depend upon the functioning of areas whose main inputs

originate in the mLGN Iles J Walsh V Richardson A Dyslexia 2000 Jul-Sep;6(3):163-77.

Visual word activation in pure alexia. Abstract: A patient with pure alexia (DM) is shown to perform rapid and accurate lexical decisions for common words without the ability to recover their complete identity. We provide evidence using a speeded decision task that DM is not forced to rely on a laborious analysis of individual letter forms when judging the lexical status of orthographic patterns varying in length, though he clearly must use this approach to fully identify a word for explicit report. By contrast, the ability to rapidly classify a word apparently does not extend to judgements of its superordinate category. Bub DN Arguin M Brain Lang 1995 Apr;49(1):77-103.

Visual-perceptual and phonological factors in the acquisition of literacy among children with congenital developmental coordination disorder. Abstract: Much research has shown that children with congenital developmental coordination disorder (CDCD) have marked impairments in the perception of visual-spatial information, a deficit which has been assumed to be causally related to difficulties that many CDCD children experience when learning to read and spell. However, current research in reading disability suggests that poor reading is mainly related to difficulties with the processing of phonological information or with metaphonological ability, not to visual-perceptual deficits, Fletcher-Flinn C Elmes H Strugnell, D Dev Med Child Neurol 1997 Mar;39(3):158-66.

Visual-spatial attention in developmental dyslexia. Abstract: Orienting and focusing of visual attention are two processes strictly involved in reading. They were studied in a group of dyslexic children and normal readers. Shifting of attention by both peripheral and central visual cues was studied by means of the covert orienting paradigm. Focusing, consisting in the ability to control the size of the attentional focus, was investigated using simple reaction times in central vision. Results showed that dyslexics had a specific disability in the shifting of attention caused by a peripheral cue at short SOAs, and were able to maintain attention focused for short periods of time only, presumably not long enough for efficient visual processing. Facoetti A Paganoni P Turatto M Marzola V Mascetti GG Cortex 2000 Feb;36(1):109-23.

Visuographemic alexia: a new form of a peripheral acquired dyslexia. Abstract: We report a single-case study of peripherally acquired dyslexia that meets the clinical criteria of "alexia without agraphia." The patient, AA, has a large infarct involving the left posterior cerebral artery. The most striking feature is a severe impairment in recognizing single visually presented letters that precludes explicit or implicit access to reading, even in a letter-by-letter fashion. AA can, however, differentiate letters from similar nonsense characters and digits, and he is able to identify alphanumeric signs when the visual channel is bypassed (through somesthesic or kinesthesic presentation). Dalmas JF Dansilio S Brain Lang 2000 Oct 15;75(1):1-16.

Visuospatial deficits with preserved reading ability in a patient with posterior cortical atrophy. Abstract: Visuospatial deficits are characteristic of posterior cortical atrophy (PCA). A 58 year old woman had progressive dressing apraxia and environmental disorientation but continued to read voraciously. Positron emission tomography revealed hypometabolism of the occipitoparietal regions bilaterally, consistent with PCA. The symptoms suggested predominant dysfunction of the dorsal ("where") stream with abnormalities in visual localization and visuospatial integration; however, the patient had a less pronounced apperceptive object agnosia Cortex 2001 Sep;37(4):535-43.

Vogel, Susan Ann. Syntactic abilities in normal and dyslexic children / Susan Ann Vogel. Baltimore: University Park Press, [1975]

Description: x, 118 p.: ill.; 24 cm. ISBN: 0839108184 LC Classification: RJ496.A5 V64 NLM Class No.: WL340 V879s Dewey Class No.: 618.9/28/553075

Voluntary saccadic control in dyslexia. Abstract: The role of eye-movement control in dyslexia is still unclear. Recent studies, however, confirmed that dyslexics show poor saccadic control in single and sequential target tasks. In the present study we investigated whether dyslexic subjects are impaired on an antisaccade task requiring saccades against the direction of a stimulus. Altogether, 620 subjects between the ages of 7 and 17 years were classified as dyslexics (N = 506) or control subjects (N = 114) on the grounds of the discrepancy between their intellectual abilities and reading/spelling achievements. Biscaldi M Fischer B Hartnegg K Perception 2000;29(5):509-21.

Wagner, Rudolph F. Dyslexia and your child: a guide for parents and teachers [by] Rudolph F. Wagner. Edition Information: [1st ed.] New York, Harper & Row [1971] Description: xi, 148 p. illus. 21 cm. ISBN: 0060145293 LC Classification: LB1050.5.W25 1971 Dewey Class No.: 371.91/4

Wagner, Rudolph F. Dyslexia and your child: a guide for parents and teachers / Rudolph F. Wagner. Edition Information: Rev. ed. New York: Harper & Row, c1979. Description: xii, 212 p.: ill.; 21 cm. ISBN: 0060145838: LC Classification: LB1050.5.W25 1979 NLM Class No.: WL340.3 W134d Dewey Class No.: 371.91/4

Waites, Lucius, 1924- Specific developmental dyslexia and related language disabilities; an interdisciplinary approach utilizing multisensory techniques for remedial language training [by] Lucius Waites and staff. Dallas, Texas Scottish Rite Hospital for Crippled Children [1969, c1966] Texas Scottish Rite Hospital for Crippled Children. Description: vii, 62 p. 29 cm. LC Classification: RJ496.S7 W3 1969 Dewey Class No.: 616.85/5

Waites, Lucius, 1924- Specific dyslexia and other developmental problems in children: a synopsis / Lucius Waites. Cambridge, Mass.: Educators Pub. Service, c1990. Description: vi, 80 p.: ill.; 23 cm. ISBN: 0838822622 LC Classification: RJ496.A5 W35 1990 Dewey Class No.: 618.92/8553 20

Walton, Margaret. Teaching reading and spelling to dyslexic children: getting to grips with words / Margaret Walton. London: D. Fulton, 1998. Description: xi, 131 p.: ill.; 30 cm. ISBN: 1853465658 LC Classification: LC4708.W35 1998 Other System No.: (OCoLC)39702781

Weber, Johannes Christoph, 1941- Die Sprache des Abwesenden: Beiträge der Psychoanalyse Freuds und der genetischen Entwicklungspsychologie Piagets zum Verständnis der behinderten Lesefähigkeit / Johannes Christoph Weber; mit einem Vorwort von Aloys Leber. Heidelberg: Asanger, 1988. Description: vi, 298 p.: ill.; 21 cm. ISBN: 3893340858 3893341390 (pbk.) LC Classification: MLCS 91/14508 (R) Series:

Weger, Ronald E. A layman's look at dyslexia: the social costs and the personal traumas and frustrations of dyslexics and their families / Ronald E. Weger. Lansing, Mich. (319 W. Genesee, Lansing 48933): Michigan Dyslexia Institute, c1989. Description: 65 p.; 21 cm. LC Classification: RC394.W6 W44 1989 Dewey Class No.: 616.85/53 20

West, Thomas G, 1943- In the mind's eye: visual thinkers, gifted people with dyslexia and other learning difficulties, computer images, and the ironies of creativity / Thomas G. West. Portion of Mind's eye Edition Information: Updated ed. Amherst, N.Y.: Prometheus Books, 1997. Description: 397 p.: ill.; 24 cm. ISBN: 1573921556 (alk. paper) LC Classification: BF426.W47 1997 Dewey Class No.: 153.9 21

What does the Ternus display tell us about motion processing in human vision? Abstract: The Ternus display is a moving visual stimulus which elicits two very different percepts, according to the length of the interstimulus interval (ISI) between each frame of the motion sequence. These two percepts, referred to as element motion and group motion, have previously been analysed in terms of the operation of a low-level, dedicated short-range motion process (in the case of element motion), and of a higher-level, attentional long-range motion process (in the case of group motion). Scott-Samuel NE Hess RF Perception 2001;30(10):1179-88.

When does a deep dyslexic make a semantic error? The roles of age-of-acquisition, concreteness, and frequency. Abstract: Semantic reading errors are the central and defining feature of deep dyslexia. This study compared the words the deep dyslexic patient LW read correctly with those she omitted and those to which she produced semantic errors in terms of their concreteness, age-of-acquisition, frequency, and length. Semantic errors were made to less concrete, later-acquired, and shorter words than were read correctly; there was no reliable effect of word frequency. More importantly, the actual semantic errors produced were later-acquired than the stimulus words, but they were not more concrete or reliably more frequent. Gerhand S Barry C Brain Lang 2000 Aug;74(1):26-47.

When reading is "readn" or somthn. Distinctness of phonological representations of lexical items in normal and disabled readers. Abstract: This paper specifies nothing less than an underlying cause of dyslexia. It is a cause which may be responsible for lacking responsiveness to both the teaching of phoneme awareness and to initial reading instruction. Can a single phonological factor explain many of the phonological deficits related to dyslexia? In this paper it is suggested that the answer may be affirmative and that indistinct phonological representations of lexical items in long term memory may be such a unifying factor. Elbro C Scand J Psychol 1998 Sep;39(3):149-53.

White, Jeffrey. Dyslexia; an introduction to causes and treatment with special reference to management in the secondary school [by] Jeffrey White and Margaret White. Perth, Alpha Print [1971] White, Margaret, joint author. Description: 28, [4] p. col. illus, tables. 21 cm. ISBN: 090949200X LC Classification: RC394.W6 W48 Dewey Class No.: 616.8/553 National Bib. No.: ANL

Why is "Red Cross" different from "Yellow Cross"?: a neuropsychological study of noun-adjective agreement within Italian compounds. Abstract: This study investigates the performance of two Italian nonfluent aphasic patients on noun-adjective agreement in compounds and in noun phrases. A completion, a reading, and a repetition task were administered. Results show that both patients were able to correctly inflect adjectives within compounds, but not in noun phrases. Moreover, they were sensitive to constituent order (noun-adjective vs adjective-noun) within noun phrases, but less Journalwithin compounds. Mondini S Jarema G Luzzatti C Burani C Semenza C Brain Lang 2002 Apr-Jun;81(1-3):621-34.

Why is learning to read a hard task for some children? Abstract: In this brief review of some of my research on reading disability, I argue that a child's development into literacy has two major ontogenetic roots, one involving early informal literacy socialization and one related to phonological awareness. Although failure in reading acquisition might be a question of cultural deprivation, the dynamic interaction between genetic dispositions and environment must be acknowledged, especially in a society providing rich sources of print exposure. Lundberg I Scand J Psychol 1998 Sep;39(3):155-7.

Wilkins, Angela. Basic facts bout dyslexia / Angela Wilkins, Alice Garside [and] Mary Lee Enfield. Baltimore, MD: Orton Dyslexia Society, c1993. Garside, Alice. Enfield, Mary Lee. Orton Dyslexia Society. Description: 20 p.; 22 cm. Variant Series: Orton Emeritus series LC Classification: MLCS 99/3370 (R)

Willie the worm and dyslexia: a 17-year follow-up. Gentry J J Child Neurol 1995 Jan;10 Suppl 1:S106-7.

Wiltshire, Paula. Dyslexia / Paula Wiltshire. Austin, TX: Raintree Steck-Vaughn, 2002. Projected Pub. Date: 0209 Description: p. cm. ISBN: 0739852213 Summary: A comprehensive look at dyslexia, a learning disability that affects up to ten percent of the population of the Western world, covering its definitions, causes, assessment, and treatments. Series: Health issues LC Classification: RC394.W6 W554 2002 Dewey Class No.: 616.85/53 21

Word decoding and picture naming in children with a reading disability. Abstract: Poor readers and reading age level matched controls performed a primed picture-naming task and a lexical decision task; their vocabulary performance was assessed. Picture-naming data showed that poor readers were slower in the repeated prime condition only. This effect could not be explained by differences in vocabulary. Semantically related primes were ineffective compared with the repeated prime condition. Lexical decision data replicated the nonword reading deficit hypothesis: Poor readers were slower, particularly on the pseudowords and nonwords. Assink EM Soeteman WP Knuijt PP Genet Soc Gen Psychol Monogr 1999 Aug;125(3):251-68.

Word length and error types in Japanese left-sided neglect dyslexia. Abstract: Seven patients who showed left-sided neglect in reading single words were examined. Neglect errors typically involved omission of initial letters in our patients. Two patients with enough errors had a tendency that longer words were more susceptible to errors than short words. Most of the patients were less affected than the patients in the previous reports. Japanese people read strings of letters written not only from left to right but from right to left. Takeda K Sugishita M Clin Neurol Neurosurg 1995 May;97(2):125-30.

Word recognition deficits in German: more evidence from a representative sample. Abstract: In a representative sample of German speaking dyslexic children, earlier findings on dyslexia in the highly consistent orthography of German were confirmed. In a sample of 78 dyslexic 3rd graders selected on the basis of their poor word recognition skills, reading accuracy for both words and non-words was deficient but high in absolute terms. This indicates that the highly consistent grapheme-phoneme correspondences of German orthography in combination with the straightforward phonics teaching approach, which is usually applied in Austrian primary schools, allows even dyslexic children to acquire the process of phonological decoding Landerl K Dyslexia 2001 Oct-Dec;7(4):183-96.

Word specific impairments in naming and spelling but not reading. Abstract: A patient, who had suffered a left-hemisphere CVA, is described. He had a major aphasic syndrome which encompassed both his propositional speech and literacy skills. However, his comprehension of both spoken and written language was intact. His superior ability to retrieve nouns as opposed to other word classes was systematically investigated. This superiority of noun processing was restricted to concrete nouns. Orpwood L Warrington EK Cortex 1995 Jun;31(2):239-65.

Word-blindness or specific developmental dyslexia; proceedings of a conference called by the Invalid Children's Aid Association, 12 April 1962, and held in the Medical College of St. Bartholomew's Hospital, London. Edited by Alfred White Franklin. [London] Pitman Medical Pub. Co. [c1962] Franklin, Alfred White, 1905- ed. Invalid Children's Aid Association (London, England) St. Bartholomew's Hospital (London, England). Medical College. Description: 148 p. facsim. 23

cm. LC Classification: RC394.W6W6 Dewey Class No.: 618.92/855

Word-centred neglect dyslexia: evidence from a new case. Abstract: Neglect dyslexia resulting from damage to word-centred representations is extremely rare. We report on a new case. A left-handed subject, SVE, presented with aphasia and neglect dyslexia/dysgraphia following a right hemisphere stroke. In tachistoscopic reading tasks, some of his errors resulted from retina-centred neglect, as he responded more accurately to words flashed in the left visual field than to words flashed in the right visual field. Miceli G CapasJournalR Neurocase 2001;7(3):221-37.

Working memory, inhibitory control, and reading disability. Abstract: The relationships among working memory, inhibitory control, and reading skills were studied in 966 individuals, 6-49 years old. In addition to a standardized measure of word recognition, they received a working memory (listening span) task in the standard, blocked format (three sets containing two-, three-, or four-item trials) or in a mixed format (three sets each containing two-, three-, and four-item trials) to determine whether scores derived from the standard format are influenced by proactive interference. Chiappe P Hasher L Siegel LS Mem Cognit 2000 Jan;28(1):8-17.

Working Party on the Needs of the Dyslexic Adult. People with dyslexia: report of a working party commissioned by the British Council for Rehabilitation of the Disabled under the chairmanship of Dr. John Kershaw / [Working Party on the Needs of the Dyslexic Adult]. London: The Council, 1974. British Council for Rehabilitation of the Disabled. Description: xvii, 160 p.; 22 cm. ISBN: 0902358014: LC Classification: RC394.W6 W63 1974 NLM Class No.: WL340 W924p 1974 Dewey Class No.: 362.2 National Bib. No.: GB75-07607

World Congress on Dyslexia (1st: 1974: Mayo clinic) Reading, perception, and language: papers from the World Congress on Dyslexia / edited by Drake D. Duane and Margaret B. Rawson; sponsored by the Orton Society in cooperation with the Mayo Clinic. Baltimore: York Press, [1975] Duane, Drake D, 1936- Rawson, Margaret B. Orton Society. Mayo Clinic. Description: xii, 272 p.: ill.; 24 cm. ISBN: 0912752076: LC Classification: RJ496.A5 W67 1974 Dewey Class No.: 616.8/553

Wuarin, Cécile. Dyslexie, que faire? / Cécile Wuarin. Lausanne [etc.]: Delachaux et Niestlé, 1979. Description: 96 p, [22] leaves of plates; 21 cm. ISBN: 2603001515: LC Classification: LB1050.5.W8 Dewey Class No.: 371.91/4 National Bib. No.: Sw79-10901

You just can't keep a good person down! Genet RM ASHA 1995 Sep;37(9):57-8.

Ziminsky, Paul C, 1962- In a rising wind: a personal journey through dyslexia / Paul C. Ziminsky. Lanham: University Press of America, c1993. Description: vii, 86 p.; 22 cm. ISBN: 0819190497 (pbk.: alk. paper)

LC Classification: LC4708.Z56 1993 Dewey Class No.: 371.91/44 20

Zimmerman, Daniel. La rééducation pour quoi faire? [Par] Daniel Zimmermann avec la collaboration d'Édith Adnet-Piat. Paris, Éditions ESF [1973] Adnet-Piat, Édith, joint author. Description: 146 p. illus. 24 cm. LC Classification: LB1050.5.Z49 Dewey Class No.: 372.4/3 National Bib. No.: F***

Zimmermann, Achim, 1945- Legasthenie und schriftsprachliche Kommunikation: Ansätze zur Neuorientierung e. fragwürdigen Konzepts / Achim Zimmermann. Weinheim; Basel: Beltz, 1980. Description: 280 p.; 21 cm. ISBN: 3407546009 LC Classification: LB1050.5.Z488 1980 Dewey Class No.: 371.91/4 19 National Bib. No.: GFR80-A

TITLE INDEX

B

C

D

E

F

J

K

L

M

O

P

S

T

U

V

W

Y

AUTHOR INDEX

E

G

H

I

J

L

M

N

O

R

S

T

U

V

W

Y

Z

SUBJECT INDEX

C

D

J

K

L

M

```
371.91    Dyslexia.
Dys
```

DATE			